Health Information Management and Technology

Health Information Management and Technology

M. Beth Shanholtzer, MAEd, RHIA, FAHIMA

Lord Fairfax Community College

Gary W. Ozanich, PhD

Northern Kentucky University

McGraw Hill Education

HEALTH INFORMATION MANAGEMENT AND TECHNOLOGY

ISBN 978-0-07-351368-3
MHID 0-07-351368-7

Senior Vice President, Products & Markets: *Kurt L. Strand*
Vice President, General Manager, Products & Markets: *Marty Lange*
Vice President, Content Design & Delivery: *Kimberly Meriwether David*
Managing Director: *Chad Grall*
Executive Brand Manager: *William R. Lawrensen*
Director, Product Development: *Rose Koos*
Product Developer: *Michelle Gaseor*
Senior Product Developer: *Michelle Flommenhoft*
Executive Marketing Manager: *Roxan Kinsey*
Digital Product Analyst: *Katherine Ward*
Director, Content Design & Delivery: *Linda Avenarius*
Program Manager: *Angela R. FitzPatrick*
Content Project Managers: *April R. Southwood/Sherry Kane*
Buyer: *Sandy Ludovissy*
Design: *Srdjan Savanovic*
Content Licensing Specialists: *John C. Leland/Ann Marie Jannette*
Cover Image: *©yienkeat, Getty images*
Compositor: *Laserwords Private Limited*
Printer: *R. R. Donnelley*

Library of Congress Cataloging-in-Publication Data

Shanholtzer, M. Beth.
   Health information management and technology/M. Beth Shanholtzer, MAEd, RHIA, FAHIMA, Lord Fairfax Community College, Gary W. Ozanich, PhD, Northern Kentucky.
      pages cm
   ISBN 978-0-07-351368-3 (alk. paper)
   1. Medical informatics. 2. Medicine—Information technology. I. Ozanich, Gary W. II. Title.
   R858.S467 2016
   610.285—dc23

                                                                        2014037955

www.mhhe.com

brief contents

part one   THE EVOLVING HEALTHCARE SYSTEM IN THE UNITED STATES

chapter 1   Healthcare in the United States 1

chapter 2   Functions, Careers, and Credentials of the HI Professional: Documenting, Maintaining, and Managing Health Information, Past and Present 32

chapter 3   Health Informatics and Health Information Management Shaping the Evolving Healthcare System 66

part two   PROCESSING HEALTH INFORMATION

chapter 4   Maintaining Health Records: An Overview 89

chapter 5   External Forces: Regulatory and Accreditation Influences 123

chapter 6   The Active Health Record in Acute Care Settings 145

chapter 7   The Post-discharge Health Record 174

part three   THE MEANINGFUL USE OF DIGITAL HEALTH INFORMATION

chapter 8   The Electronic Health Record: Meaningful Use of Patient Records 205

chapter 9   Privacy and Security of Digital Records 230

chapter 10   The Patient's Role in Healthcare 253

part four   EXPLORING NEW ROLES FOR HEALTH INFORMATION PROFESSIONALS

chapter 11   Expanding Roles and Functions of the Health Information Management and Health Informatics Professional 274

Contents

preface   ix

---

part one   THE EVOLVING HEALTHCARE SYSTEM IN THE UNITED STATES

---

chapter 1   Healthcare in the United States   1

1.1   Healthcare through the Ages—the Patient in Health and Disease   2

1.2   New Policies Transforming Healthcare   9

1.3   Healthcare in Transition   14

1.4   Health Information Empowering the Patient   23

---

chapter 2   Functions, Careers, and Credentials of the HI Professional: Documenting, Maintaining, and Managing Health Information, Past and Present   32

2.1   Documenting Healthcare   33

2.2   Traditional HIM Functions in Transition   41

2.3   The Profession of Health Information Management   52

2.4   Education and Certification of the Health Information Professional   56

---

chapter 3   Health Informatics and Health Information Management Shaping the Evolving Healthcare System   66

3.1   Health Informatics   67

3.2   New Skills in an Integrated and Wired System   71

3.3   Informatics and the Meaningful Use of Health IT   76

3.4   Accountable Care and Health Informatics   80

---

part two   PROCESSING HEALTH INFORMATION

---

chapter 4   Maintaining Health Records: An Overview   89

4.1   A Database of Patients: Building the Master Patient (Person) Index   90

4.2   Keeping Track of Every Patient and Every Encounter   96

4.3   The Concurrent Health Record, EHRs, and Maintaining Quality Health Information   100

4.4   Identifying, Storing, and Locating Records   106

chapter 5 External Forces: Regulatory and Accreditation Influences 123

5.1 Regulations versus Accreditation 124

5.2 Regulatory Agencies Affecting Health Information 125

5.3 Voluntary Accrediting Agencies 137

chapter 6 The Active Health Record in Acute Care Settings 145

6.1 The Flow of Information 146

6.2 The Use of Clinical Electronic Tools in the Documentation of Healthcare 158

6.3 Technology Used in HIM Processes 162

6.4 Integrating Clinical Systems in Acute Care Settings 164

chapter 7 The Post-discharge Health Record 174

7.1 The HIPAA-Designated Record Set and Legal Health Record 175

7.2 The Health Record in Assessing Quality 178

7.3 The Health Record in Risk Management Processes 186

7.4 Payment Models 188

7.5 The Reimbursement Cycle 197

part three THE MEANINGFUL USE OF DIGITAL HEALTH INFORMATION

chapter 8 The Electronic Health Record: Meaningful Use of Patient Records 205

8.1 The Electronic Health Record: Meaningful Use of Patient Information 206

8.2 Electronic HIM Processes 209

8.3 Standards and Interoperability for Digitized Records 215

8.4 The Role of Health Information Exchange 218

8.5 The Infrastructure Supporting Meaningful Use 221

chapter 9 Privacy and Security of Digital Records 230

9.1 Ethical Obligations 231
9.2 HIPAA Privacy Regulations 235
9.3 HIPAA Security Rule 241
9.4 Proving Compliance with Regulations and Reporting Noncompliance 243

chapter 10 The Patient's Role in Healthcare 253

10.1 Patient-centric Healthcare 254
10.2 The Patient Portal versus the Personal Health Record (PHR) 255
10.3 Mobile Health (mHealth) 261
10.4 Improved Outcomes through Patient Education and Engagement 265

part four EXPLORING NEW ROLES FOR HEALTH INFORMATION PROFESSIONALS

chapter 11 Expanding Roles and Functions of the Health Information Management and Health Informatics Professional 274

11.1 Expanding Roles in an Electronic, Patient-centric Environment 275
11.2 Health Information Professionals' New Roles and Responsibilities in an Electronic, Patient-centric Health System 286
11.3 Health Information Education and Beyond 290

abbreviations and acronyms A-1
glossary G-1
references R-1
credits C-1
index I-1

Health Information Management and Technology (HIM&T) charts a path for success in the ever-evolving health information field. This product focuses on how electronic health records (EHRs) and a philosophy of patient-centric care are currently impacting health information professionals in their everyday careers as well as the patients they serve. In a health information system that is becoming increasingly integrated and cross-disciplinary, health information students need to be equipped with the problem-solving skills to make important connections and to face the challenges and opportunities they will see in their careers. At the same time, they need to develop the soft skills to work closely with their peers to power the healthcare revolution.

HIM&T approaches foundational health information learning as an exercise in linking how complex issues fit together, all in an accessible, engaging format correlated to current health information management (HIM) standards. *HIM&T* is also available with a wide variety of digital learning tools—from Connect to LearnSmart and SmartBook—that enable instructors to easily customize their courses to craft a learning environment adapted to help every student succeed.

Key Features

- *HIM&T* is suitable for health information management and technology courses at a variety of levels, from associate degree and certificate programs to bachelor's degree programs, both in the classroom and online.

- Health information management, technology, and informatics are discussed side by side, giving the student a realistic idea of how these fields interact in today's healthcare climate and how they will become increasingly interrelated in the future.

- Over 40 "A Day in the Life" features offer extended, thought-provoking cases that link the theory behind health information management and technology to accurate real-life scenarios. Whether they are actual experiences shared by current practitioners or they cover challenges being faced in the field, "A Day in the Life" features help promote active learning and critical thinking.

- Make study time more effective and efficient for your students with McGraw-Hill Education's revolutionary new adaptive study tools, LearnSmart and SmartBook. Whether students are reviewing or reading, these products adapt to create a personalized learning experience for each student, suggesting content based on what they know and don't know.

- A variety of exercises, interactives, hands-on activities, and case studies take the approach of *HIM&T* one step further in

Connect, our online learning and assessment platform. Combined with the power of LearnSmart and SmartBook, content mastery is at the fingertips of every student.

Content Highlights of *Health Information Management and Technology* by Chapter

- **Chapter 1:** Provides an overview of the evolution of medicine, important advances of the modern age, and current factors influencing the administration of healthcare in the United States; sets the stage for transformation in digital healthcare and clarifies the current state of the US healthcare system

- **Chapter 2:** Explores the health record in paper and digital format, specifically how health information is utilized, authored, validated, stored, and processed as part of healthcare delivery by various users; outlines key roles of health information management professionals and the credentials needed to be active in the field as well as the historical roots of the health information management profession

- **Chapter 3:** Examines how the implementation of healthcare reform is evolving the complementary fields of health informatics and health information management while breaking down the differences and similarities between these two fields; details the informatics skills health information professionals will need to thrive in a healthcare system increasingly driven by accountable care

- **Chapter 4:** Discusses methods for keeping health records, tracking their location, and ensuring their completion as well as the information gleaned from data collected in each record; unpacks the differences between clinical and administrative data while showing how EHRs enable the maintenance of high-quality health data; contrasts the storage and organizational challenges of print and digital health records; outlines strategies for print and digital retention as well as disaster recovery

- **Chapter 5:** Examines the mandatory requirements of federal and state regulations as well as voluntary standards that govern record-keeping and documentation practices; explores common Conditions of Participation and state licensure requirements; compares accrediting agencies and reviews a sampling of accreditation standards

- **Chapter 6:** Delves into the types of documentation found in health records and the flow of data collection from registration through discharge; differentiates administrative versus clinical data; investigates the use of automated systems to capture documentation

- **Chapter 7:** Examines the role of health information professionals in the use of the post-discharge health record; details the use of the health record in quality assessment, risk management functions, and the reimbursement cycle; explains the difference between the legal health record and the

HIPAA-designated record set; explores external quality assessment operations by regulatory and reimbursement agencies; investigates legacy government and private payment systems, the Accountable Care Act, and value-based purchasing; introduces the concept of information governance

- **Chapter 8:** Details how the Meaningful Use of electronic health records is changing healthcare delivery and the use of health information; defines Meaningful Use requirements, relates them to their roles in clinical care, and explores their implications for health information management; describes key technical standards and their supporting health information technology infrastructure, including the role of health information exchange

- **Chapter 9:** Examines the duty of healthcare professionals to ensure patients' privacy and the security of their health information; explains HIPAA privacy and security regulations; discusses breach of privacy and tracking access to and disclosure of protected health information; explores medical identity theft as well as the use of patient portals to securely provide patients with access to their health information

- **Chapter 10:** Discusses the revolution in healthcare created by patient-centric care and patient engagement and the process of redesigning care coordination through team-based approaches and engaging the healthcare consumer through Personal Health Records and patient portals to support proactive care, including wellness and disease management; features new roles for mHealth applications and devices, including remote monitoring and wearables, the context of the implications for the health information management and health information technology professional

- **Chapter 11:** Delves into traditional roles of the health information and informatics professional and how those are evolving in a digital domain; explores new roles that have emerged and are expected to materialize as a result of the increase in digital data; investigates the reason for an impending shortage in health information professionals; addresses the current and future educational requirements for a career in health information and informatics

Health Information Management and Technology Preparation in the Digital World: Supplementary Materials for the Instructor and Student

Instructors, McGraw-Hill knows how much effort it takes to prepare for a new course. Through focus groups, symposia, reviews, and conversations with instructors like you, we have gathered information about what materials you need in order to facilitate successful courses. We are committed to providing you with high-quality, accurate instructor support. Knowing the importance of flexibility and digital learning, McGraw-Hill has created multiple assets to enhance the learning experience, no matter what the class format: traditional, online, or hybrid. This product is designed to help instructors and students be successful, with digital solutions proven to drive student success.

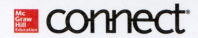

A one-stop spot to present, deliver, and assess digital assets available from McGraw-Hill: McGraw-Hill Connect® Health Information Management and Technology

McGraw-Hill Connect® Health Information Management and Technology provides online presentation, assignment, and assessment solutions. It connects your students with the tools and resources they'll need to achieve success. With Connect you can deliver assignments, quizzes, and tests online. A robust set of questions and activities, including all of the end-of-section and end-of-chapter questions, comprehensive case studies, critical thinking questions, hands-on problem-solving activities, interactives, and study questions will help students master the foundational knowledge they need to lay the framework for future success in their degree and on their credentialing exams. These activities are all aligned with the content's learning outcomes, which are in turn linked to various competencies as well as the most recent AHIMA curriculum domains.

As an instructor, you can edit existing questions and author entirely new problems. Connect enables you to track individual student performance—by question, by assignment, or in relation to the class overall—with detailed grade reports. You can integrate grade reports easily with Learning Management Systems (LMSs), such as Blackboard, Desire2Learn, or eCollege—and much more.

Connect Insight™ is the first and only analytics tool of its kind, which highlights a series of visual data displays—each framed by an intuitive question—to provide at-a-glance information regarding how your class is doing. As an instructor or administrator, you receive an instant, at-a-glance view of student performance matched with student activity. It puts real-time analytics in your hands so you can take action early and keep struggling students from falling behind. It also allows you to be empowered with a more valuable, transparent, and productive connection between you and your students. Available on demand wherever and whenever it's needed, Connect Insight travels from office to classroom!

A single sign-on with Connect and your Blackboard course: McGraw-Hill Education and Blackboard–for a premium user experience

Blackboard®, the web-based course management system, has partnered with McGraw-Hill to better allow students and faculty to use online materials and activities to complement face-to-face teaching. Blackboard features exciting social learning and teaching tools that foster active learning opportunities for students. You'll transform your closed-door classroom into communities where students remain connected to their educational experience 24 hours a day. This partnership allows you and your students access to Connect and Create right from within your Blackboard course—all with a single sign-on. Not only do you get single sign-on with Connect and Create but you also get deep integration of McGraw-Hill content and content engines right in Blackboard. Whether you're choosing a book for your course or building Connect assignments, all the tools you need are right where you want them—inside Blackboard. Gradebooks are now seamless. When a student completes an integrated Connect assignment, the grade for that assignment automatically (and instantly) feeds into your Blackboard grade center. McGraw-Hill and Blackboard can now offer you easy access to industry-leading technology and content, whether your campus hosts it or we do. Be sure to ask your local McGraw-Hill representative for details.

Still want a single sign-on solution and using another learning management system? See how **MH Campus**® (http://mhcampus.mhhe.com/) makes the grade by offering universal sign-on, automatic registration, gradebook synchronization, and open access to a multitude of learning resources—all in one place. MH Campus supports Active Directory, Angel, Blackboard, Canvas, Desire2Learn, eCollege, IMS, LDAP, Moodle, Moodlerooms, Sakai, Shibboleth, WebCT, BrainHoney, Campus Cruiser, and Jenzibar eRacer. Additionally, MH Campus can be easily connected with other authentication authorities and LMSs.

Create a textbook organized the way you teach: McGraw-Hill Create

With **McGraw-Hill Create**™, you can easily rearrange chapters, combine material from other content sources, and quickly upload content you have written, such as your course syllabus or teaching notes. Find the content you need in Create by searching through thousands of leading McGraw-Hill textbooks. Arrange your book to fit your teaching style. Create even allows you to personalize your book's appearance by selecting the cover and adding your name, school, and course information. Order a Create book and you'll receive a complimentary print review copy in three to five business days or a complimentary electronic review copy (eComp) via e-mail in minutes. Go to www.mcgrawhillcreate.com today and register to experience how McGraw-Hill Create empowers you to teach *your* students *your* way.

Record and distribute your lectures for multiple viewing: My Lectures—Tegrity

McGraw-Hill Tegrity® records and distributes your class lecture with just a click of a button. Students can view it anytime and anywhere via computer, iPod, or mobile device. It indexes as it records your PowerPoint presentations and anything shown on your computer, so students can use keywords to find exactly what they want to study. Tegrity is available as an integrated feature of **McGraw-Hill Connect Health Information Management and Technology** and as a stand-alone product.

New from McGraw-Hill Education, **McGraw-Hill LearnSmart**® Advantage is a series of adaptive learning products fueled by LearnSmart, the most widely used and intelligent adaptive learning resource proven to improve learning since 2009. Developed to

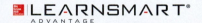

deliver demonstrable results in boosting grades, increasing course retention, and strengthening memory recall, the LearnSmart Advantage series spans the entire learning process from course preparation to providing the first adaptive reading experience found only in **McGraw-Hill SmartBook**™. Distinguishing what students know from what they don't, and honing in on concepts they are most likely to forget, each product in the series helps students study smarter and retain more knowledge. A smarter learning experience for students coupled with valuable reporting tools for instructors, and available in hundreds of course areas, LearnSmart Advantage is advancing learning like no other products in higher education today. Go to **www.LearnSmartAdvantage.com** for more information.

LEARNSMART®

McGraw-Hill LearnSmart® is one of the most effective and successful adaptive learning resources available on the market today and is now available for *Health Information Management and Technology*. More than 2 million students have answered more than 1.3 billion questions in LearnSmart since 2009, making it the most widely used and intelligent adaptive study tool that's proven to strengthen memory recall, keep students in class, and boost grades. Students using LearnSmart are 13% more likely to pass their classes and 35% less likely to drop out. This revolutionary learning resource is available only from McGraw-Hill Education; join the learning revolution, and start using LearnSmart today!

SMARTBOOK®

SmartBook™ is the first and only adaptive reading experience available today. SmartBook personalizes content for each student in a continuously adapting reading experience. Reading is no longer a passive and linear experience but an engaging and dynamic one where students are more likely to master and retain important concepts, coming to class better prepared. Valuable reports provide instructors insight into how students are progressing through textbook content and are useful for shaping in-class time or assessment. As a result of the adaptive reading experience found in SmartBook, students are more likely to retain knowledge, stay in class, and get better grades. This revolutionary technology is available only from McGraw-Hill Education and for hundreds of course areas as part of the LearnSmart Advantage series.

Instructor Resources

You can rely on the following materials to help you and your students work through the material in this book. All of the resources in the following table are available in the Instructor Resources under the library tab in Connect.

Need help? Contact McGraw-Hill's Customer Experience Group (CXG). Visit the CXG website at **www.mhhe.com/support**. Browse our FAQs (frequently asked questions) and product documentation and/or contact a CXG representative. CXG is available Sunday through Friday.

Supplement	Features
Instructor's Manual	Each chapter has • Learning outcomes and lecture outline • Overview of PowerPoint presentations • Lesson plan • Activities and discussion topics • Answer keys for end-of-section and end-of-chapter questions
PowerPoint Presentations	• Key concepts • References to learning outcomes • Teaching notes
Electronic Test Bank	• EZ Test Online (computerized) • Word version • These questions are also available through Connect. • Questions are tagged with learning outcomes, level of difficulty, level of Bloom's taxonomy, feedback, topic, and the accrediting standards of CAHIIM, ABHES, and CAAHEP.
Tools to Plan Course	• Correlations by learning outcomes to ABHES, CAAHEP, CAHIIM, and more • Sample syllabi • Asset map—a recap of the key instructor resources, as well as information on the content available through Connect

Want to learn more about this product? Attend one of our online webinars. To learn more about the webinars, please contact your McGraw-Hill sales representative. To find your McGraw-Hill representative, go to **www.mhhe.com** and click "Find My Sales Rep."

Best-in-Class Digital Support

Based on feedback from our users, McGraw-Hill Education has developed Digital Success Programs that will provide you and your students the help you need, when you need it.

- Training for instructors: Get ready to drive classroom results with our Digital Success Team—ready to provide in-person, remote, or on-demand training as needed.
- Peer support and training: No one understands your needs like your peers. Get easy access to knowledgeable digital users by joining our Connect Community, or speak directly with one of our Digital Faculty Consultants, who are instructors using McGraw-Hill digital products.
- Online training tools: Get immediate anytime, anywhere access to modular tutorials on key features through our Connect Success Academy.

Get started today. Learn more about McGraw-Hill Education's Digital Success Programs by contacting your local sales representative or visit **http://connect.customer.mheducation.com/start**.

about the authors

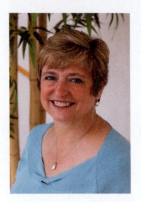

M. Beth Shanholtzer, MAEd, RHIA, FAHIMA, has been in the health information management field for 35 years. Her experience includes HIM department management positions within hospitals in New Jersey, Pennsylvania, West Virginia, and Maryland. She has been in academics for 20 years, and she is currently the program director and an assistant professor for an HIM associate degree program at Lord Fairfax Community College in Middletown, Virginia. She previously held positions as program director and instructor of associate degree programs at Kaplan University.

She is an active AHIMA member, serving on the Council for Excellence in Education (CEE) board, and is currently chairperson of the Faculty Development Workgroup of the CEE. She also serves as a student mentor. On the state level, Beth has served as president, education chair, and legislative chair of the West Virginia Health Information Management Association. She has presented at the AHIMA annual convention, the Assembly on Education (AOE), and WVHIMA conferences. In recognition of her experience as a practitioner and her advancement of the field of health information, Beth has earned the distinction of Fellow of the American Health Information Management Association (FAHIMA).

Beth has authored and co-authored the first and second editions of *Integrated Electronic Health Records: A Worktext for Greenway Medical Technologies' PrimeSUITE*, published by McGraw-Hill Education.

Beth lives in Martinsburg, West Virginia, with her husband; they have three children.

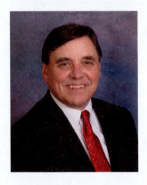

Gary W. Ozanich, PhD, is a senior research associate in the Center for Applied Informatics at Northern Kentucky University (NKU), where he was the founding director of NKU's Graduate Program in Health Informatics. He has had a career that spans both the private sector and academia. Gary has received numerous grants and contracts to conduct research in the areas of health informatics, health information exchange, and payment reform initiatives. He has served on regional and national healthcare-related committees and work-groups, including as national chair of the HIMSS Health Information Exchange Committee and chair of the HIMSS HIE Roundtable.

Gary's private-sector background includes more than 10 years as a securities analyst on Wall Street. He also has worked as a consultant at Booz-Allen & Hamilton. Relative to academic positions, he was associate director of the Institute of Tele-Information at Columbia University and has been on the faculties of Michigan State University and University at Buffalo. He holds a PhD from the University of Wisconsin–Madison.

Gary lives in Cincinnati, Ohio, with his wife and his Labrador and golden retrievers.

dedication

This book would not have been possible without the love and support of my family, Neil, Alison, J. P., and Alex. Special thanks go out to Megan McDougal, Jamie Anderson, Gary Matthews, and Marcia Sharp for sharing their experiences. My thanks to the entire McGraw-Hill team for their tireless dedication to the project. To Danielle Mbadu for your support, shoulder, ear, and inspiration. And finally, in memory of Adanya—there were so many times when I thought I couldn't write another word, and your mom would send on a funny video or a text telling me of something you said or did that would save the day for both of us. Rest in peace, little one. —Beth Shanholtzer

Dedicated to my wife, Leslie Oleksowicz, MD, with thanks and gratitude for her support and kindness. —Gary Ozanich

acknowledgments

Suggestions have been received from faculty and students throughout the country. This is vital feedback that is relied on for product development. Each person who has offered comments and suggestions has our thanks. The efforts of many people are needed to develop and improve a product. Among these people are the reviewers and consultants who point out areas of concern, cite areas of strength, and make recommendations for change. In this regard, the following instructors provided feedback that was enormously helpful in preparing the book and related products.

Manuscript Reviewers

Multiple instructors reviewed the manuscript while it was in development, providing valuable feedback that directly impacted the product.

Julie Alles, RHIA
Grand Valley State University

Mark Chustz, PhD
Alabama State University

Kristy Courville, MHA, RHIA
University of Louisiana-Lafayette

Terri Gilbert, BS
ECPI University

Kelli Lewis, MSHI, RHIA
Valencia College

Darcy Roy, CPC
Eastern Florida State College

Mona Calhoun, MS, MEd, RHIA FAHIMA
Coppin State University

Michelle Cranney, DHSc, RHIA, CPC, AHIMA-Approved ICD-10-CM/PCS Trainer
Ashford University

Laurie Dennis, AA, BS,CBCS, CCMA
Florida Career College

Lawrence Feidelman, MS, CIS
Florida Atlantic University

Elizabeth Hoffman, MAEd, CMA (AAMA), CPT
Henry Ford College

Deborah Honstad, MA, RHIA
San Juan College

Shalena Jarvis, RHIT, CCS
Hazard Community and Technical College

Barbara Marchelletta, CMA (AAMA), RHIT, CPC
Beal College

Laura J. Michelsen, MS, RHIA
Joliet Junior College

Irma Rodriguez, MEd, RHIA, CCS, AHIMA-Approved ICD-10-CM/PCS Trainer
South Texas College

Patricia Saccone, MA, RHIA, CCS-P
Waubonsee Community College

Amy Shay, CHPS, RHIT, BS
Tidewater Community College

Linda Sorensen, RHIA, CHPS, MPA
Davenport University

Christina Thomas, MHA/Ed, CPC, CBCS, CCMA, CMAA
Florida Career College

Barbara Westrick, CMA (AAMA), CPC
Ross Medical Education Center

Toni Windquist, MS-ISM, RHIA
Ferris State University

Arthur Witkowski, MEd
Chemeketa Community College

Technical Editing/Accuracy Panel

A panel of instructors completed a technical edit and review of the content in the book page proofs to verify its accuracy.

Barbara Westrick, CMA(AAMA), CPC
Ross Medical Education Center

Barbara Marchelleta, CMA(AAMA), RHIT, CPC
Beal College

Julie Alles-Grice, MSCTE, RHIA
Grand Valley State University

Brenda M. Kupecky, MSM, RHIA
Ivy Tech Community College-Central Indiana

Laura J. Michelsen, MS, RHIA
Joliet Junior College

Lawrence Feidelman, MS, CIS
Florida Atlantic University

Darice M. Grzybowski, MA, RHIA, FAHIMA
HIMentors, LLC

Study and Instructional Tool Development

Special thanks to the instructors who helped with the development of Connect, LearnSmart, and SmartBook. These include

Test Bank Development

Mona M. Burke, RHIA, FAHIMA
Bowling Green State University-Firelands

Katherine E. Baus, RHIA, CCS-P
Cardinal Medical Consultants, Inc.

Test Bank Accuracy Checking

Mark Chustz, PhD, MSW, RHIA
Alabama State University

Julie Alles-Grice, MSCTE, RHIA
Grand Valley State University

Kristy T. Courville, MHA, RHIA
University of Louisiana—Lafayette

Mary Lou Hilbert, MBA, RHIT, LHRM
Seminole State College of Florida

Amy Loskowski
Washtenaw Community College

Terri Gilbert
ECPI University

Hertencia Bowe, Ed.D., RHIA
Fisher College

Stephanie Scott, RHIA, CCS, CCS-P
Moraine Park Technical College

Connect Development

Mona Calhoun, MS, M.Ed., RHIA, FAHIMA
Coppin State University

Arthur Witkowski, M.Ed.
Chemeketa Community College

Connect Accuracy Checking

Joyce Cole
Westmoreland County Community College

Sharon K. Breeding
Bluegrass Community and Technical College

Laura J. Michelsen, MS, RHIA
Joliet Junior College

Kathy J. Ware, MCLS, RHIT, CPC, CPC-I
Lord Fairfax Community College

Mona M. Burke, RHIA, FAHIMA
Bowling Green State University-Firelands

Kristy T. Courville, MHA, RHIA
University of Louisiana—Lafayette

Amy Loskowski
Washtenaw Community College

LearnSmart Development

Shalena Jarvis, RHIT, CCS
Hazard Community and Technical College

Katherine E. Baus, RHIA, CCS-P
Cardinal Medical Consultants, Inc.

Patricia Saccone, MA, RHIA, CCS-P
Waubonsee Community College

LearnSmart Accuracy Checking

Joyce Cole
Westmoreland County Community College

Mary Lou Hilbert, MBA, RHIT, LHRM
Seminole State College of Florida

Laura J. Michelsen, MS, RHIA
Joliet Junior College

Kristy T. Courville, MHA, RHIA
University of Louisiana—Lafayette

Kelly Jeanne Fast, MS, RHIA, CMT
Missouri Western State University

Barbara Westrick, CMA(AAMA), CPC
Ross Medical Education Center

Barb Marchelleta, CMA(AAMA), RHIT, CPC
Beal College

Stephanie Scott, RHIA, CCS, CCS-P
Moraine Park Technical College

Instructor's Manual and PowerPoint Development

Michelle Cranney, DHSc, RHIA
Ashford University

Amy Shay, CHPS, RHIT, BS
Tidewater Community College

Terri Gilbert
ECPI University

Acknowledgments from the Authors

We would like to thank the following individuals who helped develop, critique, and shape our textbook and ancillary package.

We thank the extraordinary efforts of a talented group of individuals at McGraw-Hill who made all of this come together. We would especially like to thank our Managing Director, Chad Grall; William Lawrensen, our Executive Brand Manager; Michelle Flommenhoft, our Senior Product Developer; Michelle Gaseor, our Product Developer; Roxan Kinsey, our Executive Marketing Manager; April R. Southwood, our Content Project Manager; Sherry Kane, our Media Project Manager; Angela R. FitzPatrick, our Program Manager; Srdjan Savanovic, our Senior Designer; Sandy Ludovissy, our Senior Buyer; Katherine Ward, our Digital Product Analyst; and John C. Leland and Ann Marie Jannette, our Content Licensing Specialists.

We are also deeply indebted to the individuals who helped develop, critique, and shape the text's ancillary package.

We also want to recognize the valuable input of all those who helped guide our developmental decisions, especially Kate Berry, Karen Chrisman, Mary Gaetz, Phil Godel, Kevin Kirby, Pam Matthews, Ken Mitchell, Polly Mullins-Bentley, and Doug Perry.

chapter **one**

Healthcare in the United States

Copyright © 2011 R.J. Romero. www.hipaacartoons.com

"All this talk about EMRs and EHRs is just a fad - like the Internet thing."

Learning Outcomes

When you finish this chapter, you will be able to:

1.1 Describe the history of healthcare and the evolving role of patients, providers, insurers, and regulators in the delivery of healthcare in the United States.

1.2 Outline how new laws and regulations are reshaping healthcare in the United States.

1.3 Summarize the roles of key stakeholders in shaping healthcare transformation in the United States.

1.4 Explain how health information is being used to empower patients.

Key Terms

Accountable care organizations (ACOs)
Accreditation
Affordable Care Act (ACA)
American College of Surgeons (ACS)
American Hospital Association (AHA)
American Medical Association (AMA)
American Recovery and Reinvestment Act (ARRA)
Centers for Medicare and Medicaid Services (CMS)
Clinical decision support (CDS)
Conditions of Participation (CoP)
Deficit Reduction Act
Department of Health and Human Services (HHS)
Diagnosis related group (DRG)
Evidence-based medicine (EBM)

Fee-for-service
Healthcare Facilities Accreditation Program (HFAP)
Health information technology (HIT)
Health Information Technology for Economic and Clinical Health Act (HITECH)
Health Insurance Portability and Accountability Act (HIPAA)
Hill-Burton Act
Independent Practice Association (IPA)
Informed consent
Licensure
Managed care insurance plans
Meaningful Use
Medicaid

Medicare
Medicare Prescription Drug Improvement and
  Modernization Act of 2003 (MMA)
mHealth
Office of the National Coordinator for Health
  Information Technology (ONC)
Omnibus Budget Reconciliation Act of 1986
Patient-centered medical home (PCMH)
Patient-centric

Patients' rights
Physician Quality Reporting Initiative (PQRI)
Population health management (PHM)
Primary care physician (PCP)
Prospective payment system (PPS)
Quality Improvement Organizations (QIOs)
Tax Equity and Fiscal Responsibility Act of 1982
  (TEFRA)
The Joint Commission (TJC)

Introduction

In this first chapter, we will take a look at the evolution of medicine in general, important advances in the modern age, and current factors influencing the administration of healthcare in the United States. Healthcare professionals and healthcare consumers have experienced a surge in changes, particularly over the past three decades. This chapter will follow key milestones in healthcare up to the current status (at the time of writing) and will set the stage for advances to come in the foreseeable future.

1.1 Healthcare through the Ages—the Patient in Health and Disease

Through the Ages—a Brief History of Medicine

The practice of medicine has been traced back thousands of years, when disease was thought to be the result of offending the forces of nature, of being possessed, or of offending the gods. In Egypt, stone tablets, monuments, and papyri contain primitive medical records that date back as far as 2700 BCE. Edwin Smith, an American dealer and collector of antiquities, brought two of the most famous medical papyri to the attention of scholars—the Ebers Papyrus and what would come to be known as the Edwin Smith Papyrus (see Figure 1.1). The Ebers Papyrus is one of the most famous examples; it includes descriptions of ailments, the systems of the body, and the medicines, remedies, and formulas used to treat diseases at that time.

The Greeks, however, are considered the model for modern medicine. The belief that disease and its treatment were magical or spiritual was diminishing, and the scientific view of medicine was beginning to take hold. Hippocrates, a Greek physician, penned the famous Hippocratic Oath in the late 5th century BCE, which, though modernized, is still in use today.

Throughout medieval times, churches and religious orders took care of the sick, and doctors had no formal training. As a matter of fact, medicine wasn't considered a profession at all until the mid-19th century.

Medical Care and Healthcare in the United States

Science had little to do with medicine until around the mid-1800s. The belief until that time was that illnesses could be rid from the body by such things as bloodletting and purging. There were no

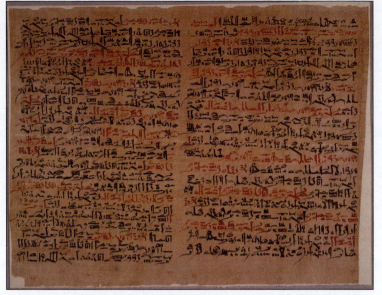

Figure 1.1 The Edwin Smith Papyrus, One of the Earliest Medical Texts (17th Century BCE)

medical schools, and doctors learned their trade by a sort of on-the-job training or apprenticeship with experienced physicians. The first formal medical school did not appear until the mid-1700s. The first four medical schools in the United States were College of Philadelphia (1756), King's College (1768), Harvard University (1783), and Dartmouth College (1797) (Shi and Singh, 2008).

The first hospital in the United States was founded by Benjamin Franklin and Dr. Thomas Bond in 1751. It was named Pennsylvania Hospital and is still in existence today (see Figure 1.2). For nearly 100 years, there was no way of ensuring that future physicians were being educated thoroughly or accurately, and the quality of their education was considered to be poor even at that time. Thus, the **American Medical Association (AMA)** was formed in 1847 to ensure quality medical education. It was founded by Nathan Smith Davis "to elevate

American Medical Association (AMA) A professional association of physicians founded in 1847 with the purpose of developing standards for medical education, improving public health, establishing medical ethics, and advancing the study of science.

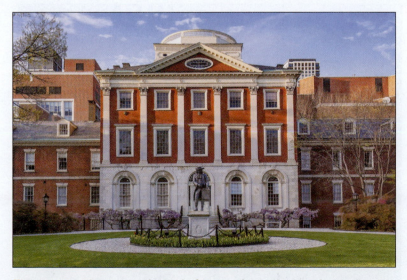

Figure 1.2 The Surgical Ward of Pennsylvania Hospital—America's First Hospital (1910)

the standard of medical education in the United States." The AMA's purpose is to develop standards for medical education, to improve public health, to establish a set of medical ethics, and to advance the study of science. Since its inception, the AMA has been an advocate for patients as well as physicians, ensuring high-quality medical care and improving the healthcare system in the United States.

Near the end of the 19th century, the **American Hospital Association (AHA)** was founded. It was committed to improving medical care by advocating for the healthcare community, educating healthcare leaders, and tracking trending healthcare-related issues, specifically for hospitals and all other types of healthcare facilities.

Some state governments also became involved in improving medical care by requiring the **licensure** of practitioners and hospitals, a result of the Medical Practice Act. In other words, if the medical school a physician attended did not meet certain standards, the graduates of that college or university were also deemed inadequate. This is much like the accreditation standards we see today for colleges and universities.

It was between 1870 and 1920 that the greatest growth in hospital openings occurred. There were fewer than 200 hospitals throughout the United States before 1870, but this number jumped to more than 6,000 in the early 1920s.

The Need for Data

The **American College of Surgeons (ACS)**, whose purpose it was to improve the quality of patient care by setting high standards for surgical education and practice, was founded in 1913 in Chicago (see Figure 1.3). Though its mission was to improve the care rendered to surgical patients, it went on to establish a system of hospital standardization as well. It was the ACS that believed that written records were essential for quality patient care and that data collected from records would lead to the information necessary to set and measure standards of care.

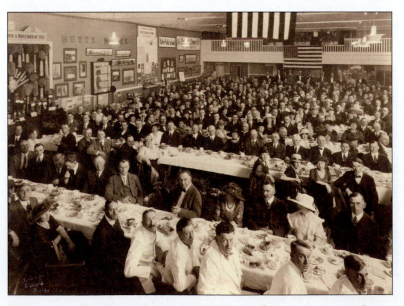

Figure 1.3 The Original American College of Surgeons at a Gala

The following is a synopsis of the 1919 ACS "Minimum Standard" document:

1. Physicians and surgeons practicing in a hospital should be organized as a group or staff.

2. Membership on the staff should include only those who are (a) full graduates of medical schools in good standing and legally licensed in their respective fields, (b) competent in their respective fields, and (c) worthy in character and in matters of professional ethics.

3. The medical staff should operate under a set of rules, regulations, and policies, and they should specifically provide that

    a. medical staff meetings are held once a month; and

    b. staff review and analyze at regular intervals their clinical experience, the clinical records of patients, free and paid, to be the basis for such review and analysis.

4. Accurate and complete written records should be kept for all patients and filed in an accessible manner in the hospital. A complete case record includes identification data; complaint; personal and family history; history of present illness; physical examination; special examinations, such as consultations, clinical laboratory, x-ray, and other examinations; provisional or working diagnosis; medical or surgical treatment; gross and microscopic pathological findings; progress notes; final diagnosis; condition on discharge; follow-up; and, in case of death, autopsy findings.

5. Diagnostic and therapeutic facilities should exist under competent supervision, for the study, diagnosis, and treatment of patients. These must include at least (a) a clinical laboratory, including chemical, bacterial, serological, and pathological services; and (b) an x-ray department providing radiographic and fluoroscopic services.

Of note is the fourth standard, which spells out the requirements for written patient records. These standards still exist and are the basis of a quality health record.

The Early 20th Century

With the advent of formal, structured medical education, standards, and professional organizations, the quality of healthcare continued to increase throughout the early 20th century. Great strides in technology were being made; physicians were choosing to specialize in particular areas of study, such as surgery, psychiatry, or obstetrics; and other medical personnel, such as nurses and technicians, were being educated on a higher scientific level.

In addition to being licensed, medical facilities were seeking **accreditation**. Whereas licensure meant that a facility was meeting minimum requirements, accreditation meant that a facility was exceeding the minimum requirements and was meeting or exceeding standards set by accrediting agencies. Licensure was and is required in order to operate a medical facility or to practice medicine.

Accreditation Voluntary assessment by an accrediting agency that proves a healthcare facility exceeds the minimum requirements set by licensing agencies.

The Joint Commission (TJC) Formerly known as The Joint Commission on Accreditation of Hospitals, a voluntary accrediting agency holding deemed status by Medicare.

Healthcare Facilities Accreditation Program (HFAP) A voluntary accreditation program used by the American Osteopathic Association, which, like The Joint Commission, holds deemed status for Medicare.

Hill-Burton Act Legislation that supplied funding for the modernization of existing hospitals and the building of new ones, in exchange for which hospitals provided care at a reduced rate or for free to patients who did not have the ability to pay.

Medicare Title XVIII of the Social Security Act of 1935; Medicare provides financial assistance for healthcare coverage to persons 65 years of age and over, to persons who are disabled, and to those with end-stage renal disease.

Medicaid Title XIX of the Social Security Act of 1935; Medicaid provides financial assistance for healthcare coverage to poor and indigent populations.

Conditions of Participation (CoP) Regulations that healthcare facilities and providers must meet in order to receive reimbursement from Medicare and Medicaid.

Accreditation, on the other hand, was and is voluntary, showing a higher level of commitment to quality. The Joint Commission (TJC) and the American Osteopathic Association's (AOA's) Healthcare Facilities Accreditation Program (HFAP) were the first of the accrediting bodies to appear on the healthcare scene.

During the mid-20th century, private insurance plans began to emerge. Corporations and businesses started offering health insurance as a benefit of employment. Healthcare for persons who were poor, sick, elderly, and mentally disabled, however, continued to be scarce, thus leading the federal government to step in and finance healthcare for underserved populations. Social Security had already come about in 1935 and provided grants to assist elderly and unemployed persons, those needing maternal and child welfare, and other underserved groups. The Hill-Burton Act was passed in 1946, supplying funding for the modernization of existing hospitals and the building of new ones. In return, hospitals agreed to provide care to patients who were unable to pay for their care for free or at a reduced rate.

The federal government also realized that there was a need for a formal and organized entity to address health issues, education, and the general welfare of its citizens. Thus, the Department of Health, Education, and Welfare (HEW) (later to become the Department of Health and Human Services, or HHS) was created in 1953.

The most influential and long-lasting change to the US healthcare system came in 1965 with the establishment of Medicare (Title XVIII of the Social Security Act of 1935) and Medicaid (Title XIX of the Social Security Act of 1935). The roots of the legislation stretch back to President Roosevelt's efforts to rebuild America following the Great Depression (see Figure 1.4). Medicare's purpose was to provide financial assistance for persons 65 years of age and over (regardless of financial need), and Medicaid was created to provide financial assistance to poor and indigent populations. With Medicare came Conditions of Participation (CoP), a set of

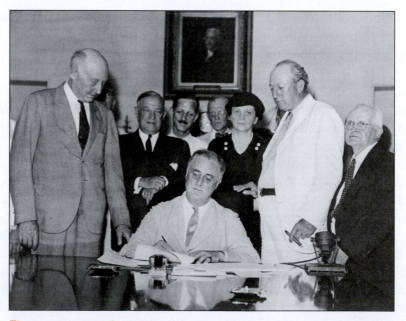

Figure 1.4   President Roosevelt Signs the Social Security Act of 1935

regulations that hospitals and providers must meet in order to be eligible to receive reimbursement from Medicare and Medicaid.

The Latter Part of the 20th Century

During the 1970s, healthcare costs grew out of control. Economic inflation was high; Medicare paid for claims on a **fee-for-service** basis—whatever a hospital or provider charged, Medicare paid. Technology and pharmaceuticals grew, and their price tags soared.

These issues brought about the Social Security Amendments of 1972, which resulted in the formation of Professional Standards Review Organizations (PSROs). PSROs were independent entities that contracted with the federal government to monitor and ensure the quality of medical care and the appropriate utilization of services provided to Medicare, Medicaid, and Maternal and Child Health recipients. PSROs were replaced by Peer Review Organizations (PROs) in the 1980s; since 2002, they have been called **Quality Improvement Organizations (QIOs)**. Another change occurred in 1977, when the Health Care Financing Administration (HCFA) replaced the Social Security Administration as claims manager and regulator of the Medicare and Medicaid programs. HCFA was later renamed the **Centers for Medicare and Medicaid Services (CMS)**.

The 1980s saw a total reform of the Medicare Part A reimbursement system. It was the **Tax Equity and Fiscal Responsibility Act of 1982 (TEFRA)**, implemented in 1983, that caused the transition from a fee-for-service reimbursement system to a **prospective payment system (PPS)**. Under a PPS, every Medicare inpatient falls into a particular **diagnosis related group (DRG)**, which is determined by the patient's principal and secondary diagnoses, the patient's age, and other factors. The amount paid to the hospital was predetermined, based on the DRG into which the patient fell. The purpose of a PPS was to control costs, and hospitals were expected to contain costs—those that were efficient and cost-effective in the treatment of Medicare patients made money; those that weren't did not. There have been several changes to the PPS system, which will be discussed in the chapter covering the records of discharged patients.

Much of the regulatory activity at the end of the 1980s dealt with healthcare quality. The **Omnibus Budget Reconciliation Act of 1986** focused on substandard care and required PROs to report such care to licensing agencies. Nursing home residents were protected by the Nursing Home Reform Act. In 1990, the Patient Self-Determination Act required that patients give **informed consent** for certain procedures and that they be apprised of **patients' rights** regarding the healthcare they receive and their end-of-life decisions.

The **Health Insurance Portability and Accountability Act HIPAA)** was a much anticipated and intensive change to the nation's healthcare system, enacted at various points beginning in 1996 and enforced beginning in 1996 and enforced beginning in 2003, with extensions and grace periods for certain entities. It consists of five rules—privacy, security, data sets and electronic transaction standards, administrative simplification, and enforcement and compliance (see Figure 1.5). Health information professionals and the jobs they do were impacted greatly by HIPAA's passage and implementation.

Fee-for-service Billing for healthcare services after the services have been provided (retrospectively) according to the facility's or office's actual fees for each service.

Quality Improvement Organizations (QIOs) Entities with which CMS contracts to review medical care, based on health record documentation, and to assist Medicare and Medicaid beneficiaries with complaints about quality of care issues and to implement improvements in the quality of care available throughout healthcare facilities.

Centers for Medicare and Medicaid Services (CMS) Formerly known as the Health Care Financing Administration (HCFA), CMS manages Medicare and Medicaid claims and regulates Medicare and Medicaid programs.

Tax Equity and Fiscal Responsibility Act of 1982 (TEFRA) Legislation that resulted in a shift from fee-for-service reimbursement to a prospective payment system.

Prospective payment system (PPS) A fixed reimbursement system based on the diagnosis related group (DRG) assigned to each inpatient stay; used by Medicare and Medicaid reimbursement and some third-party payers.

Diagnosis related group (DRG) A system that classifies patients into groups based on a patient's principal and secondary diagnoses, procedures performed, and other factors and determines the amount reimbursed to the hospital by Medicare, Medicaid, and other third-party payers.

Omnibus Budget Reconciliation Act of 1986 The act that focused on substandard care and resulted in the requirement that PROs report substandard care to licensing agencies.

Informed consent Patient consent required for invasive surgical procedures and any treatment or procedure that carries a risk to the patient; informed consent provides explanation of the procedure/treatment to be performed and the reason for it; in other words, the risks and benefits of the procedure/treatment, alternatives to the procedure/treatment and their risks and benefits, and the name(s) of the healthcare provider(s) performing the procedure/treatment.

Patients' rights Patients have the right to know who their healthcare team consists of, the right to privacy and confidentiality, the right to be informed about their diagnosis and treatment, the right to refuse treatment, the right to actively participate in their care plan, and the right to be cared for in a safe environment, free from abuse. Patients also have the right to read or have a copy (paper or electronic) of their health record, the right to know who has accessed their health record, and the right to request an amendment to their health record.

Health Insurance Portability and Accountability Act (HIPAA) A law consisting of five rules—privacy, security, data sets and electronic transaction standards, administrative simplification, and enforcement and compliance; it impacted healthcare in general and the health information profession in particular more so than any piece of legislation since Medicare and Medicaid.

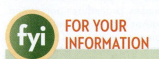 **FOR YOUR INFORMATION**

Claims data are part of administrative data collected on every patient and include identifying data as well as insurance data; clinical data are related to the diagnosis and treatment of the patient.

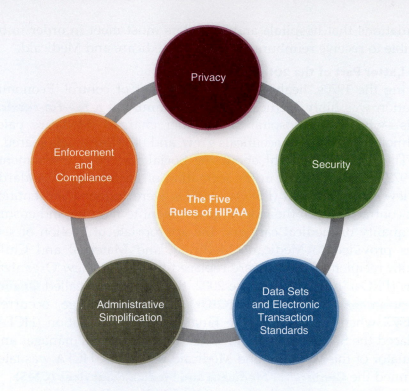

Figure 1.5 The Five Rules of HIPAA

HIPAA will be further explained in the chapter covering external forces affecting health information functions.

Though computerization had become more commonplace in healthcare settings in the latter part of the 20th century, the digital age truly hit healthcare in the early 1990s. The Workgroup on Electronic Data Interchange was created with the goal of reducing administrative costs by requiring healthcare insurance claims to be submitted and processed electronically. Financial institutions had long been "computerized," but healthcare was lagging behind in this arena. This digitization of records applied only to claims data; it did not include clinical data.

The 21st Century

The 21st century has seen a shift from episodic medical care—caring for sickness when it occurs—to healthcare—preventing sickness. Healthcare now focuses on staying healthy through preventive medical visits, a healthy diet, physical activity, and patient education.

We have seen this shift within the healthcare community with an emphasis on all patients having a **primary care physician (PCP)**, who is the "gatekeeper" of a patient's medical care and healthcare. **Managed care insurance plans**, in particular, have been a driving force behind the need for one physician who knows a patient's health and medical histories.

The population is getting older; the first members of the baby boomer generation have reached their sixties. We have become a nation of unhealthy habits and excesses—food, cigarettes, drugs, and risky behavior. The need for medical care and healthcare continues to increase, as does the technology and medical expertise necessary to care for patients. The need to control costs has become more of a challenge, since the sheer number of individuals seeking treatment is increasing, along with the cost of high-tech modalities used in diagnosis and treatment.

The cost of healthcare and the burden on Medicare have not decreased, resulting in further changes to the Medicare reimbursement system during the first part of the 21st century. In 2003, the **Medicare Prescription Drug Improvement and Modernization Act of 2003 (MMA)** was passed. Commonly known as the Medicare Prescription Drug Act, it provides Medicare beneficiaries with financial help to pay for their prescriptions. In addition, the act allows private insurance companies to bid on Medicare plans, thus introducing managed care for the first time in Medicare's history. Fraud and abuse of Medicare funds became issues of great importance, resulting in the passage in 2005 of the **Deficit Reduction Act**.

In addition, for the first time in Medicare's history, physicians were given a monetary incentive to voluntarily report quality of care indicators. This program, implemented in 2006, is the **Physician Quality Reporting Initiative (PQRI)**.

1.1 THINKING IT THROUGH

1. Why has there been increased oversight and regulation in the healthcare industry since the early part of the 20th century?
2. During the 20th century, there was a shift from inpatient care with long lengths of stay to ambulatory care, which remains the principal method of care today. Why is that?
3. Why are Medicare and Medicaid so important in shaping healthcare?
4. Brainstorm with another student or in a group what is meant by "informed" consent.

1.2 New Policies Transforming Healthcare

There has been more healthcare reform in the past decade than at any time since the passage of Medicare and Medicaid in the 1960s. Quality care, positive outcomes, and access to affordable healthcare insurance have been issues high on the priority list of government officials. In this section, we will investigate key initiatives for achieving quality, affordable, accessible healthcare. These initiatives need to be considered on the whole, not individually; they are designed to work together.

Federal Initiatives

The Patient Protection and Affordable Care Act
This is typically referred to as the **Affordable Care Act (ACA)** or "Obamacare." The ACA was signed into law on March 23, 2010. The following are the major goals of this law:

1. Improve access to care and broaden insurance coverage
2. Reduce costs by introducing new models of payment for services and improving care delivery and administrative processes
3. Improve quality of care through expanded measurement and reporting

Primary care physician (PCP) A family practitioner, an internist, or a pediatrician who manages a patient's basic healthcare needs and coordinates care with specialists under a managed care insurance plan.

Managed care insurance plans Insurance plans that promote quality, cost-effective healthcare through the monitoring of patients, preventive care, and performance measures.

Medicare Prescription Drug Improvement and Modernization Act of 2003 (MMA) This act provides Medicare beneficiaries with financial assistance in paying for prescription medications.

Deficit Reduction Act Legislation passed with the intent to reduce growth in Medicare and Medicaid spending and decrease the number of fraudulent Medicare and Medicaid claims.

Physician Quality Reporting Initiative (PQRI) A voluntary pay-for-performance incentive program.

Affordable Care Act (ACA) Healthcare reform with the goal of improving quality of care and affordable healthcare coverage through health insurance exchanges; provides healthcare consumers with stability and flexibility of healthcare coverage.

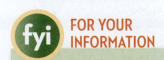

fyi FOR YOUR INFORMATION

The Affordable Care Act (ACA) is known in the media as "Obamacare" and that name is used as shorthand for the ACA.

4. Increase healthcare workforce
5. Combat fraud and abuse
6. Prevent chronic diseases
7. Improve public health

Although there continues to be debate on the merits and ultimate success of the ACA, this sweeping legislation is dramatically changing healthcare. According to the Census Bureau, 15.4% of Americans were uninsured in 2012, and the percentage of privately insured Americans fell from 73% to 63.9% as more people became eligible for the government-run programs Medicare and Medicaid. The ACA addresses both of these groups by expanding subsidized insurance as well as Medicaid for the uninsured and by supporting quality improvement initiatives combined with cost reduction goals for Medicare and Medicaid.

Key provisions of the ACA include the following:

- Mandating that all individuals acquire health insurance or face financial penalties enforced through the Internal Revenue Service (IRS)
- Requiring minimum standards for health insurance policies, including the cancellation of policies that do not meet these standards
- Requiring that the same insurance rates apply to all individuals regardless of medical pre-conditions (including chronic diseases, such as diabetes or hypertension) or gender
- Stipulating no cancellation of policies due to chronic illnesses and no limits on care
- Mandating that individuals under 26 years of age can remain on their parent's health insurance policy if they do not qualify for coverage on their own
- Establishing health insurance exchanges to encourage competition between insurance companies

Figure 1.6 offers a visual representation of the key provisions and goals of the ACA.

At the end of the first enrollment period for the ACA, HHS reported that more than 7 million individuals enrolled through health exchanges, either in expanded Medicaid programs or in private insurance plans. Some of these individuals had been covered but lost their plans under the new minimum standards requirement, and others had been uninsured. According to HHS, 85% of the individuals who purchased a plan are receiving financial assistance from the government.

HITECH and Meaningful Use

The **Health Information Technology for Economic and Clinical Health Act (HITECH)** is part of the American Recovery and Reinvestment Act of 2009 (ARRA), which was signed into law by President Obama on February 17, 2009. HITECH provisions allocated approximately $32 billion to revolutionize healthcare. This consisted of $30 billion in Medicare and Medicaid incentive payments to physicians and hospitals to adopt and use **health information technology** and EHRs

Health Information Technology for Economic and Clinical Health Act (HITECH) Legislation resulting from the ARRA that provides incentives to providers and hospitals that adopt or upgrade existing electronic health record (EHR) systems and associated technologies and use them in specified ways.

Health information technology (HIT) The framework on which health information is collected, stored, exchanged, and reported.

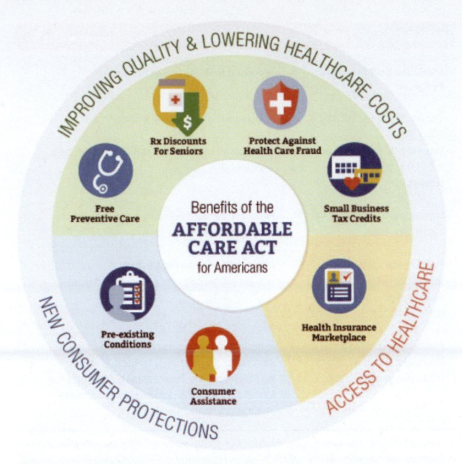

Figure 1.6   Key Features of the Affordable Care Act

Source: US Health and Human Services, http://www.hhs.gov/healthcare/facts/timeline/.

in ways defined as "meaningful," as well as $2 billion for programs administered by the **Office of the National Coordinator for Health Information Technology (ONC)** that supported the standards, infrastructure, and pilot projects for EHR use.

HITECH anticipated the passage of the ACA, as well as the act's specific goals of cost reduction through the introduction of new models of payment, improvement of care delivery and administrative processes, and improvement of quality through measurement and reporting. HITECH's principal goals, which are to increase the use of EHRs, establishment of a nationwide healthcare information system, and data analysis as well as reporting among hospitals, physicians, labs, pharmacies, clinics, public health organizations, payers, and patients, make the fundamental changes that are required by the ACA possible.

The most significant part of HITECH is the incentive payments to providers and hospitals for the adoption and use of EHRs. The idea is that these payments can be used to support an interoperable system and to ensure that providers use a certified EHR in a manner that supports the goals of healthcare reform. This is referred to as **Meaningful Use**. EHRs are capable of doing more than recording and storing information. The Meaningful Use requirements ensure that EHRs are used to achieve benchmarks in improving patient care in a way that can support payment reform and reporting requirements in the future.

Office of the National Coordinator for Health Information Technology (ONC) Located within the office of the secretary of Health and Human Services, the ONC is the federal agency promoting a national health information technology infrastructure and overseeing its development.

Meaningful Use The section of HITECH meant to increase the effective use of electronic health records through monetary incentives to adopt and use certified technology.

TABLE 1.1	Medicare and Medicaid EHR Incentive Programs
Medicare EHR Incentive Program	**Medicaid EHR Incentive Program**
The program is run by CMS.	The program is run by state Medicaid agencies.
Maximum incentive amount is $44,000 per eligible provider.	Maximum incentive amount is $63,750 per eligible professional.
Payments are made over five consecutive years.	Payments are made over six years and do not have to be consecutive.
Payment adjustments will begin in 2015 for providers who are eligible but decide not to participate.	No payment adjustments are made for providers who are eligible only for the Medicaid program.
Providers must demonstrate Meaningful Use every year to receive incentive payments.	In the first year, providers can receive an incentive payment for adopting, implementing, or upgrading EHR technology. Providers must demonstrate Meaningful Use in the remaining years to receive incentive payments.

Source: CMS, http://www.cms.gov/Regulations-and-guidance/Legislation/EHRIncentive Programs/index.html?redirect=/EHRIncentivePrograms/31_ClinicalQualityMeasures.asp #TopOfPage.

There are two Meaningful Use incentive programs, as described in Table 1.1, one administered by CMS under Medicare and one administered by state Medicaid agencies under Medicaid. Each eligible provider can receive payments of up to $44,000 and $63,750 under each program, respectively, throughout the stages of Meaningful Use. The provider or hospital elects to seek funding under one of the two programs. This is determined by the patient mix, with the Medicaid program requiring a minimum of 30% Medicaid patient volume with adjustments for pediatricians and Federally Qualified Health Clinics.

In order to encourage providers and hospitals to participate in the Meaningful Use program, penalties are applied to those that choose not to participate. At this writing, these penalties consist of a reduction in Medicare reimbursement rates by 1% beginning in 2015 and declining by 1% per year through 2017. Thus, Meaningful Use provides a "carrot" (incentive payments to purchase and use EHRs) and a "stick" (reductions in Medicare reimbursements) to motivate providers and hospitals.

There are three stages to Meaningful Use, seen in Figure 1.7. Each of these stages has specific benchmarks and requirements that must be met in order to receive Meaningful Use incentive payments. These are covered in detail in the chapter on the electronic health records and Meaningful Use.

Using an electronic health record or HIT in general will allow providers to compile more accurate and more complete health

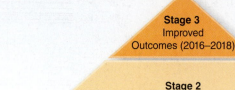

Stage 3
Improved
Outcomes (2016–2018)

Stage 2
Advance Clinical Procedures (2014–2015)

Stage 1
Data Capture and Sharing (2011–2012)

Figure 1.7   **Stages of Meaningful Use**

information about their patients. Coordination of care is also improved, because information about a patient's health status and medical care can be shared instantly rather than losing valuable time while staff makes copies of health records to be sent to potential post-acute care facilities, such as a rehabilitation facility or nursing home. Many patients are utilizing HIT by communicating with their care providers and by securely sharing information with family members, thus allowing for more **patient-centric** care.

Through health IT, care providers have access to the results of clinical trials, current treatment modalities, and **clinical decision support (CDS)** systems, which aid in the diagnosis and treatment of disease by linking structured data (such as lab results or diagnosis codes) with online clinical knowledge databases, in turn improving patient care and outcomes, reducing medical errors, and providing safer medical care at a lower cost. The US health system in general becomes more efficient as a result of the reduction in paperwork for patients, hospitals, and care providers. For an overview of the policies covered that have shaped these changes to the US healthcare system, see Figure 1.8.

Patient-centric Communications, information sharing, and decision making that includes the patient and is managed by both the patient and the provider.

Clinical decision support (CDS) Case-specific computerized alerts, clinical guidelines, and current resources regarding diagnosis and treatment options, based on the data found in individual patient records.

1.2   THINKING IT THROUGH

1. How do the Affordable Care Act and HITECH work together?
2. What are the "carrot" and "stick" components of Meaningful Use? Do you think they will achieve what they are designed to do?
3. How can technology, such as the EHR, help providers obtain more complete health information that will lead to providing better care to their patients?
4. Why do the three stages of Meaningful Use need to be rolled out in this order?

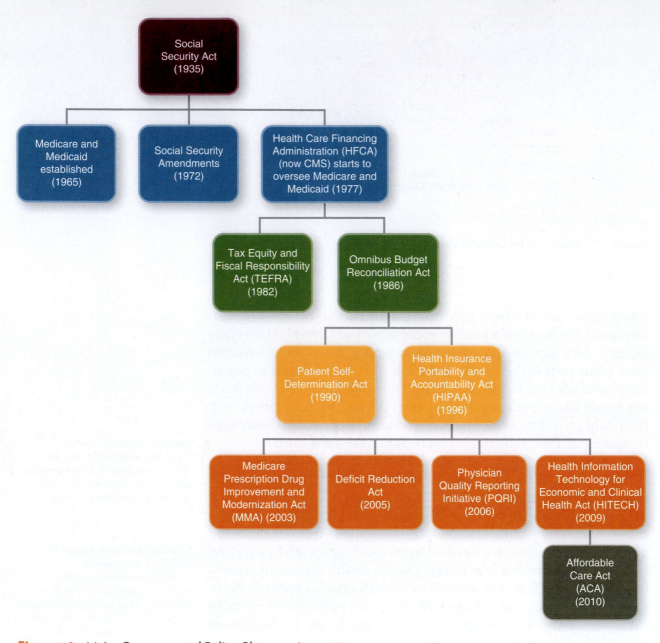

Figure 1.8   Major Governmental Policy Changes since 1935

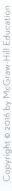
| 1.3 | **Healthcare in Transition** |

New laws and regulations have been implemented to dramatically change healthcare in the United States. This has resulted in a process of transition in healthcare delivery. Providers and other stakeholders are in the initial phase of the transition.

Healthcare Providers in the Continuum of Care

The *continuum of care* is the cycle of healthcare experienced by patients throughout their lifetime. Some patients might use all the types of providers discussed in this section, whereas others might use only one or two. *Continuum of care* can also refer to a single spell of illness. An example is a patient who has been treated by a physician for chronic ear infections. Her physician refers her to an otorhinolaryngologist, a specialist in diseases and treatments of diseases of the ears, nose, and throat. The otorhinolaryngologist's opinion is to perform an operation in which small tubes are inserted into the patient's ears. The surgery takes place in the ambulatory care department of the local hospital, and the patient's chronic ear infections resolve.

The continuum of care may follow a hierarchical path, in which the patient's care starts with *primary care*, proceeds to *secondary care* (as in the case of specialists), and then goes on to *tertiary* care in a hospital environment. Also a possibility is *quarternary* care, whereby the patient is seen in a high-level medical center environment, which may be a teaching facility and/or provide procedures that would not be performed in a community hospital setting.

1.1 A DAY IN THE LIFE

Jane was in a rehabilitation hospital from May 5, 2013, to June 1, 2013, following a stroke she had had on May 1, 2013. She had been in an acute care hospital from May 1 to May 5 for initial treatment of the stroke. She had been treated by her primary care physician, with her last visit on April 10, 2013, for treatment of hypertension. Jane is currently being seen at home by physical therapists from the local home health agency.

1. Based on the concept of continuum of care, discuss Jane's healthcare encounters in the order they would have occurred.

Private Physicians' Practices

The PCP, in the form of a family practitioner, internist, or pediatrician, has become the norm. As noted earlier, the PCP is the gatekeeper of the patient's healthcare. Managed care plans have made the use of a PCP a requirement, in many instances, but in general the notion of having a physician who knows a patient's full medical history, allergies, and current medications at all times is a prudent choice.

Specialty Care

Patients with conditions that cannot be fully addressed by a PCP are generally referred to a specialist. The major specialties include cardiology, pulmonology, urology, gastroenterology, otorhinolaryngology, orthopedics, neurology, psychiatry, gynecology, obstetrics, and pediatrics. From there, some healthcare providers choose subspecialties. For instance, a urologist may choose to specialize in diseases of the kidney and thus is a nephrologist; an obstetrician may choose to specialize in fertility issues. In all instances, specialties and subspecialties require education, training, and experience beyond that needed to become a medical doctor (MD) or doctor of osteopathy (DO).

Ambulatory Care

Fifty years ago, with the exception of private physicians' offices, patients needing healthcare went to a hospital. The provision of ambulatory care, otherwise known as outpatient care, is now more prevalent than care in a hospital setting. Ambulatory care takes several forms:

- Ambulatory clinics might have laboratory, radiology, pharmacy, or other services available under the same roof.
- Urgent care centers are popular and allow patients to be seen by a healthcare provider without an appointment. They are often called walk-in clinics.
- Ambulatory surgery centers are facilities that are either free-standing or affiliated with a hospital. They allow patients to undergo surgical procedures but still be released to return home by the end of the day.

Independent Practice Association (IPA)

A result of the managed care movement, an **Independent Practice Association (IPA)** can consist of either private physicians who have formed a medical group or a group of independent physicians who have contracted with a managed care organization to provide care at a pre-determined, pre-negotiated rate. The group can consist of only primary care physicians or can include healthcare providers from several different medical specialties.

Hospitals

When we hear the term *hospital,* a vision of a large building with an emergency room and many different departments comes to mind. We also envision patients staying overnight or for several days. Although that vision is not incorrect, more patients are treated in a hospital as ambulatory patients (outpatients) than are treated as inpatients. According to the CDC, the average length of stay in an acute care hospital is now 4.8 days. Forty years ago, a typical length of stay would likely have been six or more days.

Integrated Delivery Networks

In the past, hospitals could operate as acute care hospitals or physicians could be in solo private practices and maintain financial viability. The cost of doing business (yes, healthcare is a business) has necessitated offering a broader range of services to increase the population being served. This need has resulted in integrated delivery networks (IDNs), which might consist of a short-term hospital, a home health agency, hospice services, and a long-term care facility all under the same parent organization. Many networks also include more than one hospital in the same network. Well-known integrated delivery networks include Banner Health in Phoenix, Arizona; Bon Secours Richmond Health System in Richmond, Virginia; and Geisinger Health System in Danville, Pennsylvania.

Long-Term Care

Long-term care generally means nursing home care, which may be supervisory and custodial because the patient is no longer able to live alone. It is not covered by Medicare. *Skilled care* is long-term care in which licensed personnel are required to administer wound care, positioning, rehabilitative services, and the like. Skilled care *is* covered by Medicare. Assisted living is a type of long-term care, though the environment is more like a home, yet the patient is in a safer environment than living in his or her own home. Depending on the patient's ability, he or she may be able to leave the facility on his or her own for periods of time.

Behavioral Health

Mental healthcare is now more readily known as behavioral health. It spans the spectrum of care of persons with mental health conditions or substance abuse problems to the care of persons with an autism spectrum disorder. It is only in the past 20 or so years that behavioral healthcare has gone from mostly an inpatient care system to an outpatient and largely integrated care system.

Entities Enabling Healthcare

The **Department of Health and Human Services (HHS)** oversees healthcare in the United States. The agency within HHS that enables and manages healthcare reimbursement for persons who are elderly, disabled, or poor is the CMS. In addition to CMS, there are other HHS programs and services, such as healthcare insurance, public health programs, social service programs, and research. The following HHS entities enable the provision of healthcare in the United States.

Department of Health and Human Services (HHS) The federal agency responsible for ensuring the provision of vital human services and health protection to Americans.

Medicare and Medicaid

Implemented in 1966, Medicare is a federal program managed by the CMS. Medicare provides health insurance for persons who are elderly, disabled (regardless of age), and patients with end-stage renal disease. The patients who qualify for Medicare are enrolled in Medicare Part A. They do not pay monthly premiums, but they do have to pay a deductible. There are limits to the services and the costs that are reimbursable by Medicare.

The Medicaid program is federally funded on a shared basis with each state, and it is administered by individual states. Patients must qualify for Medicaid, which is based on income level or other eligibility factors, such as disabilities. States determine the income level, the services covered, and the amount of reimbursement. Certain services must be covered, however, in order for states to receive federal funding for their programs.

Without Medicare and Medicaid, a great percentage of the population would not have access to healthcare. In 2012, these programs accounted for 44% of healthcare expenditures, and they are estimated to exceed 50% of all healthcare expenditures in 2022. The specifics of Medicare and Medicaid will be covered in the chapter on paying for healthcare.

Health Insurance (Payers)

Health insurance comes in many different forms within many individual health insurance companies. The current picture of health insurance is in the form of managed care plans, in which insurance companies ("carriers") negotiate reimbursement rates with care providers to provide quality care to their policyholders. Managed care plans emphasize the provision of preventive care in an efficient and effective manner. The traditional health insurance plans pay on a fee-for-service basis, whereby a physician (or any healthcare facility) charges a particular amount for each service. The insurance company then reimburses that amount.

Employers

Health insurance has largely been available through employers, in what are known as group health plans. The employer contracts with an insurance carrier and offers an insurance plan (the services that are covered). The employer pays a portion of the monthly premium (the cost of the insurance), and the employee pays for the remainder.

The cost of paying for healthcare has become so high that health insurance companies are charging premiums that employers and policyholders can no longer afford. As a result, the Affordable Care Act (ACA), which entails shopping for and purchasing health insurance through health insurance exchanges, was enacted in 2010. Through these health insurance exchanges, people can search for a plan that meets their needs (for instance, coverage for a 22-year-old may be different from the coverage a 50-year-old would need) at a cost they can afford. Health insurance companies can no longer turn down an application for or drop someone's insurance because of a pre-existing or worsening medical condition.

Public Health

Public health agencies are typically administered by state governments, and each county in the state manages the local health department. Many services are offered through the public health department, such as immunizations, family planning, and women's health, and the health department monitors communicable diseases, ensures the safety of public water and food supplies, and educates the public about health and safety issues. Public health departments are another avenue for the under- or uninsured to receive care that otherwise would not be available to them.

The Critical Role of Health Information

Lowering costs and supporting a healthier population are the foundational elements of healthcare transformation. The effective and timely use of health information is required to achieve this goal. The digitization of patient records, the exchange of these records, and the analytics involved support better management with up-to-date information, clinical decision support tools such as alerts, and analyses of trends. When these digitized patient records are made available along the continuum of care, nurse managers, social workers, long-term care facilities, and other stakeholders can better manage patients by having access to a current and full range of data.

More important in the management of chronic diseases, such as diabetes or congestive heart failure, is getting health information into the hands of the patient. Patient engagement has been described as the "miracle drug of the century." By having access to health information, patients have the opportunity to take control of their healthcare. The most direct way for health information to support patient engagement is through Personal Health Records and patient portals, both of which will be covered in more detail in the chapter on the patient's role in healthcare.

Another important type of health information that will play a big role in healthcare transformation is patient-generated data. This can take the form of remote monitoring devices (such as for blood sugar levels for diabetics), fitness or other apps linked to patient medical conditions, social media support groups, educational apps, and nagging reminders (see Figure 1.9). These devices and apps are also discussed in the chapter on the patient's role in healthcare.

Improved Data Collection

ICD-10-CM/PCS

The sheer volume of possible diagnoses and procedures in the 21st century prohibits the capture and analysis of data without the conversion of diagnoses and procedures from narrative form to a numeric or coded format. The classification system used to code is the International Classification of Diseases (ICD).

The coding system used to translate diagnoses and procedures into numeric form since 1979 has been the International Classification of Diseases, 9th revision, Clinical Modification, better known as ICD-9-CM. Though it was updated yearly to reflect new diagnoses, remove obsolete ones, and capture advances in technology, it has been far overdue for a complete revision, because it could not be expanded sufficiently to capture new diagnoses and procedures. In 1990, the World Health Organization (WHO) endorsed ICD-10, and since 1994 it has been used in the majority of industrialized nations, with the United States being one of the exceptions.

At the time of this writing, the United States had not yet implemented the use of International Classification of Diseases, 10th revision, Clinical Modification (ICD-10-CM) and International Classification of Diseases, 10th revision, Procedure Coding System (ICD-10-PCS. However, the implementation date has been set for October 1, 2015. All healthcare providers must use the ICD classification system to code diagnoses, as required by the data set rule of HIPAA. All healthcare facilities use ICD to code diagnoses, and hospitals also use it to code inpatient procedures.

The need for a new coding system has been driven by the necessity for greater specificity in reporting healthcare data. For instance, in ICD-9-CM, laterality (left or right) in a diagnosis can rarely be captured in the code. Neither the location of a hemorrhagic stroke nor the severity of a patient's asthma is codable using ICD-9-CM. On the other hand, ICD-10 captures far more specificity and was designed to allow for code expansion as the need for coding new diseases, new procedures, and even greater specificity emerges.

The capturing of data leads to data warehousing and data mining—that is, housing the data and then extracting statistical

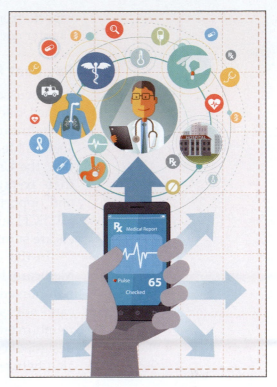

Figure 1.9 **The Future of Healthcare at Our Fingertips 24/7 through Smartphones and Other Devices**

reports from them. Both concepts will be explored in detail in the chapter covering the life cycle of health information.

Payment Reform

As discussed earlier in this chapter, the way we pay for healthcare in the United States must be transformed. The current rate of growth of healthcare costs is unsustainable, and taxpayer-funded programs, such as Medicaid and Medicare, are headed for insolvency. In addition, the United States spends almost 2.5 times more on healthcare than average for developed countries. This suggests inefficiencies and opportunities for improvement and is a core element of both HITECH and the ACA. Three key payment, or reimbursement, models are summarized in Table 1.2.

In the United States, most healthcare, including Medicaid and Medicare, has been paid for using a modified fee-for-service (FFS) reimbursement model. In effect, FFS means that the quantity of care, not necessarily the quality of care, is reimbursed. Typically, reimbursements are linked to disease and treatment-specific codes designed to describe the encounter. Reimbursement rates are negotiated between payers and providers or, in the case of Medicaid and

TABLE 1.2	Reimbursement Models		
	Fee-for-Service	**Modified Payments**	**Fee-for-Value**
Payment Process	• Traditional reimbursement based on diagnostic codes for treatment	• Traditional reimbursement adjusted for quality outcome measures for specific diagnoses	• Global payment based on patient population or capitation • Shared risk/shared savings
Model	• Fee-for-service • Concierge medicine • Prospective payment models	• Pay-for-performance (P4P) • Medicare value-based payment modifier	• Health maintenance organizations • Accountable care organizations • Population health management • Medicaid managed care organizations
Implications for Care Model	• Episodic care and preventive care • Tendency to be reactive	• Greater focus on preventive care and management for targeted diseases	• Focus on preventive care • Population health outcomes and measurement • Need to be proactive
Issues	• Payment based on quantity, not necessarily quality • Lack of transparency in pricing with wide variation • Complexity in the reimbursement cycle • Patients with low co-pay can overuse the system • Overhead costs can be inflated	• Difficult to measure and report outcomes • Limited diseases covered • Providers penalized for patient nonadherence	• Risk of care rationing or treatment based on cost, not efficacy • Providers unhappy with compensation • Difficult to measure and report outcomes • Risk adjustment for population is required but difficult • Eases paperwork and billing complexity but is complicated to set up • Providers penalized for patient nonadherence

Medicare, determined through a process that includes stakeholder input and segmented into categories of services.

There are four major criticisms of fee-for-service:

- Physicians can be incentivized to provide more services than necessary, because payment is tied to quantity or at a minimum not be incentivized to reduce costs.
- There is little transparency in pricing and wide variation in pricing for similar services and procedures at the same location, depending on the payer.
- Patients may be incentivized to overuse the system, because they often do not have any cost-sharing responsibilities.
- Fees and charges are not be linked to cost and are often inflated to allow an institution to recoup the costs of overhead or write-offs related to bad debts or charity services.

Conversely, many consider the United States to have the best health-care in the world. The debate is often framed as "value versus volume" models. The value model is that reimbursement should be based on the quality of care given, not the volume of care. The issues are how to define "value," how to measure "value," and how to structure payments for "value." The solution is based on an improved use of health information.

Migrating from a FFS model to a fee-for-value (FFV) model is referred to as payment reform. Payment reform is the strategy for reducing the rate of health expenditure growth and the principal reason for healthcare reform initiatives such as HITECH. Digitized patient records, health information exchange, and analytics in the form of health informatics provide the opportunity to measure healthcare delivery in unique and different ways.

A guiding principal of payment reform using **evidence-based medicine (EBM)** is **population health management (PHM)**. PHM is the ability to better serve a specific group of patients in a more cost-effective manner while providing better care by using digitized patient records and analytics in a proactive manner. Reducing duplicate and unnecessary tests, lengths of stay, readmissions, emergency department use, and other costly services are just a few examples of how using EHRs, preventive care, and patient engagement contribute to payment reform. The approach under PHM is that a large patient population can be statistically modeled to predict healthcare outcomes and usage patterns. This is sometimes referred to as the risk adjustment of patient population.

Typically under reimbursement models based on PHM, provider organizations receive a negotiated level of funding to provide services to the patient population. The goal is to reduce costs while improving measurable outcomes. The provider can then maximize the amount of the reimbursement it retains. Likewise, providers are responsible for any costs that exceed reimbursement levels. In some cases, as with CMS pilot programs, the payer and provider share any costs that exceed reimbursement. This is referred to as either a shared risk or shared savings program.

The use of population-based reimbursement is not new. Health maintenance organizations (HMOs) and other managed care

Evidence-based medicine (EBM) Diagnostic and treatment protocols based on proven research and documented best practice.

Population health management (PHM) Providing quality healthcare to a specific group of patients in a more cost-effective manner through the use of digitized patient records and analytics.

organizations have used capitation as a basis for reimbursement, which is a system that pays a provider for healthcare services based on a set amount of money for each patient regardless of the amount (or any) of the services used. In addition, states are increasingly turning to managed care organizations for Medicaid populations. Typically, HMOs and other managed care organizations negotiate flat-fee capitation and are not reimbursed on the risk adjustment of PHM models.

A new form of population health reimbursement, **accountable care organizations (ACOs)**, was mandated in the ACA. In the case of CMS, this is for Medicare patients. CMS is supporting ACOs: "when an ACO succeeds in both delivering high-quality care and spending healthcare dollars more widely, it will share in the savings it achieves for the Medicare program." Note the role of health information and measurement in ACOs, as compared to a pure capitation payment approach under managed care. ACOs are not limited to Medicare; private insurers and employers are also introducing and supporting them.

In addition to ACOs, other types of payment reform are under way, primarily led by CMS. Under the ACA, beginning with a phase-in 2015 and becoming mandatory for all providers by 2017, CMS is required to apply a value-based payment modifier to reimbursements. In other words, CMS must calculate both cost and quality data for providers and adjust payments accordingly. There are alternative ways to provide the data to CMS, but all require EHRs at a minimum. Once again, digitized medical records are at the center of this reform.

There are similar types of payment models, such as pay-for-performance (P4P), which links payment to minimum threshold care measures. The difference between ACOs and P4P is that P4P is often linked to specific disease measures, whereas ACOs are based on overall performance.

In making sense of payment reform, it is important to understand that all stakeholders have an interest in reducing costs and improving outcomes. CMS is leading in requiring reforms, but employers and payers typically follow CMS. Patients should have an interest in payment reform, but the way that health insurance is structured in the United States, patients often have no or minimal cost for healthcare services. This is changing under the ACA; with the exception of preventive care and some specialized drugs (e.g., contraception) and treatments, patients often have high deductibles and will subsequently have incentive to reduce their own healthcare costs.

Accountable care organizations (ACOs)
Groups of doctors, hospitals, and other healthcare providers that come together voluntarily to give high-quality care using a fixed payment model; they work collaboratively and accept collective accountability for costs and the quality of care.

1.3 THINKING IT THROUGH

1. Identify the stakeholders in healthcare and how their role is being changed by healthcare transformation.
2. What are the advantages of an integrated delivery network?
3. How will the implementation of ICD-10-CM/PCS improve healthcare data?
4. Identify the approaches to paying for healthcare. What are the advantages and disadvantages of each?

Patient Engagement

The Medical Home

The **patient-centered medical home (PCMH)** is a model developed by the American Academy of Family Practitioners for caring for patients with chronic conditions. It has evolved to cover preventive services and involves a team approach to care. The goal of PCMH is to involve the patient as well as the patient's family or caregiver(s) in the care of the patient. It is a patient-centric care model in that the patient has more of a say in what he or she sees as the goal of treatment and the type(s) of treatment he or she is willing to undergo, and the patient is well informed through communication with the physician. Care is rendered in a team approach among the PCP, the patient/family, and other healthcare disciplines. Health IT plays a very important role in the PCMH for both the physician in the form of access to clinical decision support software and for the patient in the form of a patient portal, where the patient has access to pertinent historical data, such as blood pressure measurements. For an overview of the keys to the PCMH, see Figure 1.10.

The PCMH relies heavily on the role of the primary care provider (PCP), which is a concept that grew out of the managed care insurance model. As mentioned earlier, the PCP is the "gatekeeper" of a patient's care, with the goal of reducing redundancy and overuse of testing and services. The cost of primary care is lower than that of specialists, and the PCP model results in coordinated, efficient healthcare.

Traditional models of healthcare are much different than the concept of the PCMH. Healthcare has traditionally been provided in a bubble—each physician caring for a patient according to his or her own style and, though having access to the patient's previous health history and diagnostic test results, not necessarily proceeding as part of a team. Though physicians may have attempted to contain costs, their focus was on diagnosing and treating the patient, not on efficiency or cost-effectiveness. The idea of more knowledgeable patients with an active say in their own care is a notion that has grown in the years since the passage of HIPAA, but it is even more enhanced with the PCMH model.

Physicians who adopt the PCMH model in their practices must also be willing to embrace the value of health information technology (HIT) in providing medical care as well. The use of and access to patients' health information through health information exchange (HIE) is a critical component of the coordination of care and efficiency principles. The use of clinical decision support technology,

Patient-centered medical home (PCMH) A healthcare model that involves the patient and family in the care of the patient; care is rendered in a team approach.

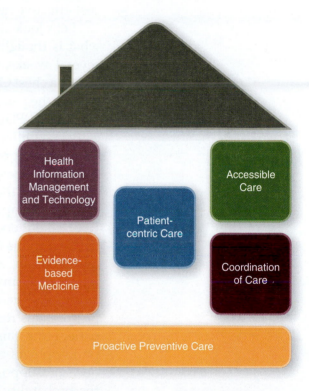

Figure 1.10 **The Keys to the Patient-Centered Medical Home**

preventive care reminders, and access to data found in disease registries all play a part in value-based medicine and the provision of care based on current, evidence-based best practice.

The value of communication among care providers, caregivers, and ancillary services is paramount in providing quality care through secure email, the patient's access to his or her test results, health and risk appraisals, and the like.

Transitions in Care and Chronic Disease Management

As noted previously, coordination of care is something that until recent years was not prevalent in healthcare. Today, because of access to electronic health information and the use of health IT, buy-in from care providers, and active participation by patients and their families in healthcare, coordination of care is a necessity in providing quality, cost-effective healthcare.

Let's look at an example. A patient has been seen by his PCP for what is thought to be bronchitis diagnosed on a chest x-ray. After several weeks, the bronchitis does not resolve and the physician orders a chest CT scan and pulmonary function studies. Based on test results, the patient is diagnosed with chronic obstructive pulmonary disease (COPD), a chronic condition of the lungs. Patients with COPD can be stabilized on medication, and perhaps oxygen, and may be able to lead a relatively normal life. But they may go through flare-ups of the disease, known as acute exacerbation, which necessitates acute care of the condition.

The example shows chronic care and acute care management. In all likelihood, a patient's medical history will also show comorbid conditions (conditions that also exist, such as diabetes mellitus, hypertension, and smoking status). The care of this type of patient requires a team effort, one that involves the patient's PCP, appropriate specialists, other healthcare disciplines (in the preceding example, perhaps respiratory therapy), and the active involvement of the patient and family. The principles noted in the PCMH and/or the philosophy of coordinated care through the use of an EHR, clinical decision support, and health IT in general will be vital in increasing the probability that this patient and others like him will be able to live productive, quality lifestyles.

Patient Engagement

Personal Health Records

The health record that has been mentioned throughout this chapter, is a legal document—it is kept by a healthcare provider or facility and is the property of the hospital. The information in it, however, belongs to the patient. Until recent years, patients did not have access to their health records, nor did they keep very good records of their own healthcare.

On the other hand, a Personal Health Record (PHR) is the property of the patient. Patients are now more active participants in their own healthcare, and part of that participation means keeping records of their own healthcare as well. Through the use of a PHR, patients can document the diagnostic studies or care they've received, keep track of medical and family health histories, document any allergies or adverse effects to medications, and keep a list of medications they are taking. In an electronic environment, patients now have access directly to their legal health record, which is kept by the healthcare facility or provider. The Personal Health Record and patient portals will be discussed in detail in the chapter on the patient's role in healthcare.

Wellness and Disease Management

The US health system has two divisions: healthcare, which focuses on wellness and prevention, and medical care, which would signify care and treatment of medical conditions, or a state of disease, rather than wellness. Both necessitate the concept of coordination of care, patient involvement, and the exchange of health information to improve patient outcomes and quality of care efficiently and effectively.

Coordination of care is more organized and streamlined when treatment plans are developed with the input of the healthcare team along with the patient and/or family. Disease management programs can be developed by independent associations, such as the Care Continuum Alliance, or by health insurance companies, federal agencies such as the Agency for Healthcare Research and Quality, or The Joint Commission.

mHealth

mHealth, or mobile health, is a relatively new concept in medicine and is discussed in detail in the chapter on the patient's role in healthcare. mHealth is the sending and receiving of health information using a mobile phone, mobile device, or other wireless device. Through the use of mobile devices, care is improved, because care providers have the information necessary to make critical, time-sensitive decisions without having to go back to the office or hospital to retrieve that information or having the information collected remotely at a patient's house. A homebound patient who needs daily blood pressure checks or a pacemaker check done remotely every few months is one example. Patients who otherwise would not receive the healthcare and monitoring necessary to achieve positive outcomes are now monitored through the use of mobile devices. Mobile health and the electronic exchange of health information will be the focus of much of this text.

mHealth The sending and receiving of health information using a mobile phone, mobile device, or other wireless device.

1.4	THINKING IT THROUGH

1. Do you have a Personal Health Record (PHR)? Why or why not? If you do, have you found it useful? If you do not, has there been a time when it would have been useful?
2. Explain how patient-centered medical homes improve patient care.
3. Why is the electronic health record the property of the physician's office or other healthcare facility, rather than the property of the patient?

chapter 1 summary

LEARNING OUTCOMES	CONCEPTS FOR REVIEW
1.1 Describe the history of healthcare and the evolving role of patients, providers, insurers, and regulators in the delivery of healthcare in the United States. Pages 2–9	• It was only in the 19th century that medicine was finally considered a profession, with the first medical schools appearing in the mid-1700s. • The 20th century saw structured education, standards, professional organizations, increases in quality of care, great strides in the use of technology, and areas of specialization by providers. • Medicare and Medicaid were established in 1965. • The 1970s saw out-of-control growth in healthcare costs. • The latter part of the 1980s saw emphasis on healthcare quality. • The 21st century brought substantial change in privacy, security, data sets and electronic transaction standards, administrative simplification, and enforcement and compliance. • Even with the vast changes in healthcare, the cost of caring for patients has continued to grow. • Medicare Prescription Drug Improvement and Modernization Act of 2003 (MMA) provides Medicare beneficiaries with financial help to pay for skyrocketing costs of prescriptions. • In the 21st century, medicine has shifted from caring for the sick (medical care) to an emphasis on preventing sickness (healthcare). • 2010—Affordable Care Act (ACA) is signed into law with the goal of making quality, affordable healthcare insurance available through a system of insurance exchanges.
1.2 Outline how new laws and regulations are reshaping healthcare in the United States. Pages 9–14	• The cost of healthcare has steadily grown out of control over the past four decades and is not economically sustainable at the current rate. • Though there has been an ongoing attempt at moving from disease management to disease prevention, chronic disease management plays a significant role in the high cost of healthcare. • Federal initiatives include the Affordable Care Act (ACA), the Health Information Technology for Economic and Clinical Health Act (HITECH), and Meaningful Use of digitized information. • Meaningful Use requirements are designed to support the ACA. • American Recovery and Reinvestment Act of 2009 (ARRA) and its emphasis is on modernization of the healthcare system and included HITECH.
1.3 Summarize the roles of key stakeholders in shaping healthcare transformation in the United States. Pages 14–22	• Health information and the professionals who manage it are key to controlling the costs through getting timelier information to providers, building and maintaining clinical decision support tools, and ensuring the digitized health information is available to all providers and facilities involved in a patient's care at any point in his or her lifetime. • Patient-centric healthcare, which involves the patient and/or family in the patient's care and decision-making process

LEARNING OUTCOMES	CONCEPTS FOR REVIEW
	• Improved data collection, particularly in the area of disease and procedure coding (ICD-9-CM to ICD-10-CM/PCS) • Payment reform movement from fee-for-service to value-based service • Evidence-based medicine and population health management allow better service to specific patient populations in a cost-effective manner. • Accountable care organizations are a form of population health reimbursement in which groups of healthcare providers and facilities work together to give high-quality, cost-effective care and assume responsibility for costs while being reimbursed on a population-based capitation rate.
1.4 Explain how health information is being used to empower patients. Pages 23-25.	• Patient-centered medical home (PCMH) is a model developed by the American Academy of Family Practitioners to care for patients with chronic conditions in a team approach. • Patients are urged to keep a Personal Health Record and/or take advantage of patient portal technology in order to be informed and actively engaged in their own healthcare. • Coordination of care involves this team approach as well as exchange of health information in order to prevent redundancy and facilitate timely, efficient healthcare, thus improving the outcome. • mHealth allows for the sending and receiving of health information digitally as well as diagnostic testing remotely.

chapter review

MATCHING QUESTIONS

Match each term with its definition.

_____ 1. **[LO 1.3]** accountable care organization

_____ 2. **[LO 1.3]** data warehouse

_____ 3. **[LO 1.1]** Conditions of Participation

_____ 4. **[LO 1.1]** accreditation

_____ 5. **[LO 1.3]** capitation

_____ 6. **[LO 1.1]** HIPAA

_____ 7. **[LO 1.4]** patient portal

_____ 8. **[LO 1.3]** Population health management (PHM)

_____ 9. **[LO 1.1]** Patient Self-Determination Act

_____ 10. **[LO 1.4]** encounter

_____ 11. **[LO 1.3]** clinical decision support

_____ 12. **[LO 1.2]** HITECH

a. Episode of care

b. Legislation that, among other things, provided monetary incentives for training healthcare professionals on health information technology

c. Providing quality healthcare to a specific group of patients in a more cost-effective manner through the use of digitized patient records and analytics

d. Secure area for individuals to access their medical information and communicate with providers

e. Linking diagnoses and healthcare treatment recommendations to databases of research and study in order to back up those diagnoses

f. Network of doctors, hospitals, and other healthcare facilities that belong to the same parent organization

g. Repository of patient information that can be accessed at any time

h. Designation that shows a facility has met strict requirements for quality and standards

i. Set of regulations that must be met by a healthcare facility before Medicare and Medicaid will reimburse for services

j. Legislation that placed stricter guidelines on the security and privacy of health information

k. Legislation allowing individuals to be informed of their care plans and to have the right to voice opinions about their medical treatment

l. Reimbursement method that pays a provider set amounts for each patient, regardless of the care and services used

MULTIPLE CHOICE QUESTIONS

Choose the letter that best completes the statement or answers the question.

13. **[LO 1.1]** Which group is considered the predecessors of modern medicine?
    a. Egyptians
    b. English
    c. Greeks
    d. Romans

14. **[LO 1.1]** One of the first medical schools in the United States was
    a. Dartmouth.
    b. Johns Hopkins.
    c. University of Chicago.
    d. Yale.

15. **[LO 1.1]** Current standards for the quality of a health record are based on the work of which organization?
    a. American Medical Association
    b. American College of Surgeons
    c. The Joint Commission
    d. Peer Review Organization

16. **[LO 1.2]** What is the overarching goal of the Health Information Technology for Economic and Clinical Health Act?
    a. Ensure that health data are being used meaningfully
    b. Encourage physicians to report quality of care indicators
    c. Modernize the healthcare system
    d. Provide universal insurance

17. **[LO 1.3]** Which is an example of long-term care?
    a. Emergency department encounter
    b. Inpatient hospital care
    c. Ambulatory surgery
    d. Skilled nursing care

18. **[LO 1.3]** What is a health insurance exchange?
    a. A website where insured individuals can swap coverage options
    b. A place where individuals can search for appropriate insurance coverage
    c. A group of providers who share information and data among themselves
    d. A network of digital medical information that is available for sharing

19. **[LO 1.2]** The purpose of healthcare reform is to achieve
    a. lower costs.
    b. improved patient outcomes.
    c. a healthier population.
    d. all of these.

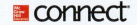 Enhance your learning by completing these exercises and more at http://connect.mheducation.com!

20. **[LO 1.2]** Which federal agency promotes a national health information technology infrastructure and is overseeing the development of it?
    a. Department of Health and Human Services
    b. Office of the National Coordinator
    c. Centers for Medicare and Medicaid Services
    d. Internal Revenue Service

21. **[LO 1.2]** Incentives earned under HITECH legislation can be used
    a. to upgrade EHR systems.
    b. for staff bonuses.
    c. to improve medical testing equipment.
    d. however a provider chooses.

22. **[LO 1.2]** Which is a goal of Meaningful Use Stage 3?
    a. Reporting clinical quality measures
    b. Improving population health
    c. Allowing more patient-controlled data
    d. Exchanging patient records electronically

23. **[LO 1.4]** An example of aggregate data is
    a. the ages of all patients seen in a facility.
    b. a report of individual patients with a diagnosis of congestive heart failure.
    c. the number of live births in the month of June.
    d. a report of all patients Dr. Smith performed an appendectomy on during calendar year 2014.

24. **[LO 1.3]** Under the Affordable Care Act, patients will have greater responsibility for their healthcare costs, *except* for
    a. preventive care.
    b. maternity care.
    c. surgical care.
    d. intensive care.

25. **[LO 1.4]** What is the difference between healthcare and medical care?
    a. Healthcare focuses on treatment, whereas medical care focuses on prevention.
    b. Healthcare focuses on prevention, whereas medical care focuses on treatment.
    c. There is no difference; healthcare and medical care both focus on patient health.
    d. There is no difference; healthcare and medical care both focus on treatment options.

26. **[LO 1.4]** If a patient is seen at a hospital with no EHR functionality, how can she guarantee that her encounter information from the hospital stay gets added to her PHR?
    a. She can email the hospital for the records.
    b. She is unable to get them; they are property of the hospital.
    c. She is required by HIPAA laws to request them in person.
    d. She can submit a written request for the records.

SHORT ANSWER QUESTIONS

27. **[LO 1.3]** Why is patient engagement referred to as "the miracle drug of the century"?

28. **[LO 1.1]** Who was Nathan Smith Davis?

29. **[LO 1.1]** Summarize the mission of the American College of Surgeons.

30. **[LO 1.1]** Outline the shift in medical care that has occurred during the 21st century.

31. **[LO 1.1]** Why is having a primary care provider (PCP) now the norm and, in some cases, a requirement in healthcare?

32. **[LO 1.2]** Why is treatment intensity one of the core elements of healthcare expense?

33. **[LO 1.4]** Other than medical treatment, what can be done to improve the care of diabetes patients?

34. **[LO 1.3]** How does HITECH create a more patient-centric model of healthcare?

35. **[LO 1.3]** List the five main provisions for insurance under the Affordable Care Act.

36. **[LO 1.3]** Why is increased specificity in coding and healthcare data a benefit to everyone?

37. **[LO 1.4]** Contrast data warehousing and data mining.

38. **[LO 1.3]** Describe one benefit and one risk of accountable care organizations.

APPLYING YOUR KNOWLEDGE

39. **[LO 1.1]** Why is it a requirement that healthcare facilities and providers be licensed?

40. **[LO 1.1]** The text mentions that health information professionals and the jobs they do were impacted greatly by the passage and implementation of HIPAA. Why is this the case? Explain, giving examples.

41. **[LO 1.1, 1.3]** Which legislation of the 21st century do you believe will have the most impact? Why?

42. **[LO 1.2]** What does it mean that chronic diseases are typically called "lifestyle diseases"? Give examples from your experience about how health outcomes could be improved for someone you know with a chronic disease.

43. **[LO 1.2]** Meaningful Use defines how providers must use EHRs and health information. What do these definitions mean in practical terms for physicians or other healthcare providers in a patient encounter? For example, digital patient records captured by an EHR can be used for clinical decision support systems. How can this or other new applications change the encounter between a patient and a physician?

44. **[LO 1.3]** Which provision of the Affordable Care Act do you believe will have the most benefit or impact? Explain your answer, giving an example.

45. **[LO 1.4]** Explain your stance in the "value versus volume" debate, giving examples as needed.

46. **[LO 1.4]** What is your opinion of pay-for-performance models? Explain.

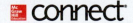 Enhance your learning by completing these exercises and more at http://connect.mheducation.com!

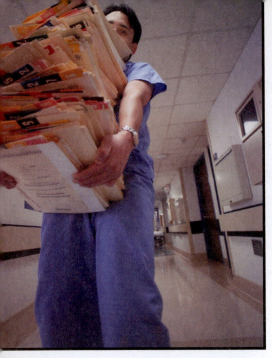

2

Functions, Careers, and Credentials of the HI Professional: *Documenting, Maintaining, and Managing Health Information, Past and Present*

Learning Outcomes

When you finish this chapter, you will be able to:

2.1 Explain the importance of documentation needed by users of health information.

2.2 Categorize the job responsibilities of health information professionals.

2.3 Discuss the development of health information management as a profession.

2.4 Evaluate the educational opportunities and certifications of health information professionals.

Key Terms

Authentication

Cancer registry

Care provider

Commission on Accreditation for Health Informatics and Information Management Education (CAHIIM)

Compliance officer

Computer-assisted coding (CAC)

Current Procedural Terminology (CPT)

Delinquent records

Digitized health records

Document imaging/scanning

eHealth management

Electronic health record (EHR)

Electronic medical record (EMR)

Encoder software

Enterprise system

Grouper software

Healthcare professional

Information (data) governance

Information security

International Classification of Diseases, 9th revision, Clinical Modification (ICD-9-CM)

International Classification of Diseases, 10th revision, Clinical Modification (ICD-10-CM)

International Classification of Diseases, 10th revision, Procedural Coding System (ICD-10-PCS)

Medical staff bylaws

Medical transcriptionist

Outguides

Physician extenders

Privacy officer

Quantitative analysis

Recovery audit contractor (RAC)

Revenue cycle managers

Third-party payer

Uniform Hospital Discharge Data Set (UHDDS)

Unit record

Voice recognition

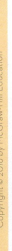

In this chapter, the health record itself will be explored in both paper and digital format. We will delve into how health information is utilized, authored, validated, stored, and processed as part of healthcare delivery. In coming to understand the nature of the health record, we will also cover the various roles of health information management professionals—both traditional and up and coming—as guardians, architects, and gatekeepers of the health record, transforming data into actionable intelligence that improves the quality of healthcare. Finally, we will take a look back at the historical roots of the health information management profession and the credentials needed to be active in the field today.

2.1   Documenting Healthcare

The Health Record

Definition

A health record is also known as a medical record or a patient's chart. It is made up of documents that accurately identify the patient and completely explain the reason for the patient's visit, including the principal or primary reason for the encounter. In addition, it documents any other co-existing or complicating diagnoses, past medical/surgical procedures, family and social histories, justification of the procedures and services performed, and the results of treatment.

Uses

Every time a patient is seen by a **care provider** or **healthcare professional**, the encounter must be documented. The health record is the source document that

- Serves as a means of communication among healthcare team members during the current episode of care and during the continuum of care
- Documents the health status of the patient, on which current and future care is based
- Protects the patient, care provider, healthcare professionals, and healthcare facility in legal matters
- Justifies reimbursement from **third-party payers**
- Provides the basis for transforming diagnoses, procedures, and services into a numeric format known as coding, to gather statistical data used for internal planning, disease and procedure registries, research, epidemiology, and public health initiatives

Care provider A physician, physician's assistant, dentist, psychologist, nurse practitioner, or midwife; these individuals can diagnose and give orders for diagnostic or therapeutic services.

Healthcare professional Generally refers to a nurse, medical assistant, or other technician who directly cares for the patient.

Third-party payer Often referred to as an insurance carrier or company; includes Medicare, Medicaid, Blue Cross/Shield, Tricare, CHAMPVA, and any of the private health insurers.

Formats

Paper Records As recently as 20 years ago, paper was the common format used to collect, maintain, and store health records. The health record is documented throughout the patient's stay or during the encounter and then, once completed by the care providers and healthcare professionals, is filed in a file room until it is needed again (see Figure 2.1).

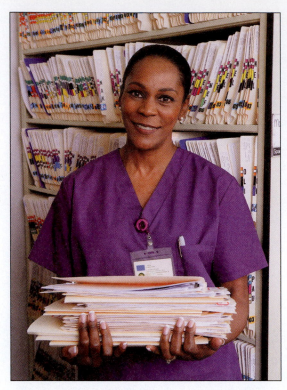

Figure 2.1   A Filing System for Paper Health Records

Paper records are convenient in the sense that they are known territory—care providers and healthcare professionals can easily pick up a pen and write their notes about a patient's progress, vital signs, or level of pain, for instance. One of the negatives, however, is the limited availability of the record. Paper records are available to only one person at a time. Case in point—a physician finishes her rounds (seeing each patient on a nursing unit) and sits at the nursing unit to document a conversation with a patient's family. She asks for the patient's health record and is told that the patient was just taken to the radiology department for an x-ray and thus the record is unavailable. The physician may not return to that nursing unit until the next day. She may not remember to document the conversation at all, and if she does the documentation may not be as detailed as it would have been, had the physician documented it shortly after the conversation took place.

Paper records are easily misplaced or misfiled, which is very serious, because they are the source documents on which future medical care is based. A misfiled record may remain lost for years, or it may never be found. Should a record be needed in legal proceedings, there would be no proof that something was or was not done for the patient or that a patient's injuries were due to an auto accident as opposed to some other cause. There is an old adage in the healthcare profession—if it wasn't documented, it wasn't done. If there is no record at all, then that is the equivalent of not being done.

The security and confidentiality of paper records is questionable. Though an authorization to release health information is needed before copies of records leave the facility, there is no way to safeguard paper records within the facility. Only staff with a need to know should have access to the health records of patients. Although that is how it is supposed to be, enforcement is very difficult with a paper record. For example, a nurse on the fifth floor notices that her next-door neighbor is currently a patient. Though she is not assigned to that patient, the record is available for her to access at any time. She could pick up the record and read it with no one ever questioning her, since she works on that unit. This scenario is surprisingly common.

Paper records consist mainly of handwritten notes. Often, these notes are illegible. Illegible handwriting is a safety concern, as errors in treatment or medication administration could result. In addition, illegible handwriting leads to wasted time on the part of healthcare professionals who are trying to find out what the documentation actually says—time that could be better spent on patient care. Some documentation is dictated, meaning that the physician dictates notes into a recorder, which is later transcribed by a **medical transcriptionist**. This is certainly a safer way of documenting, but there is sometimes a long turnaround time between the dictation

Medical transcriptionist
A healthcare professional who converts the recorded dictation of care providers into typed report form using word processing software.

and transcription of reports. Again, if the documentation was dictated but the typed report was not filed in the patient's record in a timely manner, the documentation is not of much use and could delay treatment or cause safety issues for the patient.

Paper records also require *a lot* of space to house. Once a record is complete and is placed in a permanent file, it may not be accessed again for years, if ever. Some patients' records are an inch thick, others are several inches thick, and still others are so large that they consist of several volumes. The file room seen in Figure 2.1 is a very neat one. The file folders are standing up straight, the files are of uniform thickness, and they look as if they are rarely used. A more realistic view of the file folders in a health information department is seen in Figure 2.2. In this figure, the records are of different thicknesses, some records have curled under because of the weight of the records, and the records are packed so tightly that there is little room for expansion. The red and green guides protruding from the folders are called **outguides**. They hold the place of records currently taken from the permanent file and include the date the record was taken, as well as the location of the record. The problem with outguides is that the record may have been taken out of the file for a patient's readmission, but then sent on to another department before being returned to file storage. Therefore, the whereabouts of the record are not known after it leaves the health information department.

Communication with external users of the health information found in a paper record is difficult, takes valuable time to accomplish, and is more expensive. Consider, for instance, a patient who is transferred from hospital A to hospital B. If that transfer has to occur quickly, it is very possible that copies of the patient's health record will not accompany the patient. It takes time to copy paper records—if the patient had already been at hospital A for several days, his or her record might be quite thick, making the copying process even more time-consuming. Hopefully, the attending physician at hospital A has dictated a transfer summary, but that also takes time, as does the transcription and faxing of the document to hospital B. The healthcare team at hospital B will be at a disadvantage if they do not have access to valuable information about what has been done for the patient so far and whether he or she has responded to the treatment. Not having that information could delay treatment or testing, and procedures may be unnecessarily duplicated.

Finally, paper records are expensive to maintain. Each record is maintained in at least one file folder. There may be hundreds of pieces of paper in each health record. There are copying costs each time the record is requested by outside entities, such as insurance carriers, attorneys, the patient, or other providers. It is estimated that it costs 70 cents per page in staff time to transmit a fax, compared to 10 cents per page for transmitting a digital copy electronically.

Outguides In a manual record-keeping system, these are cardboard or plastic folders that take the place of health records that have been removed from file. They include the date the files were removed and the locations to which the files were taken.

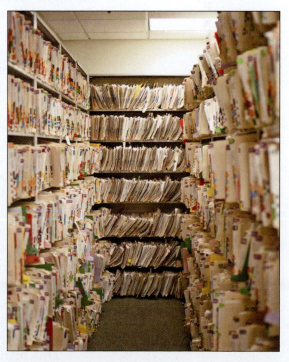

Figure 2.2 A More Realistic View of a Paper Health Record Filing System

The equipment used to house paper records is also very expensive. Every health record must be kept for a minimum of five years, even longer if required by state law or by the needs of the facility. Federal and state regulations, accreditation standards, and the needs of the facility dictate the length of time health records must be kept in some form. Later in this text, the subject of record retention will be covered in the chapter on maintaining health information.

Electronic Health Records and Electronic Medical Records An **electronic health record**, known as an **EHR**, can also be referred to as an **electronic medical record (EMR)**. Though used interchangeably in practice, *electronic medical record* and *electronic health record* have distinct definitions. According to the Office of the National Coordinator for Health IT (ONC), an EMR is "a digital version of paper charts in clinician offices, clinics and hospitals." EMRs consist of information and notes from clinicians within that one office, clinic, or hospital and have limited use, primarily diagnosis and treatment. Since they are digital documents, they are more valuable than paper records, because they can be analyzed and used to improve the quality of care.

The ONC describes EHRs, in contrast, as "built to go beyond standard clinical data collected in a provider's office and inclusive of a broader view of a patient's care." All clinicians involved in the patient's care can have access to the EHR, and the EHR is designed to exchange information with labs, public health entities, specialists, and other healthcare providers. EHRs are designed to follow the patient across the continuum of care, including long-term care or behavioral health facilities, or to providers across the country.

In summary, the first major difference is that an EMR provides a digital record of the traditional chart used within one location. An EHR captures more information, designed to be exchanged and used at any point of care, following the patient.

Additionally, under Meaningful Use, EHRs need to meet certification requirements that support this greater functionality and interoperability. As discussed in the chapter covering the evolving healthcare system, the American Recovery and Reinvestment Act (ARRA) was signed into law in 2009. Included in ARRA was the Health Information Technology for Economic and Clinical Health Act, which is more commonly known as HITECH. The financial incentives to upgrade current electronic systems or install brand-new ones, as well as the knowledge that hospitals and physicians' practices that did not go digital would be fined, convinced many physicians and hospital administrators to take the plunge into the digital age, rather than take a "wait and see what happens" approach. Those that did implement digital systems have to prove, however, that they are meaningfully using the data from their EHR systems to improve patient care and outcomes in order to receive the incentive grants. HITECH and Meaningful Use regulations will be covered in more detail in the chapter on Meaningful Use and the electronic health record.

This brings us to the second key difference between EMRs and EHRs. An EMR does not meet the certification requirements of Meaningful Use. EMRs will fade as providers adopt EHRs. Thus, for

Electronic health record (EHR) An EHR captures more information than an EMR and is designed to be exchanged and used at any point of care, following the patient. EHRs need to meet Meaningful Use standards.

Electronic medical record (EMR) An EMR provides a digital record of the traditional chart used within one location. It does not meet the certification requirements of Meaningful Use because of its limited functionality.

TABLE 2.1	Key Differences between EMRs and EHRs
Electronic Medical Records (EMRs)	**Electronic Health Records (EHRs)**
• Digital record of the traditional chart used within one location	• Capture more detailed information than the traditional chart and are designed to be exchanged and used at any point of care
• Do not meet the Meaningful Use certification requirements for greater functionality and interoperability	• If certified, meet Meaningful Use standards; support data following the patient, providing more patient-centric care
• Focused on episodes within a single specialty or single health system	• Designed to contain all of a patient's medical care and history across all specialties in one place
• Limited data analytics; used primarily for encounter capture and data viewing	• Provide a broader range of data and are designed to support advanced analytics and decision support
• Not designed to be part of a larger system	• Interoperability with other EHRs through health information exchange

the purposes of this text, the term *electronic health record* (*EHR*) will be used to refer to any health record in electronic form. For a breakdown of the key differences between EMRs and EHRs, see Table 2.1.

The keeping of health records in electronic form, also referred to as **digitized health records**, has been slowly accepted by the healthcare community. Physicians have been comfortable documenting in a paper record either through writing their notes or by dictating them. Physicians may have more confidence in a record that they can see and touch as opposed to one that is kept electronically.

Security has been a concern, yet every access to an EHR is recorded and can be tracked to see who has accessed a record, at what time, and whether they viewed, edited, entered, or deleted data. This level of tracking is impossible with a paper record. It is true that electronic records can be hacked into, but then again, paper records can be stolen and misused as well.

The initial costs of EHR implementation are very high due to the purchase price of the software, data storage costs (whether on-site or lease of cloud storage), hardware costs (additional computers, printers, modems, and the like), staff training, and loss of productivity. Once EHRs are fully implemented, however, the costs of maintenance may decline but will include the cost of support and maintenance of an in-house system.

The ability to share health information among healthcare providers, which in turn improves patient care and outcomes, is the greatest advantage of health records kept in electronic form.

The issues of illegibility are no longer of concern in an electronic system, because all the data are in typed format rather than

Digitized health records
Health records kept in an electronic binary format.

handwritten. Care is rendered more efficiently, since information is readily available about the patient's health status.

The ability to collect data for internal use and use in public health initiatives, standard health practice, research and epidemiology studies, and reimbursement far exceeds what was possible with a paper health record.

Clinical Users and Authors of Health Information

Every healthcare professional responsible for any aspect of a patient's care is a user of health information.

Physicians and Nurses

When thinking of healthcare professionals, physicians and nurses are most likely the first to come to mind. The great majority of the population has received care from a physician or a nurse. Physicians may be referred to as care providers. Nothing can be done to a patient without a physician's order. The physician's order is the instruction to a nurse or other healthcare professional of what needs to be done to or for the patient. **Physician extenders** may also give orders, and these include physicians' assistants (PAs), certified nurse practitioners (CNPs), certified registered nurse anesthetists (CRNAs) or nurse midwives, all of whom work under the supervision of a medical doctor (MD) or doctor of osteopathy (DO).

Care providers also include specialists who are not an MD or a DO, but they require specialized training; these include dentists, podiatrists, optometrists, and chiropractors. Not only do care providers document their findings in the health record, but they also rely on the documentation of others who are involved in the care of the patient, so that they are aware of the patient's status and of whether the patient is responding well to treatment. They use health information to determine or modify a plan of care.

Nurses can be registered nurses (RNs) or licensed practical nurses (LPNs). In a physician's office, a medical assistant (MA), rather than a nurse, may be employed to prepare patients for the visit, take vital signs, give medications, administer injections, procure specimens from the patient, and provide patient education based on the physician's orders.

Physicians and nurses use health information to communicate the patient's past medical, surgical, social, and family histories; history of present illness; and current status, as well as what they have done for the patient; this information is later used by themselves or other care providers. Health information also serves as protection, should there be a legal matter involving the care of the patient.

Allied Health Professionals

Allied health professionals include non-nursing personnel. Laboratory technicians are the professionals who retrieve specimens such as blood, urine, feces, and sputum and perform the tests that give the results the physician uses to make a diagnosis. Laboratory technicians, electrocardiogram (EKG or ECG) technicians, and echocardiogram technicians cannot do their jobs without knowing what kind of specimen to collect or which test(s) to perform, since a physician's order must be written in order to perform any tests on a patient.

Physician extenders Providers of healthcare who have advanced education and can diagnose as well as give orders; includes physicians' assistants, certified nurse practitioners, certified registered nurse anesthetists, and nurse midwives.

Radiology technicians also need to access the health record to determine which test(s) the physician has ordered. For instance, if a computerized axial tomography (CT scan) is ordered, it is also necessary for the technician to know whether the physician has ordered injection of a contrast material as well. Technicians may need to compare a film to previous films, for instance, in an abdominal ultrasound.

Nutritionists (dieticians) need to know how much a patient has consumed (the patient's input) as well as how much has been expelled (the output) and are an integral part of the healthcare team, since patients' diets are often restricted or need to be monitored closely due to a medical condition.

Physical, occupational, and speech therapists also need the physician's order before proceeding with therapy and to determine whether improvement, or lack of improvement, has been noted by the nursing staff.

Pharmacists rely on the information in a health record when there is a question about the dosage of an ordered drug, when a drug ordered does not make sense based on the age of a patient, or when there is concern about a drug reaction or drug allergy.

Social workers need a patient's health information when coordinating care or assisting a patient with discharge plans.

Care Coordinators and Case Managers

Care coordinators and case managers are employed by acute and chronic care hospitals as well as nursing homes and rehabilitation facilities. The position titles can be used interchangeably. Care coordinators and case managers rely heavily on the information in health records, because they are the liaison among physicians, insurance carriers, other healthcare facilities, and patients and their families.

Care coordinators do just that—coordinate the care of the patient. This process is also referred to as continuity of care. He or she is the primary point of contact and is responsible for coordinating all services provided to a patient. If a patient has just had knee surgery and needs to be transferred to a rehabilitation facility, the care coordinator will search for a suitable facility; provide the facility with access to the patient's health record, so that it can make a decision whether to accept the patient in transfer; and then communicate to the patient and family how and when the transfer will occur. Care coordinators are typically nurses or social workers.

Case managers are usually nurses, but some are health information professionals or social workers. A case manager's role is to ensure that healthcare services are not being under- or overutilized. In a hospital, this job typically begins prior to or soon after admission. Case managers first assess whether the patient's diagnosis and condition warrant acute care hospitalization. They may also contact the patient's insurance carrier to determine whether the admission is covered. The patient's medical history is very important at this point, because the insurance carrier will need to know how long the patient has been suffering from the ailment, as well as whether there are any comorbidities (chronic conditions from which the patient is also suffering—for instance, diabetes mellitus). If the admission is approved, often the insurance carrier will approve a particular number of days of hospitalization, which will then be reassessed as the case manager communicates changes in the patient's condition and any procedures that are to be performed.

The case manager also starts planning for the patient's discharge as soon as the patient is admitted. A patient who is about to undergo cardiac surgery or hip replacement surgery will most likely need the services of a rehabilitation hospital, for instance. As with care coordinators, case managers also coordinate the discharge or transfer process.

In a hospital, care coordinators and case managers may be part of the utilization management department or part of the nursing team on each nursing unit.

On the insurance carrier side, case manager is a title used as well, but the case manager's roles are to assess the patient's status from the insurance carrier's perspective and, based on what the patient's health record says (or does not say), to determine which health services are covered.

Complete, accurate, timely documentation by the physician(s), nurses, and allied health professionals is very important throughout this process.

Health Insurance Plans

Though not clinical, health insurance plans (also known as carriers), such as Medicare, Medicaid, Blue Cross, and Aetna, are very much involved in the patient's care. What the insurance plan will and will not pay for, and at what level, may severely alter the patient's plan of care as well as his or her overall health. The details of a patient's overall health, current condition(s), and plan of care, as documented in the patient's health record, is communicated to the case manager at the insurance plan. If the information is insufficient or incomplete, the care that the attending physician considers to be necessary may not be deemed so by the insurance plan. Ensuring complete documentation that accurately reflects the current health status of the patient and the medical necessity for the care he or she is receiving will certainly reduce the number of questioned or denied claims.

2.1 A DAY IN THE LIFE

Christine was recently in an automobile accident caused by another individual. She sustained injuries to her legs and suffered whiplash. Since the accident, she has also experienced some depression. She was hospitalized for 10 days, then discharged to home, where she was seen by home health physical therapists. She underwent three months of physical therapy and had to wear a neck brace for several weeks. She lost several days of pay because of migraine headaches, and she did not have any sick time remaining. She does have health insurance through her employer, but since her care was a result of an auto accident, the other driver's insurance is responsible. The responsible driver's automobile insurance company is refusing to

(continued)

pay for Christine's physical therapy and the care of her depression and migraine headaches. Christine has hired an attorney to force the other driver's insurance company to pay for her treatment.

1. How might each of the users of and contributors to health information discussed in this section be involved with Christine's healthcare for this auto accident?
2. What role will Christine's health record play in the case her attorney is planning in order to prove that physical therapy was medically necessary and that she was unable to work on several days due to migraine headaches?

2.1   THINKING IT THROUGH

1. Explain the differences between an electronic health record (EHR) and an electronic medical record (EMR).
2. What is discharge planning? At what point in a patient's hospital stay should it begin? Which healthcare professionals assist with discharge planning?
3. Discuss three disadvantages of using paper records versus electronic records.
4. Why is it important to keep track of the location of paper health records? Why is this step unnecessary in an electronic health record system?

2.2   Traditional HIM Functions in Transition

From the 1920s through the early 2000s, the role of health information professionals was to ensure that health records were completed by physicians, as well as other healthcare professionals who document in health records, within a certain time frame after discharge, to code diagnoses and procedures, to pull old records when patients were readmitted, and to run statistical reports as requested. Most of these functions were based on a paper record and manual processing, and the health information staff members were referred to as clerks. Though electronic (digital) records are becoming the norm, some facilities and offices continue to use a paper record in full or in part, and knowledge of the processes used to maintain paper records is helpful in understanding the electronic processes as well.

The next few subsections of the chapter will cover the traditional functions and how they have evolved into the 21st century.

Record Processing

During a patient's stay, under a paper record system, staff from the health information department retrieve any previous records on that patient and send them to the appropriate care unit. Then the medical transcriptionists transcribe reports as dictated by care providers.

Once a patient is discharged or his or her outpatient encounter is complete, the health record is sent to the health information

Quantitative analysis The review of a health record to ensure that required documentation is complete and a part of the record—for instance, a history and physical report or an operative report—but it does not include a review of the quality of the documentation.

Authentication In a paper record, the signature of the person who wrote an entry in a health record, showing authorship; in a digital environment, the security process of verifying an individual's right to access a system or portion of it.

Delinquent records Records that remain incomplete after 15 or 30 days post-discharge or encounter.

Medical staff bylaws A set of policies that define the code of conduct, categories of medical staff membership, rules and regulations related to individual departments with which they may be affiliated, and health information–related policies.

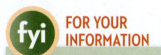 **FOR YOUR INFORMATION**

The physicians' dictation room is also referred to as the "physicians' work room," the "incomplete record room," or other titles and varies by facility.

Unit record System in which all records for one person are filed together under one medical record number in one location.

department, or the records are picked up daily by health information department staff. The records are all accounted for by checking each off the daily discharge list or outpatient list.

Individual records are assembled into a predetermined order, and then they undergo **quantitative analysis** to ensure that all of the required documents are present. Any unsigned entries in the record are **authenticated** (signed).

Specific government regulations and accreditation standards dictate what constitutes a complete and legal record; the regulations and standards will be discussed in the chapter on external forces. All incomplete records are sent to the "physicians' dictation room," where each physician signs and/or dictates his or her records.

Typically, records must be completed within 15 to 30 days after discharge (or encounter). Records that remain incomplete after that time period become **delinquent records**. The **medical staff bylaws** define incomplete versus delinquent records, and that definition is based on state requirements, CoP requirements, or accrediting requirements, whichever are more stringent. Most hospitals have policies and procedures that require physicians with delinquent records to pay monetary fines or face suspension of their hospital privileges—until their records are complete, they cannot admit non-emergency patients, perform consultations, read EKGs, and/or perform elective surgeries.

In an electronic system, the record is reviewed for completeness, but much of that work consists of running reports that show missing reports. For instance, a report might reflect a missing discharge summary or missing signatures, and the physicians involved are then notified. Electronic systems allow for automatic notifications, though the physicians or healthcare professionals with missing information may not complete the items without a "reminder" from the health information staff.

Record Filing and Retrieving

Once records are complete, a health information staff member checks again for any incomplete documents and to be certain that the documents in the record are only for that particular patient. If complete, the record is sent to the permanent file.

In a paper system, hospital records are filed by medical record number as opposed to other healthcare settings, such as physicians' offices and long-term care facilities, which most often file alphabetically by the patient's last name. In the paper system, the record is kept in a manila file folder, in a **unit record** format, meaning that all records for one person are filed together, regardless of the number of inpatient stays or outpatient encounters the patient has had (see Figure 2.3). The records for each encounter may be separated by a file guide within the folder. When the record becomes too large to house in one folder, two or more folders may be utilized, and each is considered a volume—for instance, Volume 1 of 2, Volume 2 of 2, and so on. The specific methods of numbering and filing will be discussed in the chapter on the life cycle of health information.

With electronic health records, there is no need to physically file any papers, since the images are all viewed on a computer screen. It is possible to print the images, but the full record itself is generally

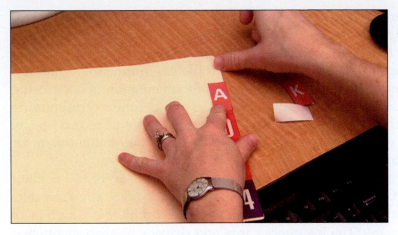

Figure 2.3 **Preparation of a Manila Folder Which Will House a Paper Health Record**

not printed unless there is a bona fide need for it. For instance, a patient has authorized her lawyer to receive a copy of her full health record. There are sometimes papers that must be merged with the remainder of the electronic record. Examples are records from other facilities or signed authorization forms. In this case, the paper document is converted to digital format and the process is known as **document imaging** or **document scanning**.

In healthcare, document scanning became common in the 1990s to archive (store) inactive records onto optical disc. Just as people now back up documents such as photos onto compact discs (CDs), health records were placed on optical discs. Five-inch discs were used, but in order to store as much media as possible in the smallest space possible, 12-inch discs are used more often. Each image is tagged (usually by medical record number, account number, and type of document), so the specific images needed are easily retrievable. Even in an electronic system, scanning at the time of registration is still common—each time a patient is seen, the patient's insurance card and some form of identification, such as a driver's license, is scanned and merged with his or her electronic health record. The scanning device used for a few images at a time is usually a portable unit connected to the desktop computer, an example of which is found in Figure 2.4.

Document imaging/scanning
The process of digitizing images of documents into computer-readable format.

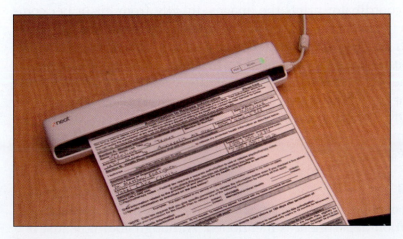

Figure 2.4 **A Portable Scanning Device**

When more than a few documents need to be scanned—for instance, an entire health record—high-speed scanners that duplex (scan on both sides in one pass through) are used.

Filing and retrieving in an electronic environment are not tangible processes. The vast majority of documentation is done using computer screens. The individual pages and records corresponding to each encounter are linked to the patient's electronic record first by medical record number and then by individual account numbers for each encounter.

Facilities and offices that use an electronic health record as their standard method of documentation, and need to scan only a few documents at a time, do not need high-volume (and therefore high price tag) scanners. The insurance cards and driver's licenses mentioned earlier, as well as consent forms, records from other physicians, and advance directives, may still be in paper form and need to be scanned.

Release of Information

All health records are confidential. The health record itself belongs to the facility where the treatment was rendered, but the information in it belongs to the patient. Health information can be released to outside entities only with the authorization of the patient/legal representative or as required by law or HIPAA regulation. Examples of disclosures required by law include the release of the names or health records of patients with communicable diseases to the local department of health and the release of a patient's current state of health to a cancer registry. HIPAA requires the release of diagnostic and procedural data for the filing of insurance claims or for patient care, for example.

The staff member who compiles and sends requested information is often called a release of information coordinator. A higher-level position, which deals with compliance with privacy laws, the investigation of potential breaches in confidentiality, and monitoring of the facility's release of information practices, is known as a **privacy officer**.

Privacy officer A higher-level position dealing with compliance with privacy laws, investigation of potential breaches in confidentiality, and monitoring of the facility's release of information practices.

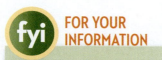

Health information is released in an electronic record format as well. With paper records, the release of information coordinator needs to physically copy the original documents found in the patient's record. If an electronic record is used, the release of information coordinator prints the images directly from his or her computer to the printer or sends the documents electronically.

With an EHR, every person who accesses, enters, or edits information in a record can be traced by the date, time, and duration that he or she was accessing the record. HIPAA requires that on request a patient be given an accounting of disclosures made internally or externally. This is a new task that was neither possible (at least not for the internal users) nor mandatory prior to the advent of the electronic record or HIPAA.

fyi FOR YOUR INFORMATION

Throughout the remainder of the text, ICD-9-CM, ICD-10-CM, and ICD-10-PCS will be referred to as "ICD."

Coding

People employed in healthcare often think of coding when the health information department is mentioned. Although coding is just one aspect of the processing of health information, it is a large part of

Copyright © 2016 by McGraw-Hill Education

it. The process of coding involves a review of each health record for diagnoses and procedures, which are then converted from narrative form into numeric equivalents. For instance, a patient with a diagnosis of left ventricular heart failure would be assigned an **International Classification of Diseases, 9th or 10th revision, Clinical Modification (ICD-9-CM or ICD-10-CM)** code (428.1 in ICD-9-CM; I50.1 in ICD-10-CM); a patient with right ventricular heart failure would be assigned code 428.0 in ICD-9-CM and code I50.9 in ICD-10-CM. At the time of this writing, the coding system used to convert narrative diagnoses is ICD-9-CM, but as mentioned in the chapter on the evolving healthcare system, the implementation of ICD-10-CM is pending and is now scheduled for an October 1, 2015, implementation date. The coding system used currently to convert narrative procedures is ICD-9-CM for inpatients, though once ICD-10 is implemented, **International Classification of Diseases, 10th revision, Procedure Coding System (ICD-10-PCS)** will be used to code procedures for inpatients. In the outpatient setting, **Current Procedural Terminology (CPT)** is used to code procedures; an example is code 77057 for a bilateral screening mammogram.

It is necessary to convert narrative diagnoses and procedures to numeric format in order to submit claims to insurance carriers, for research and epidemiologic studies, and to gather statistics for internal and external requestors.

The staff members who code are known as coders or medical coders. There are varying levels of coders, from entry-level to management positions to coding auditors. There has been no change regarding the requirement to code diagnoses and procedures—both paper and electronic records must be coded. Coders have used technology for many years in the form of **encoder software** that assists the coder through the use of computer programs that replicate actual code books. The advent of the EHR, however, has changed the coding procedure itself. Instead of having to wait for a paper record to be sent to the health information department to be coded, the coder need only access records electronically in a digital system. This change has made it possible for coders to work from home in many cases.

Grouper software works in the background of the encoder software (or in conjunction with it) to categorize each inpatient encounter into a payment classification, which will be further explained in the section on reimbursement.

In the past few years, the use of **computer-assisted coding (CAC)** has become more frequent and frees the coder from looking for codes, so that he or she can concentrate more on ensuring that all the documented diagnoses and procedures are coded accurately, completely, and with the highest degree of specificity. With the increased need for detailed, specific data and ICD-10-CM/PCS on the horizon, which is far more detailed than its predecessor, ICD-9-CM, as well as the continued need for high productivity and quick turnaround between discharge and submitting the insurance claim, coders need tools that will improve their efficiency without negatively impacting coding quality.

International Classification of Diseases, 9th revision, Clinical Modification (ICD-9-CM) A classification system used to convert narrative diagnoses and procedures to numeric form for statistical and reimbursement purposes.

International Classification of Diseases, 10th revision, Clinical Modification (ICD-10-CM) A more specific and scalable classification system for coding of diagnoses that, though approved for use in the United States, has not yet been implemented at the time of this writing.

International Classification of Diseases, 10th revision, Procedural Coding System (ICD-10-PCS) A more specific and scalable classification system for coding of inpatient procedures that, though approved for use in the United States, has not yet been implemented at the time of this writing.

Current Procedural Terminology (CPT) The coding system used to convert narrative procedures and services performed in an outpatient setting to numeric form.

Encoder software Technology used to assign ICD or CPT codes based on the coder's input of terms.

Grouper software Technology used to categorize an inpatient admission or an outpatient encounter into a payment classification.

Computer-assisted coding (CAC) Computer software that improves the efficiency and quality of coding by assessing documentation and suggesting possible code choices, which are then verified by the coder.

Abstracting

In years past, before computerization, it was necessary to collect data from paper records using manual collection forms. This resulted in an "abstract," or summary, for each encounter. The abstracts were sent to a processing company, and the facility in turn received printed statistical reports. The manual abstracting function is no longer necessary, other than for a verification process or a search for inaccurate or inconsistent data by health information personnel as the records are being processed. Computerized abstracting has nothing to do with the EHR. Rather, the administrative and demographic data abstracted through the computerized registration process and master patient index, and diagnosis and procedure codes are entered through the use of encoder software, and billing data are abstracted through the computerized billing and reimbursement functions. For hospital inpatients, the data collected are based on the requirements of the Uniform Hospital Discharge Data Set (UHDDS). The data elements that are collected include the following:

- Unique patient identifier (medical record number)
- Patient's date of birth
- Patient's sex
- Patient's gender
- Patient's race or ethnicity
- Hospital or facility identification number
- Admission (or encounter) date
- Admission source (from home, through emergency department, etc.)
- Discharge date
- Discharge disposition (to home, expired, to nursing facility, to other acute care facility, etc.)
- Attending physician identification
- Consulting physician(s) identification
- Operating physician(s) identification
- Principal and secondary diagnosis code(s)
- Principal and secondary procedure code(s)
- Date(s) of procedure(s)
- Expected source of payment (Medicare, Medicaid, Workers' Compensation, health insurance plan, etc.)
- Total charges

Administration

General health information management positions include department management and supervisory positions. A department manager/director is responsible for the overall planning, organizing, leading, and controlling of the health record processes and staff. Management or supervisory personnel lead individual divisions of a department, such as coding, electronic record processing, medical transcription, release of health information, or general operations.

Uniform Hospital Discharge Data Set (UHDDS) Defined data elements that are required to be collected on all hospital discharges.

Compliance officer positions are often held by health information professionals because of their knowledge of coding, insurance plan requirements, government regulations, and general health information policies and procedures. A compliance officer is responsible for monitoring the activities in the hospital or other healthcare facility that may be susceptible to fraud, misuse, abuse, or overutilization. The compliance officer must access health records, insurance claims, and the policies and procedures of virtually all hospital departments to ensure that the regulations or requirements of state and federal agencies and insurance carriers are being followed.

As health information department managers are responsible for the overall management of a health information department, **revenue cycle managers** are responsible for all functions that lead to an efficient and effective revenue cycle within a healthcare facility—from the point that a patient registers for an encounter to payment of the bill in full. The professional who holds this management position needs a strong accounting background and knowledge of insurance carrier requirements, as well as those of Medicare, Medicaid, and other government plans. A good understanding of how the documentation in a health record affects the choice and sequencing of ICD and CPT diagnosis and procedure codes, and the bearing those codes have on reimbursement, is also essential. Thus, the health information manager and the revenue cycle manager must work together closely.

One of the relatively new functions within a health information department is that of **eHealth management**. As the name implies, the management of electronic health information is the focus of this function. The eHealth management functions meld closely with the overall information technology functions of a hospital or other healthcare facility. The technical aspects of data integration, availability of data, data mining, and required content of the health record are all necessary if health information is kept in an electronic format. Before any of that can happen, however, an electronic master patient index is the key to ensuring that each patient in a database is listed only one time, and that all the administrative and demographic data, such as name, date of birth, unique medical record number, address, phone number(s), email address, race, preferred language, insurance carrier name, policy number, and group number (when applicable), are correct and readily available. A great number of hospitals are part of a health system, or **enterprise system**, in which the health information is shared by each facility in the enterprise. Thus, an accurate, complete master patient index is crucial.

With the surge of healthcare facilities converting from paper record-keeping to electronic record-keeping, the result is an escalation in the amount of data available regarding healthcare in this country. Tracking healthcare trends, assessing the effectiveness of diagnostic and treatment modalities, and assessing quality of care all rely on the availability of accurate, timely, reliable data. Decisions cannot be made without information, which comes from data. **Information (data) governance** ensures that the data collected are accurate and that processes and policies ensure the validity of the data

Compliance officer A position responsible for monitoring activities that are susceptible to fraud, misuse, or overutilization.

Revenue cycle managers Those responsible for the functions that lead to an efficient, effective revenue cycle from the time a patient is registered for care until the bill is paid in full.

eHealth management The processes and policies that govern the digital collection, maintenance, and archival of data.

Enterprise system A health system, made up of a hospital or hospitals, physicians' practices, long-term care facilities, outpatient (ambulatory) diagnostic and therapeutic facilities, and the like.

Information (data) governance The specification of decision rights and an accountability framework to ensure appropriate behavior in the valuation, creation, storage, use, archiving, and deletion of information; it includes the processes, roles and policies, standards, and metrics that ensure the effective and efficient use of information in enabling an organization to achieve its goals (*Gartner* 2013).

collection and the storage of it. It is also the technical ability to collect and maintain secure data. Policies and procedures, the selection of software systems that result in valid data, and the financial backing to provide for it are all part of information governance functions. This is a joint effort of many departments, but key players include the health information management staff and the information technology (IT) department.

Information security The administrative, technical, and physical safeguards put in place to ensure the validity and safety of digital data.

Although **information security** is a function that has always been of utmost importance in healthcare, it typically was incorporated into general health IT and health information management (HIM) daily operations. Recent threats to information security from computer hackers and viruses, as well as tighter federal legislation in the form of HITECH and HIPAA, have necessitated security functions that are distinct from other HIM or IT functions. Many facilities are being proactive in their information security efforts by appointing an information security manager. As with information governance, someone with a background in health information as well as health IT would be a logical candidate for the position.

College Instructor or Professor

The Department of Labor's Bureau of Labor Statistics, in its *Occupational Outlook Handbook,* has noted that the need for health information technicians is expected to increase by 21% from 2010 to 2020 (United States Department of Labor, 2013). The increase in level of education necessary to perform health information functions in an electronic environment, the increasing number of Americans seeking healthcare, and the number of Americans in the baby boomer generation expected to retire in the next 10 years all contribute to this expected increase in open jobs in the field.

This increased workforce need translates to a need for health information educational programs and the professors and instructors to educate that new workforce. The educational level of professors is most often a bachelor's or master's degree but may also be a doctorate degree. Coding certificate programs and other certification programs in specialty areas of HIM generally require at least an associate degree plus certification in the subject area being taught.

Cancer Registry

Cancer registry A database of all patients diagnosed or treated for a malignant neoplasm (cancer) in a hospital; the hospital registry data are submitted to a state cancer registry, then reported to the Centers for Disease Control and Prevention (CDC).

Cancer registries (also known as tumor registries) came about as a result of the National Program of Cancer Registries, which was established by Congress's Cancer Registries Amendment Act of 1992. Hospitals and other facilities that diagnose and/or treat patients with cancers (tumors) are required by law to collect data on each cancer case and to continue surveillance of all cancer cases until the patient's death.

The Centers for Disease Control and Prevention (CDC) administers the national program. Annual cancer statistics are published based off data submitted by healthcare facilities that ultimately reach the CDC and the National Cancer Institute. The data abstracted from each cancer patient's health records include demographic (identification) data; the patient's past medical, surgical, family, and social histories; diagnostic findings; the therapy or therapies used to treat the cancer; and follow-up information, such as the patient's quality of life, whether the patient is disease free, and any secondary cancers that have been found.

These data are then used to evaluate patient outcomes (disease free, death, etc.), quality of life (e.g., able to care for self, hospice care), and survival rates. Based on the data, researchers can better grasp the treatments that are most or least effective based on factors such as stage of disease at the time of diagnosis. Practice patterns are also analyzed, and state governments may base allocation of funds on incidence of cancer(s) by region. The professionals who collect, maintain, and report cancer statistics are *cancer registrars.* Cancer registrars are typically certified by the National Cancer Registrars Association's (NCRA's) Council on Certification, which administers the Certified Tumor Registrar's (CTR's) exam.

Other registries include trauma, birth defect, organ transplant, and disease-specific registries. The EHR has led to more efficient and timely data collection for registrars.

Auditors

Documentation, billing, and release of health information all have to be in compliance with regulations, accreditation standards, internal policies and bylaws, and requirements of third-party payers. Auditors do just that. They audit the coding, billing, and release of information—anything that has to do with the documentation of patient care. External auditors are sent in by regulators, accrediting agencies, and third-party payers. Or auditors may be internal—the facility's way of keeping tabs on its own operation. These auditors may be part of the quality assessment staff, the finance department, or the HIM department. One of the newer positions is that of **recovery audit contractor (RAC)** coordinator. Recovery audit contractors came about because of the Medicare Modernization Act of 2003, with the purpose of recovering improper Medicare payments. They do this by requesting copies of health records and then comparing the ICD and/or CPT coding to the documentation—if the facility's coding was incorrect and Medicare overpaid (in the opinion of the RAC auditor), the facility is obligated to return the overage to Medicare. This entire process is very time-consuming and labor-intensive for the facilities. The internal RAC coordinator positions came about to coordinate the process internally, to keep track of the findings of the RAC, and to verify the findings, as there is an appeal process that the facility can take advantage of if they disagree with the external RAC findings.

Recovery audit contractor (RAC) A position resulting from the Medicare Modernization Act of 2003, with the purpose of recovering improper Medicare payments.

2.2 A DAY IN THE LIFE

Megan McDougal, MS, RHIA®, CHTS-IM, is the recovery audit contractor (RAC) coordinator in the health information management department at West Virginia University (WVU) Healthcare. As RAC

(continued)

coordinator, she is responsible for the coordination of all activities associated with RAC requests, such as responding to the requests, analyzing review findings, keeping track of all RAC requests and denials to ensure compliance with regulations and mandatory deadlines, coordinating with appropriate departments to write appeal letters, following up on all open claims under review, and communicating with all affected internal and external entities involved in the RAC process. She is lead of all RAC teams in the organization and is responsible for providing education and training on RAC processes and tracking software.

Typical Day of the RAC Coordinator

Although the RAC coordinator position came about in 2003, the role of a RAC coordinator is more of a nontraditional HIM role than the traditional careers in HIM, such as coding and transcription. The RAC coordinator has many duties within HIM, such as sending records to the recovery audit contractor, auditing charts for deficiencies and ensuring that all required information is included in the charts, analyzing RAC findings, and working with other departments to guarantee data integrity. Due to the widespread nature of the role, the RAC coordinator may also work in the patient financial services department or compliance department.

It is difficult to describe a typical day for a RAC coordinator, because each day brings new challenges. The main duty that is carried out on a daily basis is reviewing the open claims under audit and checking deadlines to ensure that time frames are being met both internally and externally. If the facility is close to missing a deadline, the coordinator must work with team members to prioritize tasks, so that the deadline is met. Deadlines that must be met by the facility include sending medical records or appeal letters within the required time frame to prevent denial of the claim. If the RAC is late on meeting the deadline to respond, the coordinator must follow up with the RAC entity to learn the reason for the delay. Examples of deadlines that must be met by the RAC include record review results letters and appeal results letters.

As new RAC requests are received, the RAC coordinator analyzes the letters for issues under review and delegates tasks to various members of the RAC team for fulfillment of the requests. Fulfilling a request involves entering the request information into a tracking system, releasing the medical records for review, performing a quality assessment on the records to confirm that the required information is included, and sending the records to the RAC.

When RAC denials are received, the RAC coordinator works with the appropriate departments to determine whether an appeal needs to be written, in an effort to retain the dollars being denied. The coordinator reviews the denial and forwards it to the department that needs to review it. That department then decides whether it agrees or disagrees with the denial. Examples of denials include medical necessity denials, coding denials, and billing denials.

(continued)

Record-Keeping in Ambulatory Settings

Ambulatory healthcare settings include physicians' offices, clinics, urgent care centers, rehabilitation centers (physical and occupational therapy), and reference laboratories. Hospitals are thought of as mainly inpatient facilities, but they offer ambulatory services such as the emergency department services, outpatient diagnostic testing (radiology, laboratory, cardiac testing), ambulatory surgery, and occasionally urgent care. The requirement to keep a health record for each encounter applies to ambulatory care facilities just as it does to inpatient facilities.

Health records are the means of communication among healthcare providers and professionals. They protect the patient, care providers and professionals, and the facility in legal matters, and they prove which services were provided and the reason for them for billing purposes.

In most ambulatory facilities, there is no health information department per se. Instead, there are functions that allow for the maintenance, storage, and retrieval of health information, though the responsibility lies with positions such as receptionists, billing and coding staff, and the office manager.

Ambulatory facilities are also bound by the same privacy and security regulations as hospitals; therefore, they must have policies and procedures in place to ensure that records are secure, regardless of whether they are in paper or electronic format. Ambulatory facilities must have an authorization to release patient identifiable information to outside entities, unless required by law.

Coders are typically employed by ambulatory care facilities. The codes themselves are the same as those used in a hospital setting, but the actual coding guidelines differ in many areas.

1. What is the difference between an incomplete health record and a delinquent health record? Where in the facility is the difference documented, and what is the definition based on?
2. Why is it necessary to collect and report on data about cancer patients?
3. Celeste, a release of information coordinator, is responsible for information governance at her hospital. What additional job responsibilities would Celeste be asked to perform?

2.3   The Profession of Health Information Management

Historical Perspective

The HIM professionals of today were called "record clerks" when they first organized at Massachusetts General Hospital in 1912. By 1928, the Association of Record Librarians of North America (ARLNA) was the professional association for record clerks, and its first president was Grace Whiting Myers (see Figure 2.5).

The purpose of forming the professional association was to elevate the status of individuals who processed medical records, to set standards for the education or knowledge set held by clerks (almost entirely women at that time), and to meet as a group to network and discuss current issues.

Credentialing for HIM professionals came about in 1930; the credential was named Registered Record Librarian, or RRL. The ARLNA was a national organization, but throughout the 1930s, state and local affiliate organizations were formed. Also during the 1930s, nine schools for record librarians were established.

The first house of delegates of ARLNA was formed in the 1940s, and the title for its publication was changed to the *Journal of the American Association of Medical Record Librarians*.

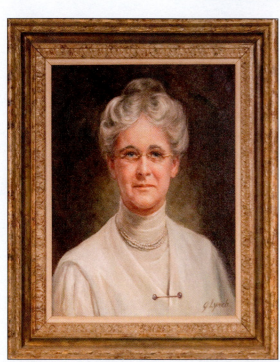

Figure 2.5   An Oil Portrait of Grace Whiting Myers, the First Librarian to Work with Medical Records at Massachusetts General Hospital and the Founder of the ARLNA

By the mid-20th century, the profession was recognized in other countries, and in the 1950s the First International Congress on Medical Records was held in London. The Joint Commission was formed in 1951, and its mission was to elevate the basic licensure requirements for hospitals. Rather than regulations, as laws are known, The Joint Commission (TJC) surveyed hospitals and compared the state of their facilities to a list of standards that needed to be met in order for the institutions to become accredited. Accreditation was and still is voluntary and shows that a hospital goes above and beyond the minimum requirements of state licensure. The medical record was, even then, used as the source document to prove compliance with the standards of The Joint Commission.

The House of Delegates voted to change the association name to the American Medical Record Association and the name of the association's magazine to *Medical Record News* during the 1960s. In the latter part of the 1960s, Medicare and Medicaid were signed into law to help pay for medical care to individuals who are elderly or disabled, or poor, respectively. The inception of Medicare and Medicaid significantly changed healthcare in general and heightened the importance of medical records.

The association was still known as the American Medical Record Association (AMRA) in the 1970s, but the name of the association magazine was again changed, this time to the *Journal of the American Medical Record Association*. It was also during the 1970s that ICD-9-CM was published, and AMRA maintained a strong presence in its implementation, as well as training for its use.

Since its inception, hospital medical record-keeping has been the focus of ARLNA and then AMRA. In practice, however, medical records, as they were then called, were required in every type of healthcare facility.

To reflect the fact that the profession pertained to all types of medical records, the association name was changed to the American Health Information Management Association (AHIMA) in 1991, a name still used today. It was also during this time that medical records became known as health records, since not all records relating to the care of a patient were due to a medical issue; patients were more and more concerned about health rather than disease, and thus the preferred terminology became *health records*, rather than *medical records*. Both are still used today; however, non-HIM professionals are more likely to use the term *medical record* than *health record*.

The 1990s was a busy time for healthcare in general and particularly for health information departments. Although individual states had laws regarding the privacy of health information and coding had been done for statistical purposes for years, the passage of the Health Insurance Portability and Accountability Act (HIPAA) tightened privacy and confidentiality laws and made the coding of diagnoses and procedures using ICD-9-CM and CPT codes a legal requirement.

The first part of the 21st century brought more name changes for credentials. The Registered Health Information Technician (RHIT®) credential replaced the Accredited Record Technician (ART) credential, and the Registered Health Information Administrator (RHIA®) credential replaced the Registered Record Administrator (RRA) credential. The credentials used today are RHIT® and RHIA®. For an overview of the development of HIM as a profession, see Figure 2.6.

Professional Associations

American Health Information Management Association (AHIMA)

As noted earlier, the American Health Information Management Association (AHIMA) is a professional organization for the health information workforce. As of this writing, there are currently more than 71,000 members of AHIMA. Membership types include active (individuals who have an interest in the profession and agree to abide by its code of ethics), student (formally enrolled in

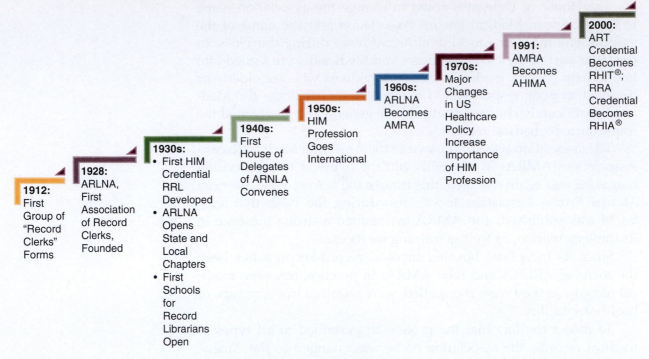

Figure 2.6 The Development of HIM as a Profession, 1912 to Present

1912: First Group of "Record Clerks" Forms

1928: ARLNA, First Association of Record Clerks, Founded

1930s:
• First HIM Credential RRL Developed
• ARLNA Opens State and Local Chapters
• First Schools for Record Librarians Open

1940s: First House of Delegates of ARNLA Convenes

1950s: HIM Profession Goes International

1960s: ARLNA Becomes AMRA

1970s: Major Changes in US Healthcare Policy Increase Importance of HIM Profession

1991: AMRA Becomes AHIMA

2000: ART Credential Becomes RHIT®; RRA Credential Becomes RHIA®

an AHIMA-approved or CAHIIM-accredited educational program), and emeritus (individuals 65 years of age and older in recognition to their service to the profession).

The AHIMA website states the association's mission:

AHIMA leads the health informatics and information management community to advance professional practice and standards.

AHIMA's role as a professional association is to provide guidance, resources, and expertise to health information professionals and to those considering the profession. It also provides current information on issues important to the industry, such as eHealth, information governance, and ICD-10-CM/PCS; advocates for the health information community to state and federal leaders; and offers career and job assistance to persons new to the profession and to experienced professionals. HIM educational standards are set by AHIMA. Finally, AHIMA has an international presence as well in the quest to create a global healthcare system.

Healthcare Information Management Systems Society (HIMSS)
The website of the Healthcare Information Management Systems Society (HIMSS) describes the association:

HIMSS is a global, cause-based, not-for-profit organization focused on better health through information technology (IT). HIMSS leads efforts to optimize health engagements and care outcomes using information technology.

Both AHIMA and HIMSS are professional associations for the health information profession; HIMSS's focus is on the technology aspect of maintaining health information as well as data analytics, consumer engagement, and general health informatics.

Individuals who have a role in health IT or group members, such as hospitals, health IT service providers, and HIM professionals, and related organizations constitute the membership of HIMSS. Health information management professionals are concerned with the content of health records, with the privacy and security of the records, and with compliance with state and federal regulations, Medicare regulations, the requirements of insurance carriers, and voluntary accrediting agency standards. They also need to have a good understanding of the technical requirements that make the electronic processes and health records possible. HIMSS and AHIMA work closely to ensure that the goals of each are being met.

HIMSS provides resources for its members, advocates for health IT–related issues, and offers career and job guidance.

American Medical Informatics Association (AMIA)

Like HIMSS, AMIA's emphasis is on the technical functions of electronic health information, known as informatics. Membership is geared more toward clinicians, such as physicians, nurses, dentists, and pharmacists, who rely on data to do their jobs as well as health researchers and educators, government officials and policymakers, and industry professionals (AMIA, 2013).

Association for Healthcare Documentation Integrity (AHDI)

AHDI was previously known as the American Association for Medical Transcription. It is an association that represents the professionals responsible for the capture of clinical documentation: medical transcriptionists. Specifically, *clinical documentation* refers to transcription of reports dictated by physicians and other healthcare providers or the editing of documentation that results from **voice recognition** software systems. AHDI promotes documentation that is of a high level of accuracy and that is private and secure.

Voice recognition Software that recognizes the dictation of a care provider or other professional and converts the speech to text.

2.3 A DAY IN THE LIFE

Michael has worked in construction for the past 10 years. His knees are giving out and he wants to change careers. He thinks he wants to go into the medical profession, but he does not want direct patient contact. He comes to you for advice, because he knows you work in a hospital as a cancer registrar.

1. What advice will you give Michael, so that he can learn about career options?

2.3 THINKING IT THROUGH

1. What was the purpose of forming an organization of record clerks? Is it similar to the reason professional organizations are still prevalent to this day? Explain.
2. Why is it necessary for AHIMA and HIMSS to maintain a close alliance?
3. Access the website of AHIMA, HIMSS, AMIA, or AHDI and explain three benefits of belonging to a professional organization.

Degrees

Associate Degree

Health information professionals can earn an associate, baccalaureate, or master's degree in health information. Health informatics has also become a degree option in recent years. Health information management is more focused on the content and requirements of a legal health record kept in any format, whereas health informatics degrees focus on the technical aspects of capturing, maintaining, and storing health information in a private and secure manner. Graduates of an HIM associate degree program approved by the **Commission on Accreditation for Health Informatics and Information Management Education (CAHIIM)** may elect to take the Registered Health Information Technician exam. Upon successful completion of the exam, the initials RHIT®, which is the acronym for Registered Health Information Technician, may be used following one's name.

Graduates of associate degree programs are typically responsible for assessing the content and quality of documentation found in health records, abstracting health data, ensuring that privacy laws are maintained when releasing health information, utilizing software while performing HIM processes, calculating statistics, and coding diagnoses and procedures used for reimbursement and statistical purposes.

Although associate degree graduates are often frontline personnel, in smaller facilities they may qualify for supervisory positions within a year or so after graduation, particularly if they had similar experience in other sectors.

Bachelor's Degree

Bachelor's degree graduates have a four-year HIM education. If the program from which the student graduated is CAHIIM accredited, he or she may sit for the Registered Health Information Administrator (RHIA®) exam.

The functions listed under the associate degree section are all part of the bachelor's degree curriculum, but at a higher level. Bachelor's programs prepare graduates to evaluate, implement, and manage electronic systems used to document healthcare and the systems used to process that documentation. Not only do these graduates need to know how to code, but they also have a higher understanding of terminologies, vocabularies, and classifications systems used to collect healthcare data. Additionally, standardization and analysis of data, the management of databases, and the validation of data are responsibilities often held by RHIAs®. Graduates of bachelor's-level programs often hold more administrative or management-type positions on or soon after graduation.

Master's Degree

The newest degree level for HIM students is at the graduate level—a master's degree in HIM. These programs may be CAHIIM

Commission on Accreditation for Health Informatics and Information Management Education (CAHIIM)
An independent accrediting organization whose mission is to serve the public interest by establishing and enforcing quality Accreditation Standards for Health Informatics and Health Information Management (HIM, 2014) educational programs (CAHIIM, 2014).

approved as well; however, there is currently no certification exam that applies at the master's level. All of the general function areas covered in the associate or bachelor's programs are also covered at the master's level, but at a higher level. Master's-level coding has to do with interpretation of clinical terminologies, vocabularies, and classification systems and the mapping of clinical terminologies and vocabularies to the appropriate classification system. Data are evaluated and presented in a meaningful way. The design of electronic systems and evaluation of network infrastructures are other examples of the level of instruction at the master's degree level. Though there is no separate certification for the master's level, practitioners with an RHIT® or RHIA® credential who have attained their master's degree and have experience in the field, as well as served their profession through volunteerism with their component state association and AHIMA, may qualify for the designation of Fellow of the American Health Information Management Association (FAHIMA).

Though few in numbers, a PhD in health information technology or management, or in the related fields of health sciences, health informatics, or health administration, is also available. Additionally, there is more of a global awareness of the need for data, population health, and the like; thus, the International Federation of Health Information Management Associations (IFHIMA) has emerged and is the global organization of HIM professional associations.

Certifications

Individuals who hold a professional certification show a high level of competence in their chosen field. AHIMA offers several certifications relating to general health information collection and maintenance, from coding competency and privacy to data analysis. Certification shows an employer that the person is current in the field and has shown that he or she has gone above and beyond education to become an expert in the field. The following certification exams are offered through the American Health Information Management Association (AHIMA). Table 2.2 summarizes the certifications and academic or experiential requirements for each AHIMA credential.

Professional Practice Experience (PPE)

A cornerstone of HIM educational programs is the professional practice experience (PPE), which is similar to an internship. It is a requirement of all HIM educational programs that the curriculum include at least one PPE setting. The PPE gives students the opportunity to translate theory into real-life situations in the healthcare field.

PPE settings include traditional healthcare sites, such as hospitals, ambulatory clinics, physicians' offices, and long-term care facilities. Or they may be nontraditional, such as consulting firms, insurance companies, government agencies, software companies, and academic institutions. Students should use the PPE to explore different jobs and settings in HIM and/or to select site(s) in the

Certification	Requirements
TABLE 2.2 **AHIMA Certifications and Requirements**	
Registered Health Information Administrator (RHIA®)	• Bachelor's-level health information degree • Successful completion of a certification examination
Registered Health Information Technician (RHIT®)	• Associate degree in health information management • Successful completion of a certification examination
Certified Coding Apprentice (CCA®)	• High school diploma or equivalent • Six months' coding experience and/or • Successful completion of a coding certificate program recommended
Certified Coding Specialist (CCS®)	• Currently holds an RHIT®, an RHIA®, or a CCA® credential and two years' coding experience or • Successful completion of a coding certificate program or • Holds a coding credential from another professional organization with one year's experience assigning codes
Certified Coding Specialist—Physician-based (CCS-P®)	• Currently holds an RHIT®, an RHIA®, or a CCA® credential or • Two years' coding experience or • Current CCA® credentials with one year of coding experience or • Completion of a coding certificate program or • Holds a coding credential from another professional organization with one year's experience assigning codes
Certified Documentation Improvement Practitioner (CDIP®)	• RHIA®, RHIT®, CCS®, CCS-P®, RN, MD, or DO and two years' experience in clinical documentation improvement or • Minimum of an associate degree and three years' experience in clinical documentation improvement (coursework in medical terminology and anatomy and physiology required)
Certified Health Data Analyst (CHDA®)	• Associate degree and minimum of five years of healthcare data experience or • Healthcare information management credential (RHIT®) and minimum of three years of healthcare data experience or • Bachelor's degree and a minimum of three years of healthcare data experience or • Healthcare information management credential (RHIA®) and minimum of one year of healthcare data experience or • Master's or related degree (JD, MD, or PhD) and one year of healthcare data experience
Certified in Healthcare Privacy and Security (CHPS®)	• Associate degree and six years' experience in healthcare privacy or security management or • Healthcare information management credential (RHIT®) and minimum of four years of experience in healthcare privacy or security management or • Bachelor's degree and a minimum of four years' experience in healthcare privacy or security management or • Healthcare information management credential (RHIA®) and a minimum of two years of experience in healthcare privacy or security management or • Master's or related degree (JD, MD, or PhD) and two years of experience in healthcare privacy or security management
Certified Healthcare Technology Specialist (CHTS)	Successfully passes a proficiency exam in one of the following areas related to the Meaningful Use of electronic health information: • The Clinician/Practitioner Consultant Examination (CHTS-CP) • Implementation manager (CHTS-IM) • Implementation support specialist (CHTS-IS) • Practice Workflow and Information Management Redesign Specialist (CHTS-PW) • Technical/Software Support Staff Examination (CHTS-TS) • Trainer Examination (CHTS-TR)

area in which they have a particular interest. For instance, a student with a high technical ability and an interest in computer applications may choose a healthcare software company. The PPE may be a combination of traditional and nontraditional sites as well.

Continuing Education

Being a lifelong learner is an important trait of a professional. Not only is it important to stay current in one's field, but it is also important for professional growth, it shows initiative, and it gives one a competitive edge when searching for a job. Healthcare is ever changing and, because the role of the HIM professional is affected by technology, changing government regulations, and new advances in medicine, ongoing continuing education is required and is a very important characteristic of the profession. Every two years, credentialed professionals are required to earn continuing education units (CEUs). See Figure 2.7 for the biennial cycle of CEUs by credential. Individuals holding more than one credential are required to earn additional credits, which vary by combination.

CEUs can be earned by attending educational seminars or workshops that are pertinent to health information or health informatics, by successfully completing college courses related to either, by conducting professional presentations or authoring HIM-related books or articles in scholarly journals, and by acting as a PPE site supervisor, to name a few.

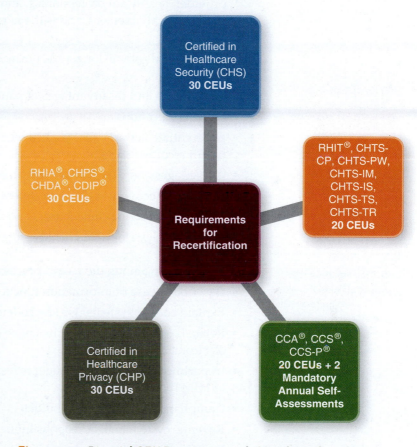

Figure 2.7 Biennial CEU Requirements by Credential

2.4 THINKING IT THROUGH

1. What does the acronym CAHIIM stand for, and why would a prospective student seek to attend a CAHIIM-approved HIM program?

2. Other than to maintain certification, what is the value of earning CEUs?

3. Explain how an associate degree would differ from a master's degree regarding the graduate's knowledge base and curriculum coverage.

chapter 2 summary

LEARNING OUTCOMES	CONCEPTS FOR REVIEW
2.1 Explain the importance of documentation needed by users of health information. Pages 33–41	• Definition of a health record • Differentiate between care providers and healthcare professionals. • The health record is a source document for communication and documentation of a patient's health status. It protects the patient, care provider, healthcare professionals, and healthcare facility in legal matters, justifies reimbursement, and is the narrative used to code diagnoses and procedures. • Paper records are no longer the norm; instead, electronic (digital) records are the norm. • Advantages and disadvantages of paper records • Filing applications • Differentiate between electronic medical records (EMRs) and electronic health records (EHRs). • Advantages and disadvantages of an electronic system • American Recovery and Reinvestment Act (ARRA) • Name and describe clinical users and authors of documentation. • Name and describe allied health professionals.
2.2 Categorize the job responsibilities of health information professionals. Pages 41–52	• Differentiate among the record processing steps. • Describe release of information functions. • Explain coding systems used by coders. • Relate how traditional functions have changed with the advent of an electronic system. • Department director or manager is responsible for the overall management of HIM functions and staff. • Compliance officer responsibilities • Revenue cycle manager responsibilities • Explain eHealth management. • Relate the role of information governance in an electronic system. • College instructor opportunities • The purpose of a cancer registry and role of the cancer registrar • Recovery audit contractors (RACs) and the role of the RAC coordinator • Explanation of the differences in record-keeping in a hospital versus an ambulatory setting
2.3 Discuss the development of health information management as a profession. Pages 52–55	• Trace the history of health information as a profession. • Trace the history of what is today the American Health Information Management Association (AHIMA). • Explain the purpose of the Healthcare Information Management Systems Society (HIMSS).

LEARNING OUTCOMES	CONCEPTS FOR REVIEW
	• How the American Medical Informatics Association (AMIA) is different from AHIMA or HIMSS • Describe the evolution of the Association for Healthcare Documentation Integrity (AHDI).
2.4 Evaluate the educational opportunities and certifications of health information professionals. Pages 56–59	• Differentiate among the degrees, certificates, and credentials available to health information professionals. • The role of the professional practice experience in the education of health information management students • Continuing education requirements for credentialed health information management professionals

chapter review

MATCHING QUESTIONS

Match each term with its definition.

_____ 1. **[LO 2.2]** information security

_____ 2. **[LO 2.2]** coder

_____ 3. **[LO 2.2]** unit record

_____ 4. **[LO 2.1]** third-party payer

_____ 5. **[LO 2.2]** information governance

_____ 6. **[LO 2.2]** quantitative analysis

_____ 7. **[LO 2.2]** enterprise system

_____ 8. **[LO 2.2]** privacy officer

_____ 9. **[LO 2.2]** compliance officer

_____ 10. **[LO 2.3]** transcriptionist

_____ 11. **[LO 2.2]** eHealth management

_____ 12. **[LO 2.2]** release of information coordinator

_____ 13. **[LO 2.1]** outguide

_____ 14. **[LO2.2]** revenue cycle manager

a. The software, policies, and procedures that ensure that medical data are accurately maintained and protected

b. Studying a bulk set of individual records to check for accuracy and completion

c. HIM professional who is responsible for monitoring information releases within a healthcare organization

d. Protection of medical record components from unauthorized access, use, or disclosure

e. A single file containing all of a patient's medical records and encounter forms

f. HIM function that ensures the accuracy and integration of the master patient index and other health record information

g. Group of hospitals or other healthcare facilities that share information among themselves

h. HIM professional responsible for the reimbursement functions from the time a patient registers for an encounter to payment of the bill

i. HIM professional who is charged with complying with requests for health information

j. HIM professional who deals with avoiding fraud and abuse in a healthcare organization

k. An entity other than the patient or healthcare provider involved in financing insurance claims

l. Tab on a paper folder that identifies the contents

m. HIM professional who converts narrative health record documentation to a numeric equivalent

n. HIM professional who converts the recorded dictation of care providers into typed report form using word processing software

MULTIPLE CHOICE QUESTIONS

Choose the letter that best completes the statement or answers the question.

15. **[LO 2.1]** A patient encounter is documented in the health record
    a. at the initial new patient visit.
    b. whenever the patient switches care providers.
    c. every time the patient is seen.
    d. if a new diagnosis is made.

16. **[LO 2.1]** Which is true of facilities that use paper records?
    a. Care providers will always have the most current record to pull.
    b. Care providers cannot share patient information among themselves.
    c. The paper files are kept securely behind the reception desk.
    d. The paper files can easily be outdated or incomplete.

17. **[LO 2.1]** Health records must be kept in some format, at a minimum for
    a. at least one year.
    b. at least three years.
    c. at least five years.
    d. forever.

18. **[LO 2.1]** Which person would be considered an allied health professional?
    a. Lab tech
    b. Medical assistant
    c. Doctor
    d. Nurse midwife

19. **[LO2.2]** Incomplete records must be completed within _____ days of an encounter or discharge.
    a. one week
    b. two weeks
    c. one month
    d. six months

20. **[LO 2.2]** What is another term for *scanning*?
    a. Copying
    b. Imaging
    c. Editing
    d. Renaming

21. **[LO 2.2]** A public health official calls your office, asking for data regarding the incidence of pertussis in your patients. What department or staff member would most likely be responsible for responding to the official's request?
    a. Information governance
    b. Privacy officer
    c. Information security
    d. Compliance officer

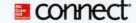

Enhance your learning by completing these exercises and more at http://connect.mheducation.com!

22. **[LO 2.1]** Which person would be considered a physician extender?
    a. HIM professional
    b. Certified nurse practitioner
    c. Doctor of osteopathy
    d. Physical therapist

23. **[LO 2.4]** A(n) _____ is awarded to someone who has demonstrated advanced expertise in his or her field.
    a. associate degree
    b. bachelor's degree
    c. master's degree
    d. professional certification

24. **[LO 2.4]** Which professional certification currently has no restriction on degrees or years worked?
    a. Certified Healthcare Technology Specialist (CHTS)
    b. Certified Coding Apprentice (CCA®)
    c. Certified Coding Specialist—Physician-based (CCS-P®)
    d. Certified in Healthcare Privacy and Security (CHPS®)

SHORT ANSWER QUESTIONS

25. **[LO 2.1]** Describe the five main uses of a health record.

26. **[LO 2.1]** Why is handwriting a safety concern with paper records?

27. **[LO 2.1]** Explain the difference between a hospital case manager and an insurance company case manager.

28. **[LO 2.2]** Name and describe three users of clinical information.

29. **[LO 2.2]** Give an example of when a health record may be released without specific patient authorization.

30. **[LO 2.3]** Explain Grace Whiting Myers's contributions to the field of HIM.

31. **[LO 2.3]** What is the purpose of The Joint Commission?

32. **[LO.2.4]** Explain the importance of professional practice experiences.

33. **[LO 2.4]** Why are credentialed HIM professionals required to maintain their credentials through earning CEUs every two years?

APPLYING YOUR KNOWLEDGE

34. **[LO 2.1]** How might EHRs have an influence on the economy, as stipulated by the HITECH Act?

35. **[LO 2.2]** Which of the HIM careers discussed in Section 2.2 sounds the most interesting? Explain your answer.

36. **[LO 2.2]** You work in a local hospital. Recently, it was alleged that a patient chart was accessed by a staff member and information was given to the girlfriend of one of your department's patients. Which staff member(s) would likely be involved in investigating this claim?

37. **[LO 2.3]** Discuss the timeline of major events in HIM. Explain how each milestone was significant to the profession.

38. **[LO 2.4]** You hold a Registered Health Information Technician (RHIT®) credential. What might your career path look like in terms of certifications and CEUs?

39. **[LO 2.4]** Are professional certifications really necessary and valuable? Defend your answer.

40. **[LO 2.4]** Arianna does not have a degree; in fact, she started working right out of high school. She currently works as a clinical documentation specialist and is interested in pursuing a certification. Is Arianna eligible for the Certified Documentation Improvement Practitioner (CDIP®) certification? Why or why not?

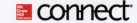 Enhance your learning by completing these exercises and more at http://connect.mheducation.com!

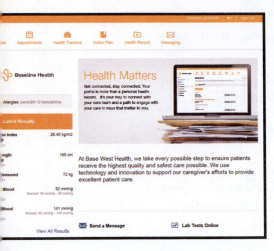

Health Informatics and Health Information Management Shaping the Evolving Healthcare System

Learning Outcomes

When you finish this chapter, you will be able to:

3.1 Differentiate between health information management and health informatics.

3.2 Explain how integrated delivery systems are changing skill sets required for health information professionals.

3.3 Summarize the informatics skills required to support Meaningful Use.

3.4 Categorize the informatics skills supporting the continuum of care under accountable care and shared savings models.

Key Terms

Change management
Data analysis
Data mining
Database management
e-Record
Health informatics
Health information exchanges (HIEs)
Integrated delivery network (IDN)
Interoperability

Legacy systems
mHealth
Patient portal
Personal Health Record (PHR)
Population health management
Project management
Regional extension center (REC)
Systems management
Workflow

Healthcare reform depends on a new system that makes better use of patient data and turns it into information that can be used by many stakeholders to improve care, lower costs, and support a healthier population. To make this happen, hundreds of billions of dollars have been spent on health information technology (HIT) since 2009. In order to use this technology and reach these goals, many existing healthcare workers need to learn new skills, and there is a need for workers in newly created positions. Health information professionals—whether they specialize in informatics, management, or technology implementation—will have to work together to make the goals outlined in recent healthcare legislation a reality.

This chapter will examine how the implementation of healthcare reform is evolving the complementary fields of health informatics and health information management while breaking down the differences and similarities between these two fields. Then, it will segue into the informatics skills health information professionals will need to cultivate to be successful in a healthcare system increasingly driven by the idea of accountable care.

3.1 Health Informatics

What Is Health Informatics?

Many of the new skills and positions in healthcare are part of an evolving area referred to as **health informatics**. *Informatics* may sound like a highly technical word, but the term itself has a long history. Originally coined in Europe in the 1960s, the term *informatique* was defined as the "science of information processing." This was Anglicized to *informatics*.

The term *medical informatics* was widely adopted in the United States in the 1980s, when physicians, scientists, and engineers began to study how computer applications could be used in medical care. In 1989, the American Medical Informatics Association (AMIA) was established. The term *medical informatics* is not in frequent use today, having been replaced by the term *health informatics*.

Health informatics is considered part of a larger field called biomedical informatics, which also includes nursing informatics, laboratory informatics, public health and population health informatics, and other evolving fields. The scope of health informatics is itself evolving, paralleling the growth in the advanced use of health information technology.

To work in health informatics, you do not have to be tech savvy. Health informatics touches every job in healthcare, whether it is a physician or nurse using an electronic health record, a coder of health records using computer-assisted coding, or case managers as they assist patients by using digitized records exchanged from several locations. At all levels of jobs in healthcare, many existing workers will need to develop new health informatics skills and knowledge. For example, medical coders with experience in working with electronic health records (EHRs) are more valuable than those with no experience using EHRs.

Many new types of positions are being created in health informatics. Some of these jobs require technical expertise, such as project

Health informatics The practice of information and knowledge management across clinical healthcare and public health domains.

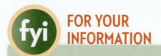 **FOR YOUR INFORMATION**

At its basic level, health informatics is the creation of new solutions to improve healthcare, using information technology.

management, **systems management**, programming, and database management. Other positions analyze and use the data created in an integrated computerized healthcare system. These include data analysts, reporting specialists, and biostatisticians.

Health Informatics versus Health Information Management

The fields of health informatics and health information management are closely linked and highly complementary. Core to both is patient data. On a basic level, health informatics focuses on the processes of electronic exchange, digital storage, and the computerized manipulation of health data; health information management (HIM) is the practice of acquiring, analyzing, and protecting medical information to provide quality patient care, and until recent years, in a hard copy format.

As more medical records are captured and stored as digital data and used electronically, the overlap between health information management and health informatics will continue to increase. The boundaries between the fields are porous and fluid, and it is not possible to say where health information management ends and health informatics begins. Educational and training programs in the two fields share many courses, and workers in both share many skills.

When electronic health records and health information exchange were introduced, some experts predicted that HIM would be less important, since all the records would be computerized and HIM traditionally dealt with paper records. This is not true. More patient information is being captured and put to an increasing number of uses both inside and outside the clinical setting. Thus, the professional management of these records has increased in importance, as has the need for HIM professionals. The scope of work has been expanded, and increasingly the skills required include working with EHRs, but the focus of HIM continues to be the management and protection of patient data, both in a clinical setting and in secondary uses.

The American Health Information Management Association (AHIMA) is the organization for HIM professionals. The relationship between AHIMA and AMIA, the informatics organization, is highly collaborative, due to their many overlapping interests. As depicted in Figure 3.1, in 2012, AHIMA and AMIA issued a joint document that provides a roadmap for understanding the larger field of biomedical informatics and defines the parameters of health informatics and its relationship to other informatics areas.

In conjunction with this process, the Commission on Accreditation for Health Informatics and Information Management Education (CAHIIM) endorsed a health informatics curriculum at the graduate level, consisting of three parts:

1. Information systems
2. Informatics principles
3. Information technology

HIM is an underlying element that shapes all parts of health informatics, allowing information to be used properly and effectively. Health informatics is built on top of this governed information and is focused on the resources, devices, and methods required

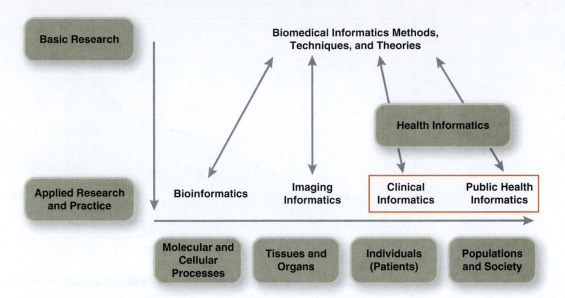

Figure 3.1   The Joint AMIA/AHIMA Definition of Biomedical Informatics

for optimizing the acquisition, storage, retrieval, and use of clinical and related patient data. The tools include not only computers but also clinical guidelines, formal medical terminologies, and information and communication systems.

The Evolution of Health Informatics

The field of health informatics began with the study of how computers could be used in clinical settings. It was narrow and specialized because of the domination of paper records. A few years ago, when you walked into a doctor's office, you would probably see a wall of file cabinets where paper patient records were stored and accessed. There were high-technology pieces of hardware for imaging and surgery, but they were used in diagnosis and treatment without being integrated into a larger hospital system. Computer screens were used for reading diagnostic tests, not for accessing entire patient records.

The adoption of information technology on the business side of healthcare, such as practice management, has been far quicker than on the clinical or patient encounter side. Many finance and business functions, such as the payment of claims by insurance companies and appointment scheduling, are highly automated. Health informatics, however, is concerned with the clinical setting and patient care, not business operations.

The best way to track the timeline for the development of health informatics is to follow the adoption of EHRs, as depicted in Figure 3.2. EHRs are needed to capture the data that health informatics professionals use. EHR adoption was given a boost in 2009, when the federal government introduced the Health Information Technology for Economic and Clinical Health Act (HITECH) program, spending $32 billion on incentive payments and supporting programs for EHR adoption and their "Meaningful Use." This legislation was described in the chapter on the evolving healthcare system in the United States. **Regional extension centers (RECs)** were established in each state to support the implementation of EHRs and HITECH requirements.

Regional extension center (REC) An organization funded by the HITECH Act to assist providers by extending EHR adoption training and support services, offering guidance in EHR implementation, troubleshooting related technical issues, and meeting Meaningful Use.

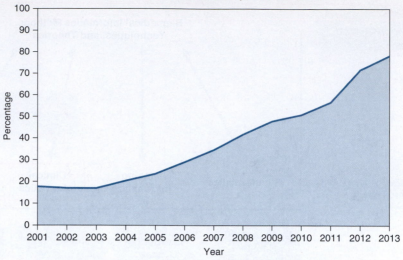

Percentage of Office-Based Physicians with EHRs

Figure 3.2 **Penetration of Electronic Health Records in Primary Care**

Source: Use and Characteristics of Electronic Health Record Systems Among Office-based Physician Practices: United States, 2001-2013, NCHS Data Brief, Number 143, January 2014. http://www.cdc.gov/nchs/data/databriefs/db143.htm.

e-Record A patient's medical history, diagnostic test results, images, and clinical notes stored digitally in a database.

According to the Office of the National Coordinator for Health IT (ONC), RECs assisted more than 147,000 providers through 2013, with more than 85% of those providers live on an EHR. In 2012, an estimated 72% of clinicians used EHRs, compared to 17% in 2002. This allows the initial capture of patient **e-records** and enables their use in other elements of health informatics.

3.1 A DAY IN THE LIFE

Under federal programs, healthcare providers are being encouraged to adopt and use EHRs. They receive funds to buy these systems and will be penalized through lowered Medicare payments if they do not have EHRs and use them in specific ways. This is a complicated process that requires selecting an EHR vendor, implementing the system, training clinical and support staff, and integrating the system into caregiving and administrative processes. Some physicians are deciding not to adopt EHRs and stay with paper-based systems. Others are deciding to retire early instead of participating in these changes. They claim that this process is too disruptive.

1. What types of problems do you think physicians and nurses will have in adopting an EHR system?
2. What issues do you think HIM professionals will have?
3. Would you go to a physician who elects to stay with a paper-based system? Do you think it matters?

3.1 THINKING IT THROUGH

1. What health informatics skills will HIM professionals need to know? What HIM skills will health informatics specialists need?
2. How do data relate to the fields of health informatics and health information management?

Just what will our future healthcare system look like? The system goes beyond the walls of a doctor's office or hospital to wherever health information is needed and useful. It might be in a patient's home or on a smartphone. Figure 3.3 shows the path of information in an integrated, wired system. Healthcare becomes far more expansive, and patient data will be used at many more locations.

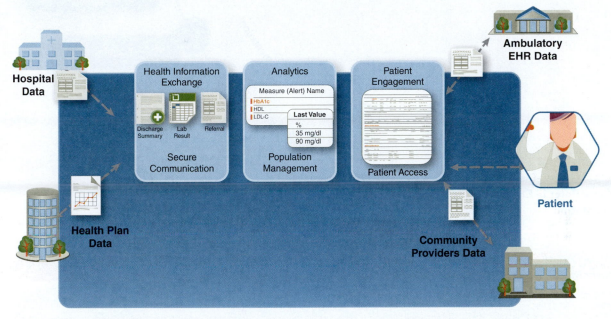

Figure 3.3   **Health Data in an Integrated System**

Changes in Workflow

In the transition to EHRs, ONC identified six areas where skilled specialists are required, as shown in Figure 3.4. These skill sets were in great demand during the early ramp-up and implementation of EHRs but continue to be needed today as systems mature.

What these positions have in common is that they support changes in **workflow**. The introduction of HIT into healthcare has disrupted the traditional workflow because technology and data are being used in what was formerly a paper-based system. Workers are needed to manage this process, especially in organizations as complex as healthcare providers. An area of expertise has developed called **change management** to support this process.

The introduction of EHRs is only the first step in the transition of healthcare. The next steps are the Meaningful Use of the technology and the migration to a patient-centered healthcare system. The new skills required to support each of these stages are listed in Table 3.1.

Thus, as the healthcare system begins to increase the use of patient data beyond the location of the clinician and patient interaction to include transitions in care and patient engagement, existing workflows will change and new workflows will need to be developed. This means new skills for existing workers and positions for new workers with the required skills.

Workflow A well-defined sequence of activities undertaken in order to achieve a work outcome.

Change management A structured approach for ensuring that changes in an organization are thoroughly and smoothly implemented and that the benefits of change are achieved.

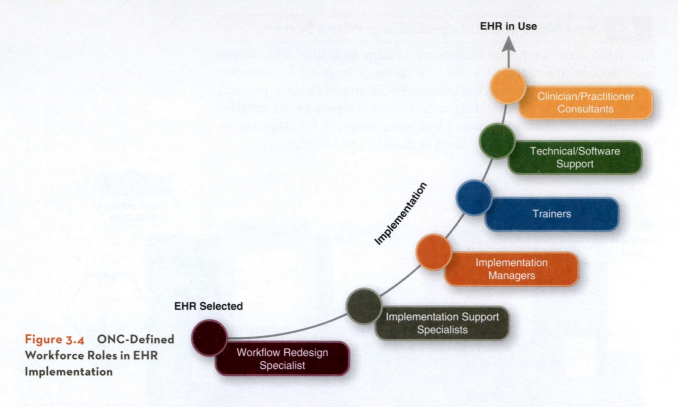

Figure 3.4 ONC-Defined Workforce Roles in EHR Implementation

EHR in Use

Clinician/Practitioner Consultants

Technical/Software Support

Trainers

Implementation

Implementation Managers

Implementation Support Specialists

EHR Selected

Workflow Redesign Specialist

TABLE 3.1	Informatics Skill Requirements by Healthcare Transformation Stage
Stage	**Informatics Skill Requirements**
#1 Enabling technology implementation	• Project management • Implementation • Systems management and maintenance • Programming • Training • Workflow redesign • Business/healthcare analysis • Health information management
#2 Meaningful Use	• Business/healthcare analysis • Project management • Data mining • Data warehousing • Programming • Health information management
#3 Patient-centric healthcare/accountable care	• Business/healthcare analysis • Data mining • Programming • Remote device management and maintenance • Health information management

Project Management

The work involved in changing healthcare is done in a series of steps or projects. All individuals involved in these projects need to understand how the projects are being managed:

- What needs to be done?
- What resources are needed?
- Who is doing what when?
- Who is responsible for meeting deadlines?
- What is the reporting structure (who's the boss)?

This is known as **project management**. The process of project management, as defined by the Project Management Institute, is shown in Figure 3.5.

Whether you are a manager or a worker, understanding project management is important, particularly given the speed with which HIT is being deployed. The details of project management change with each project, but the process is the same. Being able to manage a project's logistics, budget, and people are skills typically required to advance in careers in health informatics.

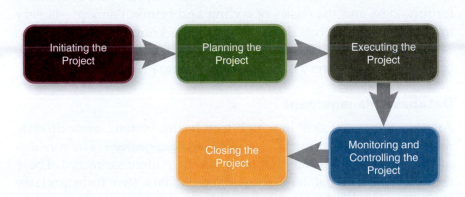

Figure 3.5   The Project Management Process

Systems Maintenance and Support

Once a project is completed and a system "goes live," the system needs to be maintained and the professionals using the system must be supported. These are important jobs, and they are growing in number, often as entry-level jobs in HIT and health informatics.

There are many parts to a wired health system and all these elements must be interconnected and **interoperable**, or able to work together. All hardware, software, and networks need to be maintained to keep them operating. Upkeep consists of cleaning, fixing, updating software, troubleshooting, and continually testing for performance. Healthcare is a mission-critical business, and any failure of technology can have serious consequences.

There is a parallel increase in the need for technical support staff in the connected health system. *Technical support* refers to helping users learn how to use HIT and assisting them when they encounter problems in using the technologies. Teaching clinicians to use an EHR, assisting a nurse in navigating through various user interfaces, and helping coders locate and extract diagnostic descriptions from digital patient records are a few examples of technical support tasks. Technical support staff roles also represent potential entry-level positions for properly trained individuals.

Project management The application of knowledge, skills, and techniques to execute projects efficiently and effectively.

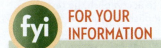

FOR YOUR INFORMATION

The Project Management Institute offers a certification for Project Management Professional (PMP). This credential is much respected in healthcare and is usually required for senior project managers.

Interoperability The ability of two or more systems to exchange data and to use the information once it has been received.

In discussing the technologies of health informatics, the focus is often on clinician/patient interaction. EHRs, computerized physician order entry (CPOE), and clinical decision support (CDS) are several examples of point of care health informatics technologies; however, other locations are equally important. An integrated system requires that all elements be interconnected and interoperable, including laboratories, pharmacies, and digital imaging. Each of these has its own HIT systems requiring maintenance and support, and they all need to be integrated and interoperable with the overall system. Figuring out how to integrate older systems—called **legacy systems**—with newer systems is a major challenge in today's healthcare. This often requires custom interfaces and programming.

The training required for positions in maintenance and support includes a basic understanding of computers, networks, and programming. However, because healthcare is a complicated business, specialized knowledge—such as HIM principles, EHRs, medical terminology, and the basics of coding and reimbursement—is very important in every role. Lack of healthcare knowledge is the main reason that individuals with a traditional information technology background find it very difficult to break into healthcare.

Database Management

Another important skill in a high-tech health system, more directly related to health informatics, is **database management**. The core element of healthcare is rapidly becoming the patient's e-record. These records reside in databases organized in data structures and are typically controlled by a database system. Database systems allow for the creation, standardization, and processing of data by multiple users. Therefore, database management requires training in one or more database systems. Databases can reside locally in a hospital, lab, or clinic as well as virtually in cloud-based systems.

Massive investments in HIT are based on the premise that getting relevant patient information to the right place at the right time will result in improved care, lower costs, and a healthier patient population. Compiling this relevant patient information means extracting data from a number of databases (e.g., patient, clinical, payer, practice management) and integrating them into a user interface while protecting HIPAA-required privacy standards and security. It is clear why database manager is an important role.

The types of skills required in database management build on those needed in system maintenance and repair, including understanding computer operating systems, server administration, and SQL (a specialized programming language designed for databases). Healthcare database managers should also have an understanding of standards, such as HL-7 and LOINC for health information exchange, coding standards such as ICD-10, and healthcare terminology systems like SNOMED.

Healthcare database management can provide an attractive career, particularly as employees refine their skills through experience and expertise. It also provides entry-level positions for individuals with core database skills and basic HIM and informatics knowledge.

Legacy systems Prior computer or business systems used to accomplish the tasks now accomplished by a new system; often, legacy systems continue to be partially used during system upgrade cycles.

Database management The maintenance of digital data stored in computer systems to ensure accuracy, access, availability, usability, and security.

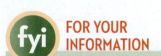
FOR YOUR INFORMATION

Across all industries, including healthcare, the growth of data has resulted in the phenomenon of "big data." Originally, *big data* was a technical term that described databases that grew so large that database systems were unable to manage them. Businesses, however, have come to realize that there is a lot of nonobvious useful information in these huge databases that improve performance and provide a competitive advantage. Database management is a very hot area for jobs and experience. Healthcare is just approaching the question of how best to use big data, but it will be an important part of health informatics. For example, by combining genetic and medical histories and pharmacological data sets, analytics will allow for "personalized medicine" and individualized treatments.

Data Mining and Data Analytics

Health informatics uses technology and data to improve the quality of care and operating efficiencies through analytical processes. Once an HIT infrastructure is in place and patient data are collected and aggregated in databases, the data use can begin. This consists of two steps: **data mining** and **data analysis**.

Through data mining, queries are established that extract formatted reports containing the needed patient data. Analysis is typically accomplished through the application of sophisticated techniques and software to compile, model, and use the information in a variety of ways. Population measurements, forecasts and projections, alerts for individual patients, and a broad array of Meaningful Use requirements are all possible through data analysis.

Jobs in data reporting and analysis include writing SQL queries, using Crystal Reports, SQL Services Reporting Services, Microsoft Access, and various statistical packages. More senior positions include writing HL-7 programming, .Net programs, and specialized encryption programs.

Data mining The search for and extraction of large amounts of data for the purpose of turning it into useful information through data analysis.

Data analysis The process of systematically applying statistical and/or other techniques to describe and illustrate, condense and recap, and evaluate data. (Source: HHS definition.)

Workforce Needs

A range of new positions are required to support the evolving wired and integrated healthcare system. Also, many existing positions will require new skills as processes and workflows change. Many of these jobs involve health informatics. The types of positions vary substantially, ranging from entry-level to senior.

3.2 A DAY IN THE LIFE

Grace has worked for Dr. Smith's Group for more than 10 years. She is RHIA® certified and is responsible for health information management at the practice. New technology is complicating her job. Grace must ensure the accuracy, standardization, HIPAA compliance, and accessibility of patient medical records. Much of the data in the medical record will now be captured electronically through the EHR and are accessible only through databases. Dr. Smith suggests Grace consider developing new skills in health informatics.

As an HIM professional, Grace knows that she needs to continue to improve her skills, but the level of new training in informatics seems like a whole new field. Grace finds that the local community college has a brand-new online certificate program in health informatics. The certificate has the technology skills she thinks she would need, including database management, basic programming, and introduction to analytics. After discussions with her family, Grace decides that she is going to enroll in the program and expand her work skills.

1. Do you think there is a conflict between traditional health information management and health informatics? How should they work together? Are they mutually supporting?

(continued)

2. Should Dr. Smith set up a health informatics department and a separate health information management department? Is this a good idea? Why or why not?
3. Grace is initially worried about learning the "technology skills" that are part of health informatics. Do you think she should be?

3.2 THINKING IT THROUGH

1. Explain the concept of change management, giving one example of how it might look in a healthcare setting.
2. What does PMP stand for? Why might 22% of organizations be seeking individuals with PMP certification?
3. Once an EHR system is in place, what health informatics skills are required to execute the stages of implementation?

3.3 Informatics and the Meaningful Use of Health IT

Data that Follow the Patient

Before EHRs and the electronic exchange of data, a patient's medical record was on paper. A medical assistant would attempt to retrieve the file before the patient visit and have it available for the clinician patient meeting. If there was an exchange of information with clinicians at another location, it would be via fax. The patient's medical history was largely limited to whatever examinations, tests, and treatments that were done at the location. Medical histories were often incomplete, and medicine reconciliation depended on the patient's knowing his or her current medications and dosage. Reliance on patients and incomplete records increased the risk of drug interactions. Tests were often repeated unnecessarily, because there was no record from earlier tests. There was also an increased likelihood of unnecessary hospital admissions or emergency department visits, because not all patient information was available. Patients usually came in only when they were sick (episodic treatment). Finally, the most important person in the process, the patient, had very limited access to his or her own medical record.

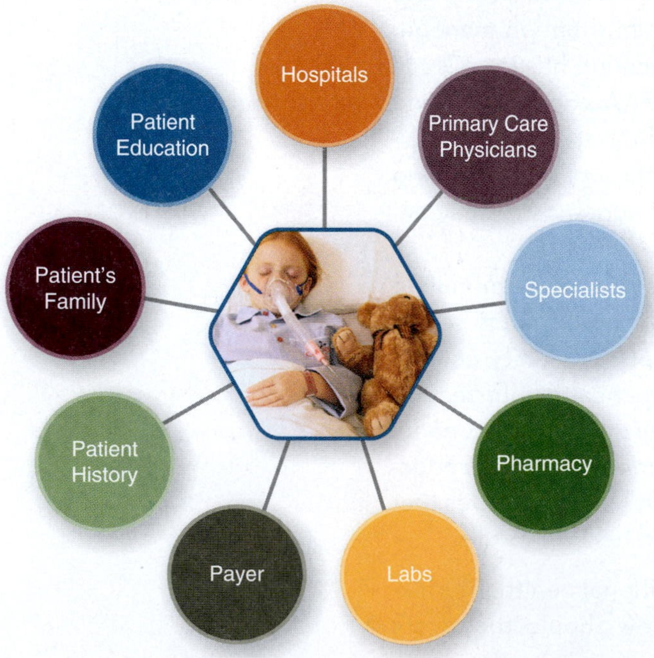

As depicted in Figure 3.6, Meaningful Use is designed to put the patient at the center of the healthcare system and to ensure that all health information is

Figure 3.6 The Patient Is at the Center of the System

available for exchange between all members of the care team as well as the patient. The objective is to get the "right information to the right place at the right time." This will solve many of the problems of paper records, will allow for better care, and should lower costs. Individuals have the opportunity to manage and become engaged in their own care through access to the most current information about their health, as well as to numerous technological tools.

What does patient-centric healthcare mean for workers' roles and skills? The core element of the whole process is health information. At every point in the system, information needs to be managed. Therefore, HIM professionals will be needed, and all team members will have to expand their capabilities and skills. The need for workers with HIT skills will grow, and as health information is used to drive healthcare reform, database managers and analysts will be needed to support the system.

Health Information Exchanges (HIEs)

Given that fixing healthcare requires getting patient information to the right person at the right place at the right time, the exchange of information across nonaffiliated stakeholders is key. Historically, healthcare systems have competed for patients and have not made it easy to exchange patient information with their competitors. Meaningful Use rules focus on the exchange of health information, requiring exchange interoperability and exchange between nonaffiliates. Also, when a patient requests information or the exchange of information between different providers, Meaningful Use requires those providers to comply.

Health information exchanges (HIEs), organizations providing exchange services, were developed to facilitate this process. There are a wide variety of HIEs, including statewide networks, regional organizations, private networks, and vendor networks. Although they have different organizational structures and use different technologies, HIEs are standards-based and evolving toward interoperability.

HIEs will play a critical role in connecting all stakeholders. There are more than 330 HIE organizations, not including the private, internal HIEs that most large hospitals are developing. The roles and skill sets required to operate these exchanges are the core health informatics positions and qualifications described earlier in this chapter. Interfaces are of particular importance in supporting interoperability and security. Thus, programmers and interface specialists are in particular demand. HIEs are a new area of employment that provide significant career opportunities.

Integrated Delivery Networks (IDNs)

In response to the increased reliance on information technology and the central role of patient e-records, many hospitals are merging. Also, hospitals are acquiring physician practices, long-term care, and other specialized facilities. The idea is for a hospital system to

Health information exchanges (HIEs) The organizations that provide the infrastructure and services allowing for the movement of health-related data between nonaffiliated stakeholders based on nationally established standards.

provide "one-stop shopping," offering all services patients need, including primary care, specialists, and acute and long-term care, along with all support services.

If hospitals are limited to a region, they may take the form of a large hospital system. Some large systems may be spread over several states or regions and have specialized relationships with insurers and other payers. These larger systems are referred to as **integrated delivery networks (IDNs)**. The reasons behind the consolidation of healthcare into large networks are seen in Figure 3.7.

In many ways, the goals of IDNs are designed to accomplish the standards of Meaningful Use, including the evolution to patient-centered care. The purpose of IDNs is to achieve better care and lower costs through productivity and efficiencies. HIM and health informatics play key roles in this strategy by supporting productivity gains through the timely and secure management of the patient record, the creation of digital records and their exchange, analytics, and the use of the data. The skill sets required in IDNs are similar to those needed as a result of Meaningful Use, except that IDNs are at the leading edge of informatics use; therefore, IDNs tend to search out workers with advanced skills. Current workers at these facilities will also need to advance their skills.

Integrated delivery network (IDN) A network of hospitals and physicians organized under a single parent company for the purpose of providing care across the full continuum of a patient population's needs.

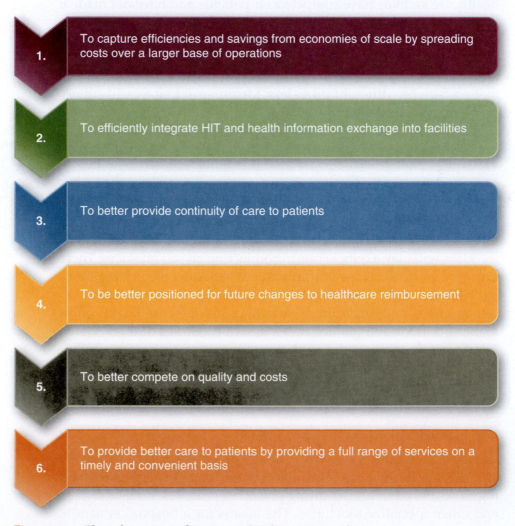

1. To capture efficiencies and savings from economies of scale by spreading costs over a larger base of operations

2. To efficiently integrate HIT and health information exchange into facilities

3. To better provide continuity of care to patients

4. To be better positioned for future changes to healthcare reimbursement

5. To better compete on quality and costs

6. To provide better care to patients by providing a full range of services on a timely and convenient basis

Figure 3.7 **The Advantages of Integrated Delivery Networks**

3.3   A DAY IN THE LIFE

Dr. Smith and her partners in a 30-physician primary care practice have selected an EHR. They now have to rely on health informatics specialists to install the system and train the staff. Consultants from the local REC and the vendor undertake an analysis of the way work is done at the clinic, or the workflow. They then determine how best to implement the new technology to minimize disruption to the ongoing practice while allowing for best practices to promote safe and efficient use of the technology in patient care.

After the implementation and testing of the new system and training of the clinical and support staff, the practice decides to use a "big bang" approach and have everyone start using all parts of the system at the same time. While work processes slow down as everyone adjusts to the new system, within several months the practice begins to notice improved efficiency. Some clinicians cannot imagine having to "go back to paper," whereas others are threatening to retire early because they don't like EHRs.

After several months, Dr. Smith's Group is able to "attest to Meaningful Use." It receives the first installment payment of more than $300,000 from CMS. Although this helps, it does not cover the total costs of the system, implementation expenses, and the lost productivity associated with learning a new system. However, this payment, combined with potential future Meaningful Use payments and the savings from the efficiencies of using digital records, should offset the cost of buying the EHR system.

1. What do you think are the types of problems that a medical practice faces when changing from paper charts to EHRs? Do you think these changes are apparent to a patient?
2. What can be done to help clinicians and staff who do not like EHRs and who want to return to paper charts?
3. Dr. Smith and her group decided to use a "big bang" approach changing to EHRs. What are the advantages of a big bang versus a more incremental approach?
4. EHRs are supposed to save money through improved efficiency. Do you think it is realistic for the practice to think it will get a positive return on its investment for the EHR systems?

3.3   THINKING IT THROUGH

1. What is the objective of Meaningful Use?
2. How do health information exchanges and integrated delivery networks use health information and health informatics in supporting Meaningful Use?

As described in the introductory chapter, the healthcare system in the United States is undergoing a massive restructuring, primarily through the Affordable Care Act (ACA). US healthcare has been based on a fee-for-service model, with care mostly given on an episodic basis (patients see doctors only when they are sick). The goal of the ACA and other policies is to move healthcare to a fee-for-value model. The hope is to reduce costs and have healthier patients through population health management, including wellness programs.

In theory, providers will be assigned a specific population of patients for care delivery. They will then be paid for achieving a set of quality-based metrics and patient outcomes for their total patient population. There are a number of ways to structure payments, but in essence if providers achieve or exceed the quality goals, they will share in the cost savings. If they do not meet the goals, then they either will be penalized in the payment or will have to meet the costs above an agreed amount. This is referred to as pay-for-performance or, more commonly, shared savings.

The ACA called for the formation of accountable care organizations (ACOs) using shared savings models that are supervised by CMS. ACOs and shared savings were discussed in detail in the chapter on evolving healthcare systems. In many cases, ACOs are established in a partnership between providers and insurance companies. At the end of 2012, there were more than 330 ACOs serving more than 31 million patients. The expectation is that by 2020 the majority of healthcare in the United States will be delivered through shared savings organizations. The shift to pay-for-performance means that measures of performance, such as patient outcomes, will be of major importance.

Health Information and Outcome Measurement

The switch to accountable care and away from fee-for-service requires the efficient use of health information and the tools of health informatics. In order to achieve their goals, ACOs are focused on providing services across the continuum of care, including transitions in care and patient engagement. It is in ACOs' financial interest for patients to be as healthy as possible. The use of health information and patient data is critical to these organizations.

The metric for provider reimbursement will shift from visits and procedures under fee-for-service to outcomes under shared savings. Measurement and performance review are part of the continuous quality improvement processes required. The switch places an emphasis on providers having the best possible patient data on demand. Data mining is a crucial support for clinical processes and for **population health management** measurement. Real-time data analysis is needed across the organization to support clinical processes, transitions in care, and patient engagement, including interventions (see Figure 3.8).

Population health management Clinical and financial activities undertaken to improve health outcomes and to lower costs for a defined group of individuals.

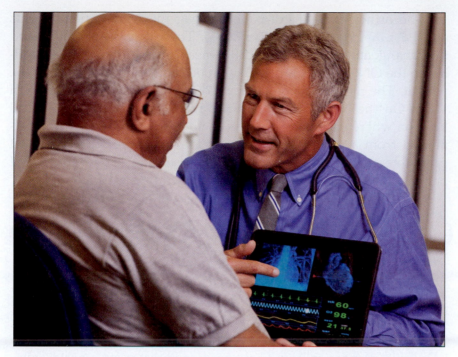

Figure 3.8 **Doctors and Other Care Providers Need Actionable Information Fast to Make Timely Interventions**

Ultimately, payment to providers will be linked to quality and outcome measurements for the total population on a risk-adjusted basis. Developing these measurements and continuously monitoring and reporting on them require informatics. It is clear that accountable care is leading to new roles in health informatics. The work of HIM and health informatics professionals provides critical support to the effort to transform healthcare. There will continue to be increased numbers of positions for individuals with these skills in these organizations.

Patient Engagement and Patient Portals

The movement to ACOs and their focus on patient quality and outcome measurements parallel the Meaningful Use initiative. As identified by the ONC, the patients are "in the best position to coordinate their care." There are consumer-oriented goals under Meaningful Use, including the following:

- Providing consumers with access to their health data
- Making it easier for consumers to use their health information
- Shifting attitudes about ownership of health data so that more information will be shared with patients and their caregivers

The ultimate goal is to empower patients to be healthier and to be proactive in their healthcare.

These goals require the use of health information and the electronic exchange of data with patients. The exchange of data with patients, as well as their use of health information, is an important and developing area for HIM and health informatics. This subject is covered in detail in the chapter on the patient's role in healthcare.

Personal Health Record (PHR) A paper record, a website, or software that contains information similar to that in an electronic health record (EHR), such as diagnoses, medications, and medical history. The patients can also add information themselves, such as notes from other clinicians (e.g., specialists), their personal notes and observations, and data from home monitoring devices or other sources. The patient or the patient's caregiver determines who has access to a PHR.

Patient portal A secure website where a patient can access information from a provider's EHR, such as diagnoses, lab results, discharge summaries, immunizations, and imaging study reports. A portal typically contains other information and functionality, such as the ability to schedule appointments, refill prescriptions, email clinicians, check insurance claims data, make payments, and gain access to online forms.

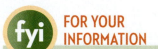

FOR YOUR INFORMATION

There are two principal differences between a patient portal and a PHR:

1. *Control:* Information in the PHR is controlled by the individual, not the provider. A patient portal is controlled by a provider.
2. *Content:* A PHR can include information from multiple sources, including multiple provider EHR data from monitoring devices, insurance company claims data, and self-sourced patient notes.

The principal means of patient engagement are patient portals and **Personal Health Records (PHRs)**. These terms are often used interchangeably but there are differences between the two. According to the ONC, a PHR is designed to be set up and managed by the patient. The most common example of a PHR is Microsoft's Health Vault. On the other hand, a **patient portal** is a secure, Web-based location where patients can access a wide range of designated information from a provider. A patient portal is the primary way that providers are meeting the Meaningful Use requirement that 5% of patients electronically view, download, or transmit their records.

3.4 A DAY IN THE LIFE

Central Hospital has offered its patient portal and PHR to Dr. Smith's practice of 30 primary care physicians at no cost. The practice would need to exchange the patient's health information with Central Hospital. The data would reside in databases at the hospital and the practice's patients would need to sign into the portal at Central's website. Dr. Smith and her colleagues are concerned that using a portal with Central's branding would weaken their relationship with their patients.

Another option is a partnership with the state health information exchange (HIE). States have received millions in grants to establish organizations that exchange health data among providers, payers, public health departments, and other stakeholders. The local HIE allows providers to re-brand patient portals as their own, even though the HIE runs them. For the first two years, there is no cost, but beginning in the third year a fee structure is established in order for the state to recoup its costs. The practice would have to share all its data with the HIE, where they would reside in a database.

The practice's final option is to develop its own patient portal website, either by using one offered by its EHR vendor at extra cost or by going with a third-party patient portal vendor. The third-party solution can be executed with contract workers. Employing contract workers, however, requires staff time for oversight, project management, and quality control. An independent project might also overrun costs and have expensive long-term maintenance. In a worst-case scenario, it might not meet all of Meaningful Use's requirements.

1. What decision should Dr. Smith make in terms of implementing a patient portal? Why is that the best choice?
2. Providers are concerned about keeping control of their patient data. Many providers do not want patient data physically located in databases outside their system. Is this justified? Is it in the patient's interest?
3. Most providers have established their own patient portals, meaning that patients who see specialists or are admitted to a hospital may have to navigate among several portals beyond their primary care physician in order to have access to their medical records. How can this problem be solved?

mHealth

The newest and most exciting area in healthcare is **mHealth**. The chapter on the patient's role in healthcare covers mHealth in detail and relative to new skills and positions for HIM and HIT workers.

The explosion of wireless communication and tech devices provides a new avenue for monitoring and engaging patients. Examples are portable devices that measure blood pressure or weight and transmit the data securely to a provider and tablet and smartphone apps that allow consumers to track diet calories and exercise (see Figure 3.9) and telehealth, where patients videoconference with clinicians. Mobile devices are also being used for alerts and communication, such as prescription refill and scheduled appointment reminders. There are more than 30,000 healthcare apps available across all mobile platforms.

As mHealth evolves, mobile devices can capture patient data and automatically send it to PHRs and EHRs. The data will be monitored electronically, with alerts and notifications sent out as appropriate. In extreme cases, the appropriate medical interventions can be initiated, such as trips to the emergency room. mHealth will support patient engagement and a healthier population. Although mHealth is opt-in—that is, participation is voluntary—engagement should lead to greater consumer wellness.

The new frontier of mHealth provides great opportunities for HIM and health informatics professionals, not only in supporting roles that enable these technologies but also as entrepreneurs developing new and exciting products and applications. The infrastructure for mHealth, however, also requires specialized skills associated with mobile technologies, wireless security, and mobile operating systems.

> **mHealth** Mobile-based or mobile-enhanced solutions that deliver healthcare.

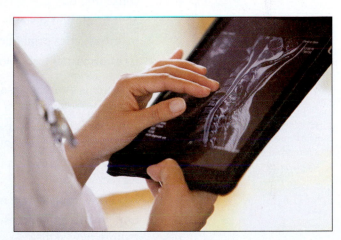

Figure 3.9 **mHealth in Action**

3.4 THINKING IT THROUGH

1. Explain how accountable care organizations and shared savings programs depend on health information management and health informatics.

2. *PHR* and *patient portals* are often used interchangeably, but there are two differences? What are they?

3. How will new reimbursement models allow the use of health records to become geographically spread out beyond the walls of a healthcare facility?

chapter 3 **summary**

LEARNING OUTCOMES	CONCEPTS FOR REVIEW
3.1 Differentiate between health information management and health informatics. Pages 67–70	• Health informatics is a relatively new field that deals with using technology for clinical information and healthcare knowledge management. 　1. Health informatics is part of a larger domain known as biomedical informatics. 　2. The use of electronic health records has increased the importance of health informatics. • Health informatics and health information management (HIM) are complementary and closely related. 　1. HIM governs the medical record, which is the core element of health informatics. 　2. Commission on Accreditation for Health Informatics and Information Management Education (CAHIIM) has defined health informatics as consisting of: 　　a. Information systems 　　b. Informatics principles 　　c. Information technology
3.2 Explain how integrated delivery systems are changing skill sets required for health information professionals. Pages 71–76	• Healthcare is evolving to an integrated, interconnected, and interoperable high-technology system. • High-tech healthcare is changing the skill sets required by current workers and creating a need for new workers with health informatics skills. • The activities undertaken in delivering healthcare, known as workflow, are being reengineered. 　1. Workflow and change management specialists are needed. 　2. Implementation and use of health information technology systems require new skills. 　3. The evolution to a patient-centered system as shaped by federal rules will create a growing need for informatics specialists. • System maintenance and support are critical roles and represent potential entry-level positions. • Patient e-records require workers skilled in database management and data analysis. • Interoperability requires workers skilled in healthcare-specific standards, such as HL-7, for programming and interface development.
3.3 Summarize the informatics skills required to support Meaningful Use. Pages 76–79	• The three stages of Meaningful Use are based on health informatics functionality. • The goals of Meaningful Use are: 　1. Improve quality, safety, and efficiency 　2. Engage patients and families 　3. Improve care coordination 　4. Improve public and population health 　5. Ensure privacy and security for personal health information

LEARNING OUTCOMES	CONCEPTS FOR REVIEW
	• Meaningful Use requires data to be available "at the right place and at the right time." This requires a robust health information technology (HIT) infrastructure supported by workers with informatics skills. • Health information exchanges (HIEs) provide interconnection and data support to all stakeholders in this process. HIEs require HIM and workers with the full range of informatics skills. • Integrated delivery networks (IDNs) are large systems encompassing hospitals, clinics, specialized care, and most other facets of healthcare. These networks are at the forefront of meeting Meaningful Use. They are created based on advanced health IT and cutting-edge informatics.
3.4 Categorize the informatics skills supporting the continuum of care under accountable care and shared savings models. Pages 80–83	• Accountable care organizations (ACOs) and shared savings programs are based on pay-for-performance (also known as fee-for-value) reimbursement as opposed to traditional fee-for-service reimbursement. • Health informatics in the forms of population management, outcome measurement, continuous quality improvement, and patient-centered delivery are central to ACOs. • Patient portals and Personal Health Records (PHRs) are key parts of ACOs and will need to be supported for interoperability, security, data management, and consumer-source data. • mHealth is a rapidly growing area of HIT. Mobile devices, such as smartphones and tablets, will bring healthcare and wellness directly to the consumer. These require technical support, data management, and analytics.

chapter review

MATCHING QUESTIONS

Match each term with its definition.

_____ 1. **[LO 3.2]** interoperability

_____ 2. **[LO 3.4]** portal

_____ 3. **[LO 3.1]** health informatics

_____ 4. **[LO 3.2]** data mining

_____ 5. **[LO 3.1]** HITECH

_____ 6. **[LO 3.3]** integrated delivery network

_____ 7. **[LO 3.3]** Meaningful Use

_____ 8. **[LO 3.4]** Personal Health Record

_____ 9. **[LO 3.2]** database management

_____ 10. **[LO 3.1]** e-record

_____ 11. **[LO 3.2]** project management

_____ 12. **[LO 3.1]** regional extension center

a. Joint medical history maintained by a patient and his or her provider

b. Patient's medical information stored digitally in a database

c. Application of knowledge, skills, and techniques to execute projects efficiently and effectively

d. Organization to assist providers by extending EHR and implementations services

e. Legislation that requires healthcare facilities to meet certain criteria to become eligible for incentive payments

f. Process of maintaining data to ensure their quality, security, and integrity

g. Multiple systems sharing and using data

h. Managing health data across clinical and public domains

i. Legislation aimed at expanding and rewarding electronic health record use

j. Networked group of hospitals and providers dedicated to providing solid continuity of care

k Process of searching data to identify trends and other useful information

l. Website that enables patients to securely access their medical records

MULTIPLE CHOICE QUESTIONS

Choose the letter that best completes the statement or answers the question.

13. **[LO 3.1]** According to CAHIIM, health informatics includes all of the following *except*

   a. information technology.

   b. informatics management.

   c. information systems.

   d. informatics principles.

14. **[LO 3.1]** Which of the following work activities is considered health informatics?
    a. Analyzing monthly billings by procedure
    b. Doing computer-assisted coding
    c. Developing an interface between an EHR and a cancer registry
    d. Managing secondary uses of a health record

15. **[LO 3.1]** _____ is (are) central to both health informatics and health information management.
    a. Data
    b. Patient care
    c. Coding
    d. Flow

16. **[LO 3.2]** Which of the following is the best example of a workflow?
    a. An office manager creates a checklist outlining which staff member is responsible for each part of patient flow.
    b. A care provider enters a patient's information into the EHR in the order in which it is listed on the screen.
    c. A medical assistant takes vital signs in the same sequence for every patient.
    d. A hospital administrator mandates that the coding department follow her specific protocol for processing claims.

17. **[LO 3.2]** Data mining will be most important to which stage of healthcare reform?
    a. Implementation of enabling technologies
    b. Meaningful Use of new technologies
    c. Accountable patient-centric care
    d. Fee-for-service care

18. **[LO 3.2]** A wired health system must be
    a. simplistic.
    b. virtual.
    c. interoperable.
    d. adjustable.

19. **[LO 3.2]** In addition to having a strong knowledge of healthcare, which of the following skills must a health systems database manager possess?
    a. Repairing computer hard drives
    b. Understanding programming language
    c. Writing computer code
    d. Maintaining a computer's operating system

20. **[LO 3.3]** Which of the following is the biggest benefit of forming integrated delivery networks, from a patient perspective?
    a. Lower operational costs through economies of scale
    b. Improved positioning for changes in reimbursement
    c. Fewer opportunities for information exchange
    d. Improved continuity of care

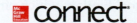 Enhance your learning by completing these exercises and more at http://connect.mheducation.com!

21. **[LO 3.4]** Which of the following best describes an accountable care organization?
    a. Fee-for-service
    b. Fee-for-value
    c. Episodic care
    d. Public utility

SHORT ANSWER QUESTIONS

22. **[LO 3.1]** Explain the difference between health informatics and health information management. How do the two fields overlap?

23. **[LO 3.1]** Describe how the field of health informatics has evolved and what the introduction of EHRs and health information exchange means to the future of the field.

24. **[LO 3.2]** Outline the workflow process for EHR implementation.

25. **[LO 3.2]** Identify the types of informatics skills that will be required under a patient-centric healthcare model.

26. **[LO 3.2]** What are "big data"? Explain how they can be used in healthcare.

27. **[LO 3.3]** Compare and contrast a health information exchange (HIE) organization and an integrated delivery network (IDN).

28. **[LO 3.4]** Assess the importance of outcome research to accountable care organizations (ACOs). What types of work roles are required to support ACOs?

29. **[LO 3.4]** Explain the role of mHealth in healthcare reform.

APPLYING YOUR KNOWLEDGE

30. **[LO 3.1]** Do you think health informatics should be a separate field of study? Is there a need for specialized degree programs and certifications? Support your answer.

31. **[LO 3.2]** How will the use of EHRs and digital patient records affect the workflows of physicians, nurses, HIM professionals, and other staff? Give examples as needed.

32. **[LO 3.2]** The ONC identified the worker roles required for the implementation of EHRs. How would those roles be incorporated in a project management plan? Identify the key steps that would be part of the plan.

33. **[LO 3.3]** Patient-centered medicine seems like a good idea in theory. What are the major barriers to reaching this goal? Which of these barriers are related to health information management or health informatics?

34. **[LO 3.4]** What elements should be incorporated into a patient portal? Will patient portals and Personal Health Records work? Will they lead to a healthier population? How can wellness programs be incorporated into patient portals?

35. **[LO 3.1, 3.2, 3.3, 3.4]** Access AHIMA's career map at http://hicareers.com/careermap/. Using the map as a guide, address the following questions: What are the emerging positions in IT/infrastructure? What types of skills do you think those positions would require? Do you believe the Informatics/Data Analysis category adequately represents the importance of informatics under Meaningful Use and payment reform? Why or why not? Explain which emerging career path interests you the most.

chapter **four**

Maintaining Health Records: *An Overview*

Learning Outcomes

When you finish this chapter, you will be able to:

4.1 Discuss the purpose of a Master Patient Index.

4.2 Contrast patient tracking in manual and electronic record-keeping systems.

4.3 Explain how EHRs enable the maintenance of higher-quality health data.

4.4 Organize patient records according to various numbering and filing systems.

Key Terms

Administrative data
Centralized registration
Client/server
Clinical data
Clinical documentation improvement (CDI)
Cloud-based solution
Decentralized registration
Demographic data
Disaster recovery planning
Electronic signature (eSignature)

Hybrid record
Jukebox
Legal health record
Master Patient (Person) Index (MPI)
Medical record number
Record retention plan
Reimbursement cycle
Straight numeric (sequential) filing
Terminal digit filing
WORM technology

Introduction

The health record serves as proof of everything that was done, and consequently what was not done, to each patient. Every healthcare facility that cares for or performs testing on patients must keep a record of each patient treated, which is then further divided into individual encounters. In this chapter, the methods for keeping health records, tracking their locations, and ensuring their completion, as well as the information gleaned from the data collected in each record, will be explored.

4.1 A Database of Patients: Building the Master Patient (Person) Index

The Registration Process

In a hospital setting, the registration process begins when the patient presents to the emergency department, is directly admitted from home or a physician's office, is pre-admitted for an elective surgery, or presents to the registration area for outpatient laboratory, radiology, or other testing or outpatient service.

The registration process is either **centralized registration**, meaning all patients presenting for any type of care are registered through one central area, or **decentralized registration**, meaning the emergency department has its own registration area, as do the inpatient admission area, ambulatory surgery, and outpatient diagnostic testing.

At registration, the following data are gathered from the patient:

- Full name
- Date of birth
- Marital status
- Former surname, if applicable (for instance, change of name due to marriage/divorce), also known as an alias
- Sex
- Race
- Primary language
- Religion
- Home address
- Home phone number
- Cell phone number
- Occupation
- Employer
- Employer phone number
- Email address
- Insurance name
- Insurance policy number
- Insurance group number
- Subscriber

Centralized registration Type of hospital registration in which all patients presenting for any type of care are registered through one central area, regardless of the type of care being sought.

Decentralized registration Type of hospital registration in which there are multiple points of patient access, depending on the type of care being sought—inpatient admission, emergency department, outpatient diagnostics, ambulatory surgery, and so on.

- Patient's relationship to the subscriber
- Name of secondary insurance, if applicable
- Secondary insurance policy number
- Secondary insurance group number
- Secondary insurance subscriber
- Patient's relationship to the subscriber of secondary insurance
- Person to notify in case of emergency
- Relationship to patient
- Phone number(s) for person to notify
- Reason for visit (this may be a diagnosis found on a physician's order or a symptom as stated by the patient)

With the exception of the reason for the visit, these data elements are all **administrative data**. The patient's name, date of birth, address, and phone numbers are administrative data as well, but they are specifically **demographic data**, because they help identify the patient. **Clinical data** include the patient's diagnosis or presenting symptoms. Clinical data continue to be documented once the patient's care begins. You may recognize many of these data elements as part of the requirements of the Uniform Hospital Discharge Data Set (UHDDS) from the abstracting section of the chapter on documenting, maintaining, and managing health information.

It is at the time of registration that patients also sign consent forms, such as consent to treatment and the HIPAA notice of privacy practices form. Consents may be general, as in the consent to treatment, which is signed when the patient is registered for services, or they may be specific, such as in the case of surgery. Figure 4.1 shows a general surgery consent form.

Registration is typically an automated process. Though healthcare has been slow to adopt an electronic health record, the automation of admission (registration), discharge, and transfer transactions, as well as the reimbursement process, has been in place for at least the past 30 years. The registration process is necessary to account for every patient treated in the facility and to ensure that each patient has only one master registration, which is done through the Master Patient Index.

The Master Patient (Person) Index

The registration process results in the **Master Patient (Person) Index (MPI)**, which is the database where the previously listed data elements are entered. Each patient has only one master entry in the MPI in each facility or healthcare organization (enterprise). To that master entry, however, many single encounters are connected.

The first time a patient is seen at a facility, all the data elements must be entered, and a unique identifier, known as a **medical record number** or health record number, is assigned; medical record numbers are assigned sequentially by the computer system or manually during the registration process.

During the registration process on a patient's subsequent visit, the database is first searched to determine whether the patient already has a record at that facility. If the patient has never been seen

Administrative data
Nonmedical data, such as patient identifiers, insurance-related data, authorizations, and business correspondence.

Demographic data Administrative data that identify the patient—name, date of birth, address, and gender.

Clinical data Data found in a health record that are of a medical nature—past medical or surgical history, vital signs, test results, physician progress notes, nurses' notes, and so on.

Master Patient (Person) Index (MPI) A permanent listing of all patients who have been admitted to or received care in a healthcare facility; it is the key to locating patient records in a facility and is maintained permanently.

Medical record number A unique numeric identifier for each patient seen in a health facility; sometimes referred to as a health record number.

Memorial Hospital

PATIENT'S CONSENT FORM

(Please read this form and the notes overleaf very carefully)

A. TO THE CONSULTANT

TYPE OF OPERATION, INVESTIGATION, OR PROCEDURE

....

....

(i) I confirm that I have explained the nature of the surgery or other procedures to be performed upon the patient named below, as well as other appropriate options as are available and the possible risks involved. I have also advised them of type of anesthetic (if any) proposed. No assurance has been given that the procedure will be performed by a particular individual. The explanation I have given is in my judgment suited to the understanding of the patient and/or the parent(s) or guardian of the patient.

Signed ....   Date ....

(ii) Non-English Speakers-English Interpretation

I confirm that the explanation stated in (i) above was to the best of my knowledge and belief truly and faithfully interpreted to the patient.

Signed ....   Date ....

Witness Signature & Print Name ....

B. TO THE PATIENT/GUARDIAN/RESPONSIBLE PERSON

1. If you do not understand the explanation of the surgery or other procedures to be undergone, or if you require further information you should ask your consultant/medical practitioner.

2. Please check that all information on the form is correct. If it is and you understand the explanation, then sign the form.

I.. of .... hereby consent to undergo the proposed operation to be performed upon myself (upon ....), the nature and purpose of which has been explained to me by Mr./Mrs./Ms./Dr. ....

I also consent to such further or alternative operative measures as may be found necessary prior to, during the course of, and after the operation, and to the administration of a general, local, or other anesthetic for any of these purposes.

(Please delete as applicable)

Signed .... Patient/Parent/Guardian/Responsible Person

Address ....

....

Figure 4.1   A General Surgery Consent Form

there before, a new entry is made. If that patient already exists in the MPI, the patient is asked to review the screen, which includes the administrative data, or the registration coordinator prints a copy for the patient to review. The index is then edited with the new data. Certain data elements, such as the patient's date of birth and usually the first name, are static (they do not change). A patient's last name may change due to marriage or divorce, or a woman may begin using her maiden name rather than her given middle name, once she has married. Of course, addresses, telephone numbers, employers, and the like may change several times throughout a patient's lifetime, and therefore this type of data may be edited in the MPI.

Because the registration process has been automated over the past three decades, the MPI has also been automated. Prior to automation of the registration process and the MPI that resulted from it, healthcare facilities maintained the MPI manually, often on 3 × 5 or 4 × 6 index cards. The data found on them were scant compared to the data collected today. Figure 4.2 shows a typical manual MPI card, and Figure 4.3 depicts an automated MPI showing potential MPI matches for a patient.

MEMORIAL HOSPITAL 7652 HORIZON WAY ANYWHERE, TX 44555			
Last Name, First Name, Middle Name Philips, James Bernard		**DOB** 07/31/1990	**Gender** Male **Race** Caucasian **Medical Record Number** 07-45-85
Home Address 1234 Oriole Way, Anywhere, TX 44555			**Telephone Number** 555-555-3333
Previous Name n/a			**Social Security Number** 123-45-6780

ADM/ENCOUNTER DATE	DISCHARGE DATE	TYPE OF SERVICE	PROVIDER
1/15/2010	1/28/2010	IP	Howard Hinkins, MD
6/22/2010	6/22/2010	ED	Sylvia Crowell, MD
9/30/2010	9/30/2010	OP	Lloyd Wright, MD

Figure 4.2 A Manual MPI Card

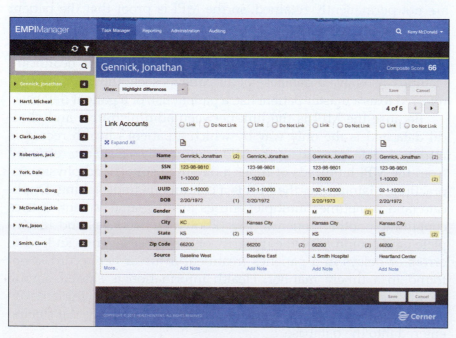

Figure 4.3 An MPI Entry from an Electronic Record

Enterprise-wide MPIs are more the norm in the 21st century, now that hospitals, physicians' practices, retail pharmacies, and outpatient services are commonly part of a health system, or enterprise. An enterprise may include one hospital and several ambulatory facilities, or it may include three or four hospitals and a hundred or more ambulatory facilities. The larger the enterprise, the more difficult the task of ensuring the integrity of the MPI database.

The MPI links a patient's administrative data to the patient's clinical data, found in the EHR. Decisions regarding patient care and reimbursement hinge on the information found in a patient's record.

The individual encounter entries also include data elements, such as the following:

- Facility identification number (particularly if referring to an enterprise-wide MPI)
- Account number linked to the encounter
- Admission or encounter date
- Discharge date of the admission or date of departure, in the case of an outpatient
- Encounter or service type—inpatient, emergency department, outpatient laboratory, and so on
- Encounter or service location—room and bed number for an inpatient, room or bed number in the emergency department, and so on
- Primary physician—the physician who is responsible for the patient's care, in the case of an inpatient or emergency patient, or the physician who has ordered an outpatient test
- Discharge/departure disposition—home, transfer to other acute care hospital, transfer to long-term care, expired, and so on

The MPI is a permanent database, because it is the record that shows each visit to a particular facility. Health records themselves are not permanently retained, so the MPI is proof that the patient was treated at a given facility on one or more occasions.

Long-term care facilities, hospices, home health agencies, physicians' practices, outpatient laboratories, and all other healthcare facilities also have a database of all patients seen, though it may be referred to as a master patient list, a patient list, or a patient database.

Because the MPI is the link between administrative and clinical data and is the only way by which a patient's health record is retrieved, data integrity of the MPI is imperative. Data are retrieved from the MPI hundreds of times a day in hospitals and physicians' practices. Maintaining the MPI is a continuous undertaking. Duplicate (and sometimes multiple) entries for the same patient, entries containing another patient's data (known as overlays), and incomplete data compromise the integrity of the database and can lead to errors or delays in a patient's treatment if his or her record is not found in a timely manner. Health information is shared among healthcare providers and healthcare facilities, thus placing an even greater importance on complete, accurate, and timely data being entered into the database.

4.1 A DAY IN THE LIFE

Jamie Anderson, RHIT®, CHTS-IM, CPC-A is a data integrity coordinator in the Health Information Management Department at West Virginia University (WVU) HealthCare and is part of the Information Governance Team. This is a diverse and challenging nontraditional HIM role. Her responsibilities include

- Maintaining the integrity of the facility and the Enterprise Master Persons Indices (EMPI)
- Leading the Enterprise Duplicate Record Merge Team and Enterprise Record Correction Team
- Providing resolution to EMPI duplicate records, overlays, and documentation errors
- Facilitating and coordinating process improvement initiatives
- Developing and revising policies and procedures impacting the EMPI and integrity of the medical record
- Writing education and training materials
- Developing reports to audit, track, trend, and resolve duplicate records, overlays, and copy/paste/cloning
- Testing system upgrades
- Participating in various health information governance projects

Jamie considers her position rewarding because it is a nontraditional, evolving HIM role. Her role as data integrity coordinator provides diversity and the opportunity to have a positive impact on patients and facilities. She sees every day as a new adventure that presents new challenges, and she particularly looks forward to the opportunity to dabble in different areas, including information governance, leadership, project management, information technology, and analysis. The WVU Health System has an enterprise electronic health record (EHR) and MPI (multiple hospitals and clinics that share one health record and MPI), and her team is the hub for the enterprise. The biggest challenges they face include managing duplicate records and overlays, developing prevention techniques at the front end, and auditing to discover and resolve duplicates and overlays on the back end. To overcome these challenges, Jamie and her team work closely with multiple individuals, teams, application systems analysts, and departments throughout the enterprise to identify potential risks and problem resolutions and to develop and revise policies and procedures that impact the EMPI, as well as the integrity of the medical record.

4.1 THINKING IT THROUGH

1. What is the justification for making the Master Patient Index a permanent index?
2. Why is patient registration such a critical component of healthcare?

Once the Master Patient Index is established and being maintained, each facility will develop its own system for tracking and building the health records of its patients. Each facility has its own needs. The black-and-white split between paper and electronic health records that was laid out in the chapter on the health record and the basic functions of the health information professional is in reality less cut-and-dried.

Systems for Building the Heath Record

Though electronic systems are becoming more commonplace, it is not unusual to find **hybrid record** systems, in which the health record is kept electronically as well as on paper, as in the following examples:

1. Facility A has an EHR but prints each record in its entirety and files it just as it always had before—in a manila folder in the HIM department.

2. Facility B has an electronic record, but consent forms, documentation from the emergency department, physicians' orders for outpatient diagnostic testing, and records from other hospitals are kept in paper form and filed in the HIM department.

3. Facility C follows the same system as Facility B, but all the paper is scanned into the EHR; then the paper copies are filed in a manila folder in a permanent file.

4. Facility D does not print any electronically maintained records; old records remain in paper, and the tracings generated by EKGs, fetal monitors, echocardiograms, and other diagnostic tests are not merged with the remainder of the electronic record.

Therefore, in all of the facilities, some of the documentation is electronic and some is not.

The cost of maintaining dual systems of record-keeping is incredibly expensive—more staff is needed to maintain both systems, physical space is necessary for both, and very detailed policies and procedures are necessary to sustain a dual system. There is a great chance that important health information will be missed by a care provider if he or she assumes the record provided for review is complete when in reality it is not. It is possible that amendments or corrections are found in the paper record but were never merged with the electronic record, and vice versa.

Hybrid records will be the norm for some time to come, at least until all disparate systems, such as EKG or fetal monitoring technology, integrate with EHR technology, as explained in the previous example of "Facility D."

The Legal Heath Record

The hybrid record, in whatever form, brings into question what a facility considers to be its **legal health record**. A facility, whether it be

Hybrid record Health record maintained in paper, electronic format, and/or in the form of recordings or tracings derived from diagnostic tests.

Legal health record The health record, identified by facility policy, that is considered the official business record and that would be presented if subpoenaed.

a hospital, nursing home, or physician's practice, must have a policy that identifies its legal health record—the record that would be presented in response to a subpoena.

The definition of the legal health record will vary from facility to facility, and is affected by state and federal laws. The American Health Information Management Association's position statement on the legal health record is an excellent resource when writing the definition of legal health record. For instance, a hospital that not only has an EHR but also prints it and places it in a permanent file may consider only the digitally filed records as the legal health record, whereas another facility with the same procedure may consider the paper version to be its legal health record. When records are in paper format, documentation is written or dictated by physicians, nurses, therapists, and other healthcare professionals. Other documents are added, such as laboratory, pathology, or radiology reports. A written record may consist of less than 20 to well over 100 pages just for one encounter.

The Developing Health Record

Paper

Recall that the chapter on documenting, maintaining, and managing health information, past and present, included a discussion of the processing functions, including the assembly of all documents into a predetermined order and analysis for deficiencies in documentation. Once assembled and analyzed, paper records are made available to physicians for completion, and then as the records are completed, they are permanently filed by the patient's medical record number. Manual processes are long and laborious. Each step of the process is done individually; thus, it may take weeks or months for the record to make it to the permanent file. Figure 4.4 depicts the typical flow of the major steps in compiling, processing, and filing health records in a hospital.

A record may be handled hundreds of times before and after it is permanently filed. Table 4.1 shows just a few of the reasons a record may be retrieved before or after permanent filing. The chance of the record's being misplaced or misfiled is high. Lost records are a liability for the hospital as well as the physician(s), because a record that is not available equates to missing information necessary for patient care, as well as missing evidence in legal cases.

Electronic

Electronic systems include the capture of all the clinical and administrative data gathered on each patient, as well as the processing of each record (see Figure 4.5). With the exception of record assembly, the steps shown in Figure 4.4 are necessary in an electronic environment, although they are handled differently.

As with manual systems, each patient has a master record with individual encounters within that record, so a unit record is maintained. The unique identifier remains the medical record number in an electronic system.

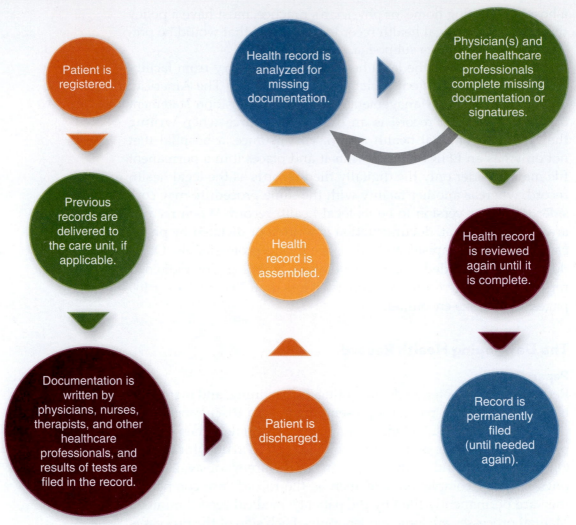

Figure 4.4 The Flow of Health Records from Admission to Permanent Filing

TABLE 4.1	Reasons a Record May Be Retrieved
Readmission of a patient	Routine quality review
Completion by *each* physician or healthcare professional who has been notified of an incomplete report or signature	Correspondence request (request for a record by the patient, an insurance company, workers' compensation, an attorney, and so on)
Risk management review	Quality assessment study
Billing inquiry	Addition of "loose" documents that were separated from the remainder of the record
Insurance audit	Research study

In a totally electronic record (not hybrid), the assembly function is not necessary, since there is no physical record in which to find a particular set of documents; rather, the document needed is found

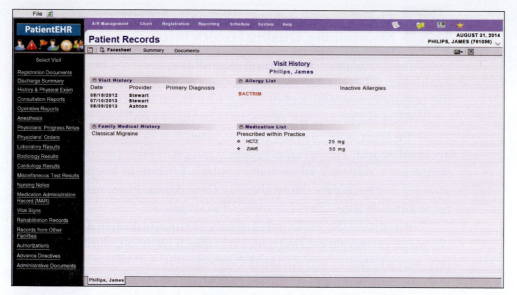

Figure 4.5 A Master Entry Page in EHR with Visit History and Electronic Health Record Sections

through the click of a button. Figure 4.5 shows a typical layout of the sections of a record. The portion of the record needed is clicked, and the report appears to the user.

If a physician were interested in a patient's vital signs over a period of time, he or she would click on the Vital Signs section and would have the option of viewing each vital sign, including temperature, pulse, respiration, blood pressure, and body mass index (BMI). These vital signs could then be viewed over time (for instance, from admission to the last recorded vital signs), in list view, or by a particular date and time. A sample vital signs page from an EHR can be seen in Figure 4.6.

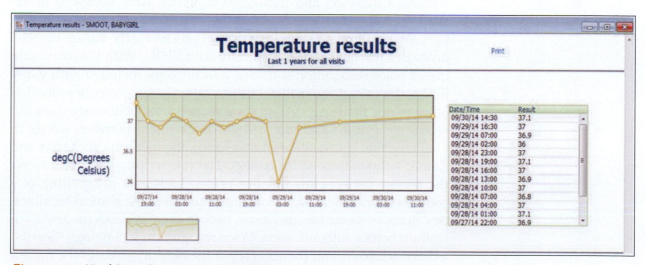

Figure 4.6 Vital Signs Progression in an EHR

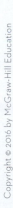

4.2 THINKING IT THROUGH

1. Why do facilities define the legal health record differently?
2. What factors influence a facility's definition of a legal record?

4.3 The Concurrent Health Record, EHRs, and Maintaining Quality Health Information

Concurrent means "happening simultaneously." The concurrent health record is the developing health record that is compiled while the patient is hospitalized or being seen in an ambulatory setting.

With a paper record, physicians or other healthcare professionals write their notes as they see the patient or immediately after—in an ideal world. However, consider a surgeon who performs several surgeries a day. It will be hard enough for her to keep the details straight for each procedure the day they occur. How much will she remember in three days? A week? Two weeks?

With an EHR, concurrent analysis (quantitative analysis) for record documentation deficiencies is much more efficient. An operative report that is not dictated immediately following surgery not only is noncompliant with regulations and accrediting standards but also brings into question the quality of care. If concurrent analysis is performed, that elapsed time is shortened; otherwise, the deficiency may not be caught until after discharge. At that point, one has to question the value of the documentation so long after the event occurred.

Ensuring that quality data are being gathered is an essential part of maintaining health records. Poor health data can have far-reaching implications for everyone from the patient and healthcare personnel to the healthcare facility itself. EHRs and some hybrid systems offer a number of opportunities that paper record-keeping does not to positively impact the maintenance of an accurate health record.

Dictation and Transcription

Although dictation and transcription, which were reviewed in the chapter on documenting, maintaining, and managing health information, are traditional health information processes, the nature of these processes has changed dramatically with EHRs. With the increasing use of voice recognition software, a technology included with many EHRs, the role of the medical transcriptionist has become more that of an editor than of a typist. Voice recognition technology does not recognize every word and cannot differentiate between words in medicine that sound alike—for instance, the medications Xanax and Zantac—thus the need for editors. The transcriptionist first reviews the report, corrects any obvious errors, such as a misspelling of a common nonclinical word, or routes questionable clinical terminology, such as *Xanax* versus *Zantac,* back to the physician for any clarification before authentication. Voice recognition technology "learns" a dictator's voice, and the accuracy of the output increases the more it is used by the dictator. The training process for physicians is lengthy, which is a deterrent to some. Others prefer it and are able to edit as they dictate (front-end speech recognition); others do not care to edit their own dictation, and that is done after a transcriptionist has completed the dictation (back-end voice recognition). Dictation and transcription with voice recognition technology is one example of EHRs' allowing for the concurrent analysis of medical records.

Deficiency Reporting

Like paper records, EHRs are reviewed for completeness. Rather than looking for an individual report on paper, the analyst searches in the particular section to determine if the required report was present. The analyst may not have to review each individual record if automated record completion software is used. This may be stand-alone software that interfaces with the EHR, or it may be a part of the EHR software package. In either case, incomplete or missing documentation or reports are identified electronically, which then allows health information staff to track the deficiencies by type of deficiency or by physician. Figure 4.7 depicts a portion of a typical record deficiency report—in this case, for discharge summaries only.

Manual signatures are all but obsolete in an electronic system, thanks to **electronic signatures**, also known as **eSignatures**.

Through the use of eSignature technology, physicians are alerted to the entries in the electronic record that need to be signed. For instance, a history and physical report, as seen in Figure 4.8, was dictated by the physician but transcribed by a medical transcriptionist; thus, the physician needs to authenticate that documentation by reviewing it for errors and signing it to show that he/she indeed was the author and did approve the content of the report or chart entry. In order to eSign a document, the physician enters a code (much like a password) that only he or she uses, which in turn "signs" and date stamps the documentation.

Electronic signature (eSignature) A digitized signature placed on a chart entry through the use of a personal identification number (PIN).

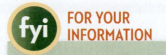

FOR YOUR INFORMATION

The term *chart* is often used to refer to the record while it is in use during the patient's stay.

FIGURE 4.7 — An Automated Record Deficiency Report

RECORD DEFICIENCY REPORT AS of 05/31/2014		
DEFICIENCY TYPE: Missing discharge summary		
Records missing discharge summary:		
Medical Record Number	**Physician Responsible**	**Date of Discharge/ Encounter**
101856	Garner, Robert	04/28/2014*
101601	Garner, Robert	05/05/2014
810185	Thomas, Carolyn	05/08/2014
190105	Thomas, Carolyn	05/08/2014
101075	Zimmerman, Felix	05/16/2014

*Denotes a delinquent record.

Nurses and other healthcare professionals enter their own documentation, so the time and date stamp is applied to the chart entry based on that person's UserID and serves as authentication of that entry.

Simultaneous Data Entry and Usage

Unlike paper records, records kept in electronic format can be used by two or more people simultaneously, and data are entered in real time—as the data are gathered. The high risk of loss is not inherent in an electronic record, unless a patient has previously registered under another name and does not notify the hospital staff of that fact at the time of registration. There is a risk of a computer crash or tampering, though this problem is no greater than the loss of a paper record through misfiling or because someone has taken a paper record without permission. Best practice dictates security measures to protect against tampering and backup of data to mitigate the possibility of data loss. Security of electronic records will be further discussed in the privacy and security chapter.

Electronic records can be shared with other healthcare providers who have a need to know, improving patient safety and outcomes as well as ensuring fewer duplicate tests. For instance, Kay Matthews is seen in the emergency department following a fall. An x-ray of her elbow reveals a fracture. The emergency department physician refers her to an orthopedic surgeon for possible surgery. Since she lives on the other side of the city, Kay prefers to see an orthopedic surgeon nearer her home. She

MEMORIAL HOSPITAL

41056 Hospital Drive
Anywhere, MN 10856

HISTORY AND PHYSICAL EXAM

Patient: Roberts, Alexandra   MRN: 081650

DOB: 08/15/1955   ATTENDING PHYSICIAN: Mark A. Stewart, MD

ADMISSION DATE: 09/12/2014

CHIEF COMPLAINT: Right lower abdominal pain with nausea and vomiting.

HISTORY OF PRESENT ILLNESS: The patient was awakened early this morning with severe right lower quadrant abdominal pain and nausea. She put a heating pad on her abdomen and fell back to sleep. Approximately three hours prior to admission, she experienced vomiting and chills. The pain continued to worsen, which she describes as a stabbing feeling that radiates around to her right buttock. She did not take any OTC medications.

ALLERGIES: The patient has **no known drug allergies.**

PAST MEDICAL/SURGICAL HISTORY: The patient has mild hypertension and arthritis in her right knee. Previous surgery includes a cesarean section in 1980.

CURRENT MEDICATIONS: HCTZ 25 mg daily and OTC ibuprofen for mild to moderate arthritis.

PAST FAMILY HISTORY: Mother has CAD and has undergone coronary artery bypass; father had colon CA and is deceased.

VITAL SIGNS: The patient's respiratory and heart rates were within normal limits in the ED. The patient's temperature upon arrival to the ED was 102.0.

LABORATORY FINDINGS: Urinalysis done while in the ED was within normal limits. The white count is elevated at 16,000. CBC is otherwise within normal limits.

RADIOLOGY FINDINGS: CT scan showed inflamed appendix.

IMPRESSION: Appendicitis.
PLAN: Prep for appendectomy.

Mark A. Stewart, MD
Electronically signed on 09/12/2014 at 8:20 AM

MAS/acm

Figure 4.8   **A History and Physical of a Patient in an EHR**

is taken to the orthopedic surgeon of her choice, and on arrival, he has already reviewed the x-ray films electronically as well as the documentation from the original emergency department. Because her health information was shared immediately, there was no delay in treatment, and her orthopedic surgeon did not need to repeat any x-rays, because he/she was able to see not only the radiologist's impression but also the films themselves. Simultaneous data entry, in particular, means more positive outcomes for patients.

Coding and Clinical Documentation Improvement

In a paper system, coding is most commonly done retrospectively (after discharge), mainly because of logistics—the paper record can be used by only one person at a time, and patient care outranks coding. It is more efficient to begin the coding processes concurrently with an electronic record. Rather than waiting for a record to be complete after discharge, coders begin the process during the patient's admission. A coder's role may be that of coder as well as **clinical documentation improvement (CDI)** specialist.

Coders know the level of specificity needed to accurately and completely code a patient's diagnoses and procedures. By having the coder and/or CDI specialist review the record while the patient is still admitted, he or she is able to speak directly with the physician or query the physician in writing immediately. If the coder waits until after discharge to review the record, it may take days or weeks to receive an answer. Concurrent coding is a more efficient process, which results in faster turnaround time from discharge to the submission of an insurance claim, and the CDI process ensures that the diagnosis and procedure codes on the claim are supported by the documentation in the health record. For consistency, hospitals may have a CDI plan in place that also includes flagging of missing documentation.

Coding is part of the **reimbursement cycle**, since diagnosis and procedure codes are required in order to file an insurance claim. The reimbursement cycle begins when a patient is registered—that is when insurance information is gathered.

From there, insurance verification takes place (is the patient really covered, and if so are there any limitations to the health coverage?). Diagnoses and procedures are converted to codes as a means of collecting data for research studies, education, submission on insurance claims, and statistics. The timely coding of all diagnoses and procedures affects the cash flow of the hospital. All healthcare facilities are businesses; as such, they have bills to pay. Without a constant source of cash flow, the financial well-being of the facility is compromised. An efficient reimbursement cycle is possible through concurrent coding, complete health records, a sound CDI program,

Clinical documentation improvement (CDI) The review of health records, usually concurrently, to ensure that the documentation in the health record is at the level of specificity that allows for code assignment that accurately depicts the patient's diagnoses and procedures performed.

Reimbursement cycle The processes that take place from the time a patient is registered for care to the time the services are paid, whether paid by the patient or through insurance.

and a final review of the health record to ensure that the final coding is supported by the documentation in the health record.

The Evolution of Data to Information

Thus far in this section, we have primarily covered how EHRs and some hybrid systems are allowing for the creation and maintenance of higher-quality health data than ever before. Data consist of individual facts—a patient has a blood pressure reading of 160/110; she is 5 feet, 3 inches tall; and she weighs 180 pounds. Individually, these facts perhaps don't seem important. However, the physician needs all these individual facts to make a conclusion. There is a fine line between data and information—putting all of the data together paints a picture or tells a story from which conclusions can be drawn. Data must come together to form information, and information is knowledge—about a single patient, a group of patients, or a population.

The inability to locate previous records about a patient, a missing physical examination report prior to a surgery, a diagnosis that cannot be coded because the physician was not specific in his or her documentation—all of these leave holes in an otherwise full picture. All necessary data have to come together completely, accurately, and in a timely manner in order to evolve into information—information that is used first and foremost for the care of the patient but also for reimbursement; for the legal protection of the patient, physicians, and facility; for research and the education of current and future physicians and healthcare professionals; and for internal and external statistics. It is not enough, therefore, to just maintain health data. All healthcare professionals—and especially health information professionals—should strive to ensure that the *best* possible data are maintained.

4.4 A DAY IN THE LIFE

Dr. Carlisle, an emergency department (ED) physician, is about to see a patient who was brought in by ambulance after being found unconscious in a parking lot. On arrival, the patient is still unconscious, and no family, friends, or witnesses have accompanied him. The emergency medical technician's notes state that on arrival the patient's blood pressure was 90/50, his respirations were 16, and his heart rate was 82.

1. At this point, does the physician have data or information?

4.3 THINKING IT THROUGH

1. Why is clinical documentation improvement important to the financial well-being of a hospital?
2. What is meant by querying a physician?

4.4 Identifying, Storing, and Locating Records

After quality health data and information have been captured and maintained during a patient encounter, how do you make sure that information is retained for future encounters? Paper or manual systems of identifying, storing, and locating health records present more challenges than electronic systems. Still, electronic health record systems have their own hurdles to overcome. In this section, we will compare and contrast identifying, storing, and locating health records in paper and electronic systems.

Numbering and Filing Methods in a Manual System

Numbering Systems

Though some facilities and offices utilize a paper health record, generally they have automated registration systems, and the MPI is electronic as well. The medical record number is assigned by the computer in sequential order and is typically five or more digits in length. In years past, some facilities used the patient's Social Security number as a unique medical record number, but that practice has not been used in many years, since a Social Security number in the wrong hands can lead to a data breach or breach of confidentiality. Veterans Administration Hospitals, however, continue to use Social Security numbers.

If an automated registration system is not employed, medical record numbers are assigned manually. To ensure that each number is used only one time, an ongoing register of each number is kept, with the corresponding patient's name. In the manual MPI card seen in Figure 4.2 earlier in the chapter, James Bernard Philips's medical record number is 07-45-85. Various numbering systems are used by healthcare facilities, as seen in Table 4.2.

TABLE 4.2	Numbering Systems
Numbering System	**Description**
Unit numbering	The patient is assigned a medical record number on his or her first visit; that number is maintained on all future visits.
Serial numbering	The patient is assigned a new medical record number on each visit.
Serial-unit numbering	A new medical record number is assigned on each visit, but the patient's records under the previous number are brought forward to the current number.
Family numbering	All members of one family are filed under the same number, but the records for each family member are kept together. This numbering system may be used by clinics or family practice offices but is not popular due to patient privacy concerns.

Filing Methods

The filing of paper health records in a hospital is generally by medical record number. The record is stored in a manila folder, then housed in a filing unit. Filing methods include **straight numeric (sequential) filing** and **terminal digit filing**.

In straight numeric filing, the folders are filed sequentially by counting up. For instance, in Table 4.3, when gathered by the HIM staff, health records would be in a random pile, with no distinct order to their medical record numbers, as seen on the left-hand side of the table. The staff would then reorganize the files, putting them into straight numeric order by medical record number, as seen on the right-hand side of the table, before taking the files to refile.

In a straight numeric filing system, there is a good chance of misfiling, since the entire number must be taken into consideration when filing. Also, the filing units themselves must be rearranged on an ongoing basis, since records grow in size with each admission and file space on each shelf becomes limited.

Terminal digit filing is a popular method, in which the medical record number is broken into sections—for instance, groups of two numbers. The filing units themselves are separated into sections 00–99, and the records are evenly distributed throughout the filing units, which decreases the ongoing redistribution of folders that is necessary in a straight numeric system. Often, the medical record numbers are separated into increments of two or three digits. The last two digits (or sometimes three) are the *primary* filing digits, the middle digits are the *secondary* filing digits, and the first digits are the *tertiary* digits. Some may think of terminal digit filing as "filing backward." As illustrated in Figure 4.9, breaking the number into sections before filing is less confusing and cuts down on misfiles. Color coding the last digits and sometimes the middle digits where all of the 1's are a particular color, all of the 2's another, and so on, also helps cut down on misfiles.

In the terminal digit filing example in Table 4.4, the medical record numbers on the left-hand side of the table have been filed in random order. Note that the tertiary digits, the secondary digits, and the primary digits do not follow ascending or descending order. On the right-hand side of the table, however, the medical record numbers are in ascending order based on their primary digits, or their final two numbers. These medical record numbers are said to be in terminal digit order.

Straight numeric (sequential) filing Records are filed in sequential numeric order.

Terminal digit filing Breaking a medical record number into segments of single or multiple digits, with filing based on the last segment as the primary file placement, followed by the middle segment, and then the first segment.

TABLE 4.3	Sequential Filing
Random Order	**Straight Numeric Order**
123456	123454
123459	123456
123454	123458
123462	123459
123458	123462

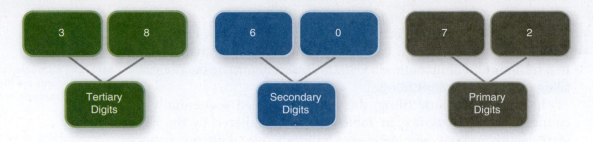

Figure 4.9 Terminal Digit Filing

TABLE 4.4	Terminal Digit Filing
Random Order	**Terminal Digit Order**
22-19-77	38-60-72
12-21-77	45-60-72
07-21-77	15-18-74
38-60-72	22-19-77
22-20-77	22-20-77
15-18-74	07-21-77
45-60-72	12-21-77

Often, there are gaps in the numbers once the records are filed, as some have become inactive due to the patient's death or because a record was destroyed because the patient had not been readmitted or received any other type of treatment within a certain period of time.

Many physicians' practices and long-term care facilities use *alphabetic filing* rather than numeric filing, because their patient population is much smaller than a hospital's. There are various resources regarding the rules of alphabetical filing, including the American Library Association (ALA), the American Record Management Association (ARMA), and the National Information Standards Organization (NISO). The important thing is that a practice selects a single set of rules, then incorporates those rules into its filing procedures. This way, all staff members who file records (or anything else in the office) are using the same set of rules, resulting in filing consistency.

To guard against misplaced records, or records that are "missing in action," it is imperative that each time a record is taken from file for any reason it is replaced with an outguide, which we first saw in the chapter on maintaining and managing health records. An outguide should include a paper that contains the location of the record, the person taking the record, and the date it was taken; the outguide then takes the place of the health record. Should it be needed for a readmission or other reason, its location will be known. Also, if it is not returned to the file within a certain period of time, it can be retrieved. Some facilities use particular colored guides for records pulled from file due to readmissions, another color for records being removed for quality assessment activities, still another for release of information, and so on.

"Numbering and Filing" in an Electronic Health Records System

Much of what was just covered regarding the ordering of a paper record system does not apply to electronic health records. When using an EHR, there is no need to "file" records, because the images are retrieved online. There is also no need for outguides or tracking records, because the records don't "leave" the computer. Recall that an advantage of using an EHR is the retrievability of the health record by more than one person at a time. That is not to say, however, that best practices to ensure a complete, accurate, timely health record cannot be learned from a paper record system and then applied to an electronic health record-keeping setting.

The EHR, like the paper record, is a legal document. It must be available at all times; it must consist of all reports and documentation required by federal and state agencies, accrediting bodies, third-party payers, and internal policies; and each entry must be authenticated to prove authorship and ensure accuracy.

Regarding the location of each electronic record, as with a paper record, each patient is entered once into the MPI, and each encounter is linked to that one MPI entry. Each patient also has a unique identifier—the medical record number. As with a paper system, the number is assigned by the computer in sequential order and is typically five or more digits in length. Whereas the medical record number is used as a means of locating a physical record and serves as a unique identification for each patient, in an EHR, the medical record number links the patient to all of his or her encounters, each of which is assigned an account number. Each "page" in an EHR includes both the medical record number and the account number. If the MPI was computerized prior to conversion to an EHR, it is possible that the existing MPI can also be converted to the new software program. A sampling (10% to 20%) of entries should be audited to ensure that the conversion was successful.

With many facilities currently converting from a paper record-keeping systems to a fully electronic health records system, one of the challenges is how to convert and then file paper records into a patient's electronic health record. Due to the high cost of conversion and the time involved, a facility may choose to leave the paper records in paper format. Others choose to convert their paper records to a format that is readable by the EHR software by scanning each record.

Hospitals may choose to contract with an outside vendor to convert their paper records into digitized images rather than scanning individual records internally. Doing so will save staff time (or the need to hire temporary staff), and there is no need to find the space necessary for the preparation and scanning of such a large number of records.

The scanned images must be protected from tampering or editing; thus, the technology used to store images on optical disk is known as write once, read many, or **WORM technology**: scanned records added to the EHR from optical disks cannot be altered, added to, or deleted. The process of verifying each scanned image is very important, as it ensures that each image is attached to the correct patient for the correct encounter date. Otherwise, the records of all previous encounters may not be available when needed. In a true EHR, documentation can be altered or hidden, but the original documentation is always retrievable. Typically, the altered documentation is labeled as version 1, version 2, and so on. Hidden documentation is retrievable at all times but is noted as having been deleted, by whom, and the date and time. Without the ability to retrieve the original documentation or a hidden image, the EHR could not be used as the legal health record.

Storing Paper Health Records

Health records consume a lot of valuable floor space in a hospital or an office. They are heavy, generate a lot of paper dust, and need to be maintained on a frequent basis. There are ways to minimize the space taken up by paper records, however. The most common equipment used to house paper health records are filing cabinets, compressible files, and open shelf filing units.

One type of filing cabinet is a vertical drawer-type cabinet. These are rarely used in hospitals or other large facilities but may be seen in physicians' practices and long-term care facilities.

Advantages	Disadvantages
• Security from theft (locking) • Security from fire (enclosed and made from heavy-duty, fireproof metal)	• Inconvenience of opening and closing drawers • Only one person at a time can file or retrieve • Requires a lot of space to open the door and for the person who is filing or retrieving—the cabinet itself is typically 36″ deep, and an additional 36″ needs to be added to open a drawer, plus space for the person filing or retrieving the records from the cabinet

A common filing system used in hospitals and larger outpatient facilities is the compressible filing unit, which is seen in Figure 4.10. Though they are expensive compared to filing cabinets, they are much more efficient and space-saving.

Advantages	Disadvantages
• Security from theft (locking) • Security from fire (when closed) • Take up less overall floor space	• Only one, possibly two, people can file at one time • More expensive than traditional cabinets • Installation time

Open shelf filing is the most common filing system used in physicians' practices. Records are easily accessed and are fairly space-efficient.

Advantages	Disadvantages
• If the office area includes ample wall space, are more space-efficient or can be placed back to back • Can be used as dividers between departments/areas of offices • Easily installed • Relatively inexpensive	• No protection from theft • No protection from fire

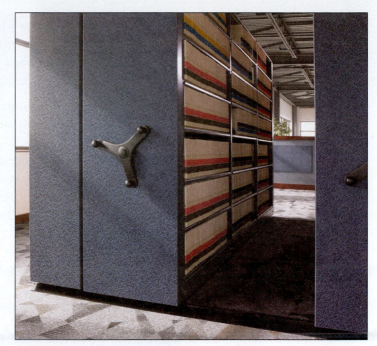

Figure 4.10 Compressible (Movable) Files

When selecting filing systems, the office supply vendor will assist with measurements and calculations; however, it is still the HIM director's responsibility to verify that the estimates will meet the needs of the department. The following should be taken into consideration:

- Current filing space used (in linear inches)—is it sufficient and will it allow for expansion, or is space lacking?
- The average size (in inches) of the current records (found by measuring a sampling)
- The number of patients seen each year as well as the number of readmissions (readmission rate)
- The number of outpatient records (emergency department and outpatient diagnostics) compiled each year and the average size of each record
- The retention period—the amount of space that is opened up each year due to the purging of inactive records

4.5 A DAY IN THE LIFE

Dr. Kramer's office currently uses 15 open shelf filing units. Each unit houses 7 shelves, and each shelf holds 36 inches of records. That accounts for 3,780 inches of file space (7 shelves × 36 inches each × 15 units = 3,780). The shelves are just about full, and another physician is joining the practice. Over the next two years, there are plans to convert to an electronic record system, but the staff anticipates the need to house an additional 1,000 inches of records. To calculate the additional filing space needed, one would add 3,780 currently used inches plus the 1,000 anticipated inches, for a total of 4,780 inches.

(continued)

Each filing unit holds 252 inches. To determine the total filing units needed, divide 4,780 by 252 = 18.9 (19) filing units needed. The office currently has 15 open shelf filing units; thus, it needs 4 more units to meet anticipated filing needs

1. If the anticipated need were for an additional 3,000 inches of file space, how many additional filing units would need to be purchased?
2. If the anticipated need were for an additional 1,000 inches of file space, but the office manager only wants to use 6 of the shelves on each unit for filing of records and use the additional shelf for storing reports and items that are not needed often, how many units would be necessary?

Health records are legal documents, important to the patient, the facility, and the healthcare providers and professionals. It is the responsibility of the HIM director to ensure that records are kept in a secure area that is accessible to authorized personnel only, that the location is not prone to flooding or fire, and that the flooring is adequate to support the weight of the records. The HIM director should work closely with the facilities management (maintenance) director before any changes in filing equipment or methods are considered.

Storing Electronic Health Records

Numerous benefits are associated with using EHRs. One is the fact that they require significantly less space for storage. There are two models for storing these records:

1. On-site client/server solutions
2. Cloud-based solutions

Client/server configurations are the traditional solution for computers used in most businesses, including healthcare. A network of computers linked to a server is the typical configuration for EHR systems. The client computer runs the EHR software in a clinic, and the patient data and additional software supporting the EHR are stored on the server. In this case, patient records are stored on a server in a secured area at the hospital or doctor's office. Hospitals and most clinics use this model.

A **cloud-based solution** serves as an alternative to the client/server model. EHR vendors offer two types of cloud-based products. Most offer a hosted version of their EHR. Under this model, the client software is more or less the same, but the health data and application software is "in the cloud," being hosted on remote servers by the vendor and accessed via a secured Internet connection. The provider does not have to maintain, secure, and back up a local server but does have to pay monthly fees to the vendor.

The second type of cloud solution is an EHR that is available only over the Web. This is a "pure" cloud-based solution and is accessed through a browser. Very little customization can be done

Client/server The use of computers in a network where functions are split between server tasks and client tasks; the client computer makes requests of the more powerful server computer in order undertake local processes.

Cloud-based solution Service in which software and data are stored on remote computers and accessed by a local computer through the Internet, typically using a browser.

with this type of EHR, and it is simpler than the cloud solutions offered by traditional client/server vendors. This pure cloud EHR is a cost-effective solution for smaller practices that cannot afford the EHR, server, maintenance, and customization expenses of the other solutions.

As far as storage is concerned, the place where the digital health record is stored depends on the EHR solution selected. Most hospital and large practices use a client/server solution, with the records stored on one or more computers in a secured and environmentally controlled room. If a cloud-based solution is used, the digital health record is stored at a secured and controlled location established by the vendor; these locations are typically referred to as "server farms." If a provider is using a pure cloud solution, patient data will likely be on servers shared by all the vendor's clients. If a provider is using the cloud solution of the traditional client/server vendor, there will likely be dedicated servers for each client. Each of these approaches to storing EHRs must meet all HIPAA requirements for security and integrity.

Paper and Electronic Health Record Management Plans

Each medical facility should have a written plan that addresses the length of time that health records will be considered active and housed in the active files, whether those active files are paper or electronic. Inactive files take up valuable space, and there are more efficient, economical retention methods available. Paper files present the most challenges for long-term storage and retention; however, EHRs have issues of their own.

Defining the Active Record

The length of time a record is considered active is a decision to be made collectively by the HIM director, the medical staff leaders, the quality assessment department, and the administration. This decision is based on a number of factors, including the amount of space available for filing or for a database, the medical staff's professional opinion of what is useful in terms of patient care, the use of health records for quality assessment and risk management activities, and the period of time within which records may be requested by third-party payers and licensing or accrediting bodies. For some facilities, this may be 5 years from the last date the patient was seen; for others, it may be 10 years or more. Once an active record has been defined, a long-term record retention plan can be developed for both print and digital health records.

Developing a Record Retention Plan

Whether referring to active or inactive health records, paper or digital, a **record retention plan** must be in place. The nature of the plan is determined by the factors noted previously, and the HIM director must ensure the retention plan is in accordance with state law, Medicare Conditions of Participation regulations, HIPAA and other federal laws, and accreditation standards.

The Medicare Conditions of Participation require health records to be kept for a period of 5 years; state laws vary, but if the facility

Record retention plan
A written policy that documents the length of time a healthcare facility retains its health records, the form (medium) in which the records will be kept, and the location(s) of the records.

receives federal monies (in the form of Medicare or Medicaid reimbursement, for example), the facility has to retain health records for a minimum of 5 years. Statutes of limitations for filing lawsuits vary, and insurance plans may require that records be maintained for a certain period of time. If these require a longer retention period than the Conditions of Participation, it is logical to keep all records for the longer period of time rather than purging only certain records. Many facilities opt for a 25-year retention plan, which also takes into account the requirement to keep minors' records for a certain period after they reach the age of majority (18 years old). Some states require that a record be retained for 1 or 2 years after the age of majority; others require 7 years past the age of majority, or 25 years.

The time period begins on the date of the patient's last visit. Thus, if a facility has a retention period of 25 years, the records of a patient who was first seen in 1987, who was seen again in 1992, and whose last visit was in 1994 would be retained until 2019. AHIMA's record retention guideline is 10 years after the most recent encounter. Record retention requirements apply to both paper and electronic records.

Whichever format is used, the facility should take the following into consideration:

- How long the records are needed for care of the patient
- Whether the facility is a teaching hospital that may need old records for educational or research purposes
- The internal use of health records for quality assessment and risk management activities
- The state's legal requirements and statute of limitations
- The federal laws and regulations for retention
- Available storage space in the facility
- The requirements of third-party payers

Strategies for Paper Record Retention and Destruction

Paper Record Archiving Techniques

Now that we have covered how facilities create record retention plans, let's explore the options for paper record retention as well as the timeline and techniques for record destruction.

The most economical, space-saving, and efficient method for storing paper records long-term is optical disk, which is most often used to store scanned images. One disk holds thousands of images, which cannot be altered because of WORM technology, discussed earlier in the chapter. The images are in a digitized format that is read by the computer. The images are each indexed to link to the patient's medical record number and the specific encounter. Each type of form (history and physical, discharge summary, nursing notes, etc.) is also indexed for ease of retrieval. Images on an optical disk can be printed, if needed, or are viewed on a computer screen.

Optical disks often reside within a **jukebox** or cabinet, which holds many disks that are delivered to the reader, much the same

Jukebox A means of storing multiple optical disks using a robotic arm that loads and unloads optical disks for delivery of requested health records.

way as a record is requested from a music jukebox. The disk(s) on which the requested patient's medical record resides is (are) loaded, and the data are then sent directly to the requestor's computer screen. Once paper records have been scanned onto optical disk, the need for filing supplies and cabinetry is reduced.

Records that are scanned and stored on optical disk are not electronic records. True electronic records are compiled in real time through data entry—that is, automated forms processing. Also, an EHR contains longitudinal health data (data over time on the same patient) and can support clinical decision making and spot potential safety issues (for instance, a drug ordered for a patient, where the record contains notation of an allergy to that drug). Think of scanned records as electronic photocopies of a record that has already been compiled and an electronic record as the "paper" on which the documentation is made.

Another major method of archiving records once they become inactive, but before the retention period expires, is warehousing. With this method, health records are placed in boxes, usually in order by medical record number, and sent to a warehouse. Archiving is very time-consuming for the HIM staff, and the warehouses may not be temperature-controlled or free of rodents and bugs. Furthermore, because the records are often housed in boxes, usually stacked on shelving units that are very high, retrieval is difficult at best. Security is of major concern when warehousing is used; the confidentiality and security of records in any form or kept in any location continue to be the responsibility of the HIM director and the hospital itself.

Until optical disk storage gained widespread acceptance and became an affordable option, in the 1980s, microfilm, or microfiche (now referred to as a microform), was the archival medium of choice. Given the varying time frames for record retention, it is still possible to encounter this legacy system while on the job, especially at smaller healthcare facilities. Miniature images of each document is taken using 16-millimeter film; they were either left in roll format, which is not very efficient, because each roll contains multiple patients' records, or were separated into 6-inch strips and inserted into flexible plastic sleeves. The advantage of the sleeves is that each contains only one patient's records, though one patient can have many sleeves of microfilm. Microfiche is similar to microfilm in jackets, but the images are embedded in the plastic jacket rather than inserted into the jacket (see Figure 4.11).

The process of microfilming is done in a department (often the HIM department) in the hospital, or the records are sent out to a microfilming company. Either way, it is a time-consuming and expensive undertaking. Microfilm is also very heavy, and though it certainly requires far less floor space than

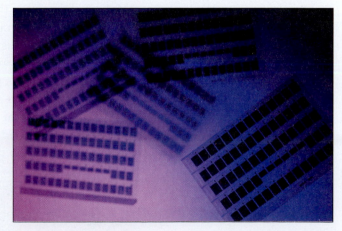

Figure 4.11   Microfiche

the original health records, the cabinets themselves take up a great deal of space. To view images on microfilm, a microfilm reader/printer is needed.

Record Destruction

Once the retention period expires, records may be destroyed. State and federal regulations as well as the facility's record retention and destruction plan govern the destruction method, which must ensure no possibility that the records could be reconstructed. The methods of destruction for paper records are often incineration, pulverization, or shredding. Microfilm is destroyed either by recycling or by pulverizing the film.

HIPAA also governs record destruction and requires that when records are destroyed by an organization hired by a healthcare facility, also known as a business associate, the following must be included in the contract with the facility:

- The method used to destroy and dispose of the records
- The length of time between acquisition of the records and actual destruction or disposal
- How the organization intends to safeguard the records against breach of confidentiality
- A statement that indemnifies the facility or provides for loss that occurs due to unauthorized disclosure
- The liability insurance the business associate obtained at a specified amount
- The damages, or indemnity, the organization must pay in the event of unauthorized disclosure

As you can see, many factors must be taken into consideration to maintain paper records. It is something that the HIM director or office manager must stay on top of, and he or she should consider the efficiency of operations, the cost, and the requirements of various regulators when developing a record retention or management plan.

4.6 A DAY IN THE LIFE

Melissa Johnson is the chief information officer for a large hospital in Southern California. Among her many responsibilities is planning for the event of a disaster, such as an earthquake, that could disrupt the hospital's EHR and connected clinical systems. Melissa develops a disaster recovery plan that includes a data backup system. She decides to establish a backup data center that is fully equipped with servers and data that can support critical functions within a few hours. This center is located outside of the region, in a neighboring state. An out-of-state backup center is very expensive, but she believes that it is necessary and must justify the expense to her board of directors.

1. How can she justify this approach?
2. Why is she locating the center in another region?
3. What might be her other alternatives?

Record Retention and the Electronic Health Record

Record retention and the EHR, at the point of this writing, is a debated issue in the health information management and technology community. EHRs are governed by the same principles, regulations, and standards as paper medical records, even though these standards were developed in a principally paper and hybrid environment. Both state laws and Centers for Medicare and Medicaid Services (CMS) determine the length and characteristics of patient record retention. As mentioned earlier in this chapter, state requirements vary for record retention for adults, minors, and special needs patients and have different requirements for medical doctors and hospitals. Though a 25 year retention period is common, the longest period is in Massachusetts, which requires hospitals to keep records for 30 years after a patient's discharge.

CMS requires that medical records be retained for 6 years from the date of creation or the date the record was last in effect, while providers in the Medicare managed care programs must keep records for 10 years. CMS is indifferent to the media format of storage with records in their original form or in a legally reproducible electronic or digital format that may be reviewed or audited. In fact, many providers retain records in excess of the CMS requirements, primarily due to the requirements of state laws, liability insurance, and concerns of malpractices claims.

There are numerous logistical and financial problems in record retention. The introduction of EHRs has made this more complicated for two reasons. First, as discussed earlier in this chapter, there is the problem of hybrid systems with patients having both a paper and a digital record. The typical, but expensive, solution is to scan these paper records into the EHR record. These scanned records are not usable for analytics or manipulation, but at least all the records are in one location. Alternatively, the patient's record will be stored in two locations, one physical and one virtual.

The second problem is the exponential growth in digital imaging studies that are becoming part of the patient record. These are huge files and add up very quickly. Although digital storage costs are dropping, storing patient records, including their imaging studies, requires servers with huge capacities, and the expenses can be significant.

A subcategory of record retention is that of archiving—the storage of nonactive patient records, records that have become too old to be useful, and records kept for liability purposes. Archived records may or may not be covered by record retention laws. In the days of paper records, archived records were typically boxed and shipped to an off-site warehouse. Archived digital records will likely be segregated but kept in manners similar to those for active digital records. There are three ways that digital health records can be stored for the purposes of retention or archiving:

1. Server storage
2. Magnetic tape storage
3. Optical storage

With these methods, records can be stored on-site, off-site, or in the cloud. Cloud storage is initially less expensive, because a provider doesn't have to purchase servers, storage media, or recording devices, but monthly charges and mounting fees for storing rising volumes of data can increase costs rapidly. As a result, the use of local servers or storage devices or the off-site storage of physical media is more cost effective and flexible. Cost/benefit analyses need to be carefully considered when deciding how to store retained and archived records.

Disaster Recovery Planning

Whether Hurricane Katrina, Tropical Storm Sandy, or a flood in the basement of a hospital strikes, disasters can affect medical records. The protection and recovery of patient records are critical, and disaster recovery planning is required under HIPAA. This requirement was strengthened under HITECH, with increased oversight of disaster recovery plans and increased financial penalties for performance failure. Meaningful Use also requires that in the event of a disaster a patient's digital record must be recoverable within a provider's information system.

For paper records, disaster recovery focuses on the physical storage location, such as fireproofing, and the development of protocols for record use during a disaster, such as those in AHIMA's Disaster Planning and Recovery Toolkit. EHRs and digital patient records support improved disaster recovery planning, but at a high price tag. Servers housing patient records must be backed up whether due to a natural disaster or a technical failure. Referred to as data redundancy, EHR disaster planning usually consists of a mirrored data center operated by the provider, but it can also be a third-party solution. A backup data center should be in a different geographic location in the event of a natural disaster.

Data redundancy supporting disaster recovery can also be provided through cloud solutions, particularly for smaller offices. Health information exchanges have also provided effective disaster recovery in the past, for Staten Island during Hurricane Sandy and in Kentucky when tornados struck a hospital. It was possible to reconstruct a patient's record through the exchange's Master Patient Index and Record Locator from other physicians' offices and hospitals.

EHRs and their related infrastructure also face new types of disaster: cyber attacks and data breaches. These require a different type of disaster prevention and recovery, one that is far more proactive in identifying threats. Cyber attack and data breach prevention also requires parallel backup systems that are ideally not subject to the same security lapses. Data security is a continuously evolving problem that must be constantly monitored.

Disaster recovery planning
Consists of having a backup infrastructure to support business continuity after a disruptive event. In healthcare, minimal recovery service levels are defined, such as access to patient records within a targeted time frame.

4.4 THINKING IT THROUGH

1. Why is terminal digit filing known as "backward filing"?
2. Explain what is meant by WORM technology. Why is it beneficial?
3. Why are there so many restrictions and stipulations governing the destruction of medical records?

chapter 4 summary

LEARNING OUTCOMES	CONCEPTS FOR REVIEW
4.1 Discuss the purpose of a Master Patient Index. Pages 90–95	• Why do patients need to be registered? • Differentiate between centralized and decentralized registration. • Define administrative, demographic, and clinical data, and give examples of each. • Explain the general consent to care process. • Define Master Patient Index (MPI) and state its purpose. • Why is the MPI necessary in a manual system and in an electronic system? • Explain the importance of data integrity of the MPI.
4.2 Contrast patient tracking in manual and electronic record-keeping systems. Pages 96–99	• What is a hybrid health record system? • What is a legal health record? • Why might the definition of legal health record vary from facility to facility? • Chart the flow of information from registration through permanent filing in a paper system. • Which functions are not necessary in an electronic system (or are handled differently than in a manual system)?
4.3 Explain how EHRs enable the maintenance of higher-quality health data. Pages 100–105	• Compare traditional dictation and transcription to voice recognition systems. • How are record deficiencies tracked in paper and electronic systems? • Discuss the relationship between quality of documentation and accurate, complete coding of diagnoses and procedures. • Explain the difference between data and information.
4.4 Organize patient records according to various numbering and filing systems. Pages 106–118	• Compare numbering systems—unit, serial, serial-unit, and family. • Compare filing methods—straight numeric, terminal digit, alphabetic. • Why are outguides necessary to track paper records but unnecessary in electronic record-keeping? • Discuss record storage in a manual system and compare to record storage in an electronic system. • Define active versus inactive records. • Discuss the types of storage media—optical disk, microfilm/fiche, paper. • Explain cloud storage. • Why is it necessary to develop a record retention plan? • What is the purpose of a jukebox in the storage of health records? • What considerations should be addressed before compiling a policy on retention and destruction of health records? • Discuss the need for a disaster recovery plan.

chapter review

MATCHING QUESTIONS

Match each term with its definition.

_____ 1. **[LO 4.4]** WORM technology

_____ 2. **[LO 4.3]** authenticate

_____ 3. **[LO 4.1]** centralized registration

_____ 4. **[LO 4.4]** jukebox

_____ 5. **[LO 4.1]** clinical data

_____ 6. **[LO 4.2]** unit record

_____ 7. **[LO 4.1]** enterprise

_____ 8. **[LO 4.4]** outguide

_____ 9. **[LO 4.1]** demographic data

_____ 10. **[LO 4.1]** decentralized registration

a. Collected patient information, such as symptoms and diagnoses

b. Registration format in which patients check in at a desk in the department at which they are seeking care

c. Data that identify the patient

d. Colored tab that aids in the filing and organization of paper records

e. System of health providers and facilities that are under the same ownership

f. Process of reviewing, verifying, and approving documentation

g. Large cabinet for storing optical disks

h. Registration format in which patients are registered in one common location

i. Security feature that prevents EHRs from being altered, no matter how many times they are accessed

j. Master record that houses each individual encounter record

MULTIPLE CHOICE QUESTIONS

Choose the letter that best completes the statement or answers the question.

11. **[LO 4.1]** Helene Jones presents to the hospital and tells the information desk that she is there for an ultrasound test. The receptionist directs Helene and her husband to the radiology department for check-in. This hospital must have a _____ registration process.
    a. centralized
    b. common
    c. decentralized
    d. deferred

12. **[LO 4.1]** Which of the following is true of the Master Patient (Person) Index?
    a. Each patient is entered once, and only the patient's clinical information is stored.
    b. Once a patient is entered, his or her information is static and cannot change.
    c. Each patient is entered twice, on the clinical and administrative sides.
    d. Once a patient is entered, his or her information is reviewed each visit.

13. **[LO 4.3]** Healthcare facilities can increase the efficiency of reimbursement cycles through which of the following?
    a. Performing high-quality, timely coding of diagnoses and treatments
    b. Ensuring the legality of their release of information practices
    c. Creating a multiple-department record review process
    d. Submitting insurance claims immediately on patient discharge

14. **[LO 4.4]** In the terminal numbering sequence 15-11-72, 15-14-72, 16-14-72, which number would be next in order?
    a. 17-15-72
    b. 17-14-72
    c. 16-15-72
    d. 16-14-73

15. **[LO 4.4]** Of the following, who would have the most input on the final selection of a filing system used to house paper health records?
    a. The staff members who work with the records daily
    b. The facilities/maintenance staff who oversee office layout
    c. The HIM manager who oversees record security
    d. The supply vendor who is selling the systems

16. **[LO 4.4]** Determining the difference between active and inactive records is typically
    a. done by the administration of a healthcare facility.
    b. based on state and regional guidelines.
    c. addressed and modified on an annual basis.
    d. dictated by a facility's Master Patient Index.

17. **[LO 4.4]** Though there are varying state guidelines and federal regulations, taking into consideration retention of records of pediatric patients, some facilities choose to store their inactive health records for
    a. 7 years.
    b. 10 years.
    c. 20 years.
    d. 25 years.

18. **[LO 4.3]** Concurrent documentation takes place
    a. while a patient is being seen or treated.
    b. after a patient is discharged.
    c. during code verification.
    d. after the transcriptionist edits the EHR.

SHORT ANSWER QUESTIONS

19. **[LO 4.1]** Contrast administrative and clinical data, giving an example of each.

20. **[LO 4.1]** Summarize the importance of the Master Patient (Person) Index.

21. **[LO 4.1]** Discuss a benefit of centralized registration and of decentralized registration.

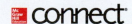 Enhance your learning by completing these exercises and more at http://connect.mheducation.com!

22. **[LO 4.2]** Why would a lost record be a liability for a healthcare facility? Explain, giving at least two examples.

23. **[LO 4.3]** Why do facilities continue to monitor electronic records for deficiencies, even though the records are documented in real time on computers?

24. **[LO 4.3]** How is an electronic health record different from a paper record that has been scanned and stored on an optical disk?

25. **[LO 4.3]** How has the medical transcriptionist's role changed as new dictation and transcription technologies have emerged?

26. **[LO 4.3]** Why is the process of record completion more efficient with EHRs than with paper?

27. **[LO.4.4]** Name and describe two logistical/financial problems in EHR record retention.

28. **[LO 4.4]** What role does data redundancy serve in EHR disaster planning?

29. **[LO 4.4]** Discuss the two models for storing electronic health records.

APPLYING YOUR KNOWLEDGE

30. **[LO 4.1]** Why is it necessary to collect so many pieces of data for each patient (during registration, for the MPI, etc.)?

31. **[LO 4.1]** Nina Valadez presents to County Hospital complaining of chest pains. Country Hospital has a centralized registration format. Walk through the administrative processing of Ms. Valadez as she is admitted to County Hospital.

32. **[LO 4.2]** Discuss some of the unique factors to consider when creating the definition of a legal health record for a facility that uses hybrid records; give examples to justify your answer.

33. **[LO 4.3, 4.4]** Create a brief scenario that shows how data become information and how the accuracy of those data is critical for patient outcomes.

34. **[LO 4.4]** Of the medical record numbering systems discussed in the text, which makes the most sense? The least sense? Does it depend on the type of healthcare facility using the records? Explain, using examples as necessary.

5

External Forces:

Regulatory and Accreditation Influences

Learning Outcomes

When you finish this chapter, you will be able to:

5.1 Differentiate among regulations, standards of documentation, and record-keeping practices.

5.2 Outline the health information regulations of various government agencies.

5.3 Justify the need for accreditation.

Key Terms

Accounting of disclosures
Accreditation
Business associate
Clearinghouse
Compliance
Covered entity
Critical Access Hospital (CAH)
Deemed status

Health Plan Identifier (HPID)
Individually identifiable health information
National Provider Identifier (NPI) number
Notice of Privacy Practices (NPP)
Omnibus Final Rule to the HITECH Act
Privacy
Protected health information (PHI)
Security rule

Introduction

Healthcare is a highly regulated industry, influenced by both federal and state mandates, as well as the requirements of third-party payers. These requirements are not optional. In order to provide healthcare, certain regulations (laws) must be followed, and participation in most healthcare plans (receiving payment for treating patients covered by the plan) requires adherence to their policies and procedures. Government regulations are mandatory minimum requirements. Policies and regulations set by third-party payers may exceed government regulations and are mandatory in order to participate in the plan. Accreditation is voluntary, and many standards exceed the minimum requirements of government regulations. Health information and health information technology regularly intersect with these external forces, and this chapter will map out the various ways in which these factors influence health information professionals.

5.1 Regulations versus Accreditation

Regulatory Agencies

Each state requires all healthcare facilities and healthcare providers, such as physicians, nurses, physicians' assistants, therapists, dentists, podiatrists, and chiropractors, to be licensed to provide medical care or practice their profession in that state. Licensure is mandatory, and regulations vary from state to state. Many healthcare practitioners and professionals hold licensure in more than one state.

Federal regulations apply to any healthcare facility that treats (and therefore expects payment for services) patients covered by Medicare and Medicaid. The regulations apply to the entire facility and all patients, not just Medicare/Medicaid patients. The set of regulations with which the facility must comply is the Conditions of Participation (CoP). For hospitals, the official reference is 42 CFR Part 482 and its associated parts and subparts. CFR is the abbreviation for Code of Federal Regulations, but in print only *CFR* is used.

Accrediting Bodies

Unlike mandatory state licensure and federal regulation, accreditation is voluntary and applies to an organization or a facility, rather than individuals. The requirements are known as *standards,* and they may be more stringent than the regulations of licensure or the CoP. Specific accrediting agencies will be covered later in this chapter.

Third-Party Payer Requirements

Insurers are in the business of paying for the healthcare of their subscribers; however, they pay only for quality, medically necessary healthcare. Particularly with managed care plans, healthcare providers and organizations must prove they are providing both. The proof is found in the massive amounts of data that are gleaned through the coding and abstracting functions performed by health information professionals. Any healthcare provider, facility, or organization that participates in managed care plans can qualify as a Center of

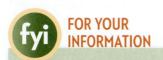

FOR YOUR INFORMATION

The full text of 42 CFR Part 482 can be found at http://www.cms.gov/Regulations-and-Guidance/Guidance/Manuals/Downloads/som107ap_a_hospitals.pdf.

Regulatory Agencies	Accrediting Bodies	Third-Party Payers
• State requirements • Federal regulations • Medicare and Medicaid • Licensure for medical professionals • Mandatory	• Voluntary standards • Apply to organizations, rather than individuals • Often more stringent than mandatory regulations and requirements	• Insurers • Managed care plans • Apply to both facilities and providers • Meet goals to qualify for special status • Certain level of compliance mandatory

Figure 5.1 Differentiating among Regulatory Agencies, Accrediting Bodies, and Third-Party Payers

Excellence if it can prove (through data) that it has met certain quality of care goals and/or offered competitively priced services. Board-certified physicians are a requirement, and credentialing criteria must be met by the facility and any support services, such as laboratory or pharmacy services, and its personnel. Compliance is monitored through periodic re-examinations of the facility or provider (Managed Care Answer Guide). For an overview of the differences among regulatory agencies, accrediting bodies, and third-party payers, see Figure 5.1.

The Role of Health Information

Health records are the source documents that prove what was and was not done to each patient seen in any type of healthcare facility. Thus, health records play a very large role in **compliance** monitoring by state and federal agencies, accrediting bodies, and third-party payers. The documentation found in health records is the only proof that facilities are operating within the scope of regulations and standards.

Compliance Adherence to rules—for instance, regulations and standards; also refers to the culture of an organization to provide high-quality, cost-effective, efficient healthcare that operates within the requirements of regulatory, accreditation, and other requirements.

5.1 THINKING IT THROUGH

1. Why is licensure mandatory but accreditation is voluntary?
2. Why do health records play such a huge role in compliance?

5.2 Regulatory Agencies Affecting Health Information

Keeping up with the many regulations that apply to health information, whether state or federal, is a daunting task. Not only does an HIM professional need to know which regulations apply to documentation as a whole, but he or she also needs to know which regulations apply only to certain areas—for example, mental health or surgical services. The breadth and complexity of health information regulations is an excellent example of how HIM touches the entire organization (and vice versa), since the records are the source documents upon which healthcare is based, reimbursement is paid, statistics are extracted, and legal decisions are made. In this section, the more common, specific regulatory and accrediting agency requirements will be discussed.

State Licensure

As noted earlier, state licensure requirements vary from state to state; however, all states require all healthcare providers to be licensed within that state. Each state publishes its licensure requirements. Let us look at two examples—Rhode Island and Virginia.

Rhode Island's hospital licensure requirements are published by the State of Rhode Island and the Providence Plantations Department of Health. They are titled *Rules and Regulations for Licensing of Hospitals*. Section 27.0 contains the medical records–related regulations. The first three are:

27.1 The medical record service shall be under the full-time direction of a registered medical record administrator or a registered health information administrator (RHIA®) who is certified by the American Health Information Management Association or who possesses equivalent training and experience.

27.2 The medical record department shall be adequately staffed and equipped to facilitate the accurate processing, checking, indexing, filing and retrieval of all medical records.

27.3 A medical record shall be established and maintained for every person treated on an inpatient, outpatient (ambulatory) or emergency basis in any unit of the hospital. The record shall be available to all other units.

Virginia's licensure requirements come under the control of the state department of health. However, unlike Rhode Island's regulations, Virginia's licensure requirements do not address the direction (management) of the medical records functions specifically. *The Regulations for the Licensure of Hospitals in Virginia* state:

12 VAC 5-410-370. Medical records. (revised 1/25/2006)

A. The medical record department shall be staffed and equipped to facilitate the accurate processing, checking, indexing, filing and retrieval of all medical records.

B. A medical record shall be established and maintained for every person treated on an inpatient, outpatient (ambulatory) or emergency basis in any unit of the hospital. The record shall be available to all other units.

There are general medical record regulations, such as the fact that medical records must be maintained for every patient encounter, and then there are specific regulations that focus on certain care units, such as obstetrics or the surgical suite, and the documentation

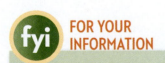

FOR YOUR INFORMATION

The Rhode Island licensure requirements for hospitals are found in full at http://sos.ri.gov/documents/archives/regdocs/released/pdf/DOH/7022.pdf, and the Virginia licensure requirements for hospitals are found in full at http://www.vdh.virginia.gov/OLC/Laws/documents/2011/pdfs/2011%20complete%2012vac5-410%20hospital.pdf.

of care given in each unit. The health information manager is responsible for knowing and understanding the specific regulations as well as those that are more generic.

The following are general medical records regulations that would likely be seen in the licensure regulations of all states:

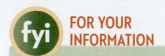

- A medical record must be kept for each patient encounter, regardless of the service provided (inpatient, emergency department, outpatient diagnostics, etc.).
- The medical record must be available at all times.
- The medical record department is staffed adequately.
- Written policies and procedures are in place regarding the content and completion of medical records.
- Only authorized individuals (as spelled out by facility policy) shall document in any medical record.
- Medical records shall be completed within a certain period of time following the date of discharge or date of the outpatient encounter.
- Medical records shall be safely stored (though most do not specify in what medium the records must be maintained).
- Medical records shall be preserved (regardless of the medium) for a certain period of time, known as the retention requirement.

Specific areas of the regulations may also contain requirements for the content of certain reports—for instance, a discharge summary or an operative report—and the length of time within which the report must be completed.

Healthcare facilities other than hospitals—such as home health agencies, hospice organizations, long-term care facilities (nursing homes), and mental health agencies—are licensed and regulated by the state as well. The regulations are contained in the department of health licensure requirements, just as they are for hospitals. Searching for licensure regulations is accomplished by using the term "licensure regulations hospitals" or "code of regulations home health agencies," for example, and the state you are interested in. The general requirements listed earlier are fairly standard regardless of the setting. One example of a difference is the requirement for the patient's psychosocial and spiritual needs to be assessed in a nursing home or in hospice care. Because hospitals provide short-term care focused on a particular healthcare issue and patients are discharged or transferred to different levels of care (e.g., outpatient rehabilitation), a state might not require that patients' psychosocial and spiritual needs be met in a hospital. A psychosocial and spiritual needs assessment of patients who are dying or are facing the reality of life in a nursing home is very important to the overall care of patients and their physical well-being.

It is very important for HIM professionals to thoroughly read and understand all the licensure requirements for the type of facility in which they work, and in the state in which the facility is located.

Licensure survey visits vary in method and frequency from state to state. Some states survey each facility yearly; others have a less frequent schedule. This being said, states are required to investigate any complaints filed against an institution outside the normal review period.

Conditions of Participation

The Conditions of Participation (CoP) apply to all facilities that diagnose or treat Medicare and Medicaid patients and, in turn, expect payment from either. The CoP regulations apply to the entire facility, not just the care, treatment, and resulting health records of that patient population. All records are subject to review, not just Medicare and Medicaid records. Formal complaints must be investigated, resulting in a survey. The survey team reviews the facility for compliance with all the regulations, not just those that pertain to the topic of the complaint.

The opening section of the *Hospital Interpretive Guidelines of the State Operations Manual of the Center for Medicare and Medicaid Services* (*CMS*) is shown in Figure 5.2. This begins the general requirements for the collection and maintenance of medical

---

A-0431

§482.24 Condition of Participation: Medical Record Services

The hospital must have a medical record service that has administrative responsibility for medical records. A medical record must be maintained for every individual evaluated or treated in the hospital.

Interpretive Guidelines §482.24

The term "hospital" includes all locations of the hospital.

The hospital must have one unified medical record service that has administrative responsibility for all medical records, both inpatient and out patient records. The hospital must create and maintain a medical record for every individual, both inpatient and out patient evaluated or treated in the hospital.

The term "**medical records**" includes at least written documents, computerized electronic information, radiology film and scans, laboratory reports and pathology slides, videos, audio recordings, and other forms of information regarding the condition of a patient.

Survey Procedures §482.24

- Review the organizational structure and policy statements and interview the person responsible for the medical records service to ascertain that the service is structured appropriately to meet the needs of the hospital and the patients.

- Review a sample of active and closed medical records for completeness and accuracy in accordance with Federal and State laws and regulations and hospital policy. The sample should be 10 percent of the average daily census and be no less than 30 records. Additionally, select a sample of outpatient records in order to determine compliance in outpatient departments, services, and locations.

Figure 5.2 Conditions of Participation: *Hospital Interpretive Guidelines of the State Operations Manual*

records, as well as the instructions for the surveyors regarding what they are to review and how they are to go about it.

The interpretive guidelines in Figure 5.2 are used by surveyors when performing on-site visits. These guidelines should also be used during internal quality reviews of documentation to ensure compliance with the regulations, whether they are state or federal.

Specifics regarding the content of the medical record, the length of time within which the medical record must be completed, retention requirements, and the like are covered in specific sections of the interpretive guidelines, such as surgical services or emergency services.

The HIM director and staff are responsible for not only knowing the CoP regulations but also ensuring compliance. Appropriate hospital policies cannot contradict state or federal mandates. The HIM director is responsible for reporting noncompliance by individual physicians or by staff to the Medical Record Committee, which is a standing committee of the medical staff. Any physicians or other personnel who are noncompliant may face suspension of privileges, fines, suspension of privileges, or dismissal.

In the event that CoP and state licensure regulations are contradictory, the more stringent of the two must be followed. For instance, the CoP require that medical records be completed within 30 days of discharge (or encounter). If the state regulations require the record to be completed within 15 days of discharge (or encounter), the hospital must comply with the 15-day limit.

Some of the major conditions and standards of the CoP that directly impact health information processes are the following:

- The Governing Body (including that of the medical staff and chief executive officer)
- Care of Patients
- Emergency Services
- Patient's Rights
- Privacy and Safety
- Confidentiality of Patient Records
- Restraint or Seclusion
- Death Reporting Requirements
- Quality Assessment and Performance Improvement (including scope, data, activities, and projects)
- Composition of the Medical Staff
- Medical Staff Organization and Accountability
- Medical Staff By-laws
- Nursing Services (including organization, staffing, and delivery of care)
- Medical Record Services (including organization and staffing, form and retention of the medical record, and content of medical records)
- Utilization Review (including applicability, composition of the Utilization Review Committee, scope and frequency of review, and admissions, continued stay, and extended stay review)

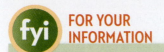
- Discharge Planning (including identification of patients in need of discharge planning, discharge planning evaluation, discharge plan, transfer or referral, and reassessment)
- The Organization, Staffing, and Delivery of Services for Individual Services (such as surgery, anesthesia, rehabilitative medicine, emergency services, outpatient services, nuclear medicine, and respiratory services)

The influence of the CoP on health information processes is summarized in Figure 5.3.

Health Insurance Portability and Accountability Act (HIPAA)

The Health Insurance Portability and Accountability Act of 1996 (HIPAA) is most commonly known, particularly by healthcare consumers, as "the privacy law." It is far more than that, however, and its original intent was, as the name implies, portable healthcare coverage. Prior to HIPAA, people who left a job where health insurance was provided also lost their health insurance coverage. Under HIPAA, individuals can retain their healthcare coverage or obtain

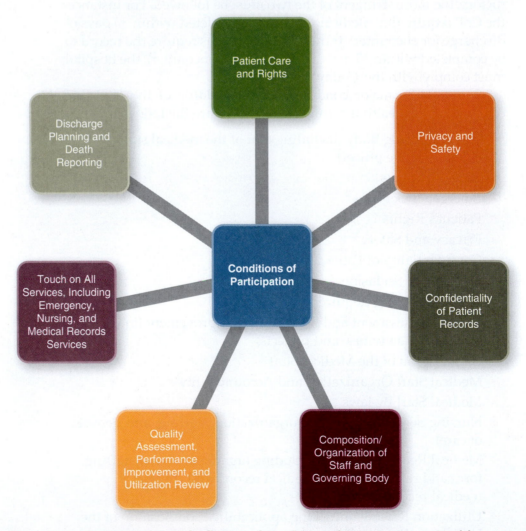

Figure 5.3 The Vast and Varied Influence of Conditions of Participation on Health Information Processes

new coverage, even with a pre-existing condition. The individual is responsible for paying for the coverage but is not left without insurance or with the prospect of not being able to find coverage because of a pre-existing condition.

The rules of HIPAA apply to all **covered entities** that electronically process, store, transmit, or receive medical records, claims, or remittance advices (which accompany payments from any third-party payer). Thus, a covered entity is any physician, hospital, or other healthcare facility, health insurance company, **clearinghouse**, and **business associate** of a covered entity that has access to **individually identifiable health information**. The HIM professional is often responsible for obtaining Business Associate Agreements (BAAs) from vendors or contractors that have access to patient records.

In the next sections, we will explore the privacy and security rules, code sets, unique identifiers, and enforcement and compliance.

The Privacy Rule

A patient has the right to expect **privacy**—the right to be left alone—and the right to expect that only persons with a need to know a patient's health history or status have access to it. Information about the patient is known as **protected health information**, or **PHI**. PHI includes any piece of data that identifies the patient—name, address, date of birth, email, phone number, account numbers associated with the patient, medical record number, Social Security number, fingerprints, photographs, and any piece of information that would automatically identify a patient. PHI also includes clinical information tied to that patient

Prior to HIPAA, there were laws regarding the release of health information, and most disclosures were the responsibility of the health information department, but the laws were not standardized, nor did they specifically address electronic transactions. As a result of HIPAA, authorizations to release health information have to contain certain elements in order for PHI to be released. Those elements are covered in detail in the privacy chapter. Limits were placed on the uses and disclosures of PHI, and patients were given the right to access their own health information, including the right to examine and obtain a copy of their health records and to request amendments or corrections.

HIPAA requires covered entities to present patients with a **Notice of Privacy Practices (NPP)** form, which tells patients how their PHI is used, disclosures that are made without authorization, their rights regarding their PHI, the persons to whom PHI may be released, and the covered entity's legal duties with respect to that information. As a general rule, a patient/legal representative signs the NPP on the first visit to a provider. It is not a requirement of the rule that patients re-sign the NPP after the first visit; however, if any changes have been made in how the covered entity uses PHI or if the patient chooses to change who may receive his or her PHI, a new form must be signed. The patient/legal representative may ask for a copy of the NPP at any time, and it must be provided. A revised NPP was implemented in 2013 and will be discussed in the section on the Omnibus Final Rule in this chapter.

Covered entity Any healthcare provider or contractor that transmits in electronic form any individually identifiable health information.

Clearinghouse An organization or entity (public or private) that processes data into a standardized billing format and checks for inconsistencies or other errors in the claims data.

Business associate An individual or organization with which a covered entity contracts to perform functions or duties that involve the use or disclosure of individually identifiable health information.

Individually identifiable health information Data that identify a patient, such as name, address, date of birth, and gender.

Privacy The right to be left alone and to expect that one's health information is available only to those who have a need to access it.

Protected health information (PHI) Any piece of data that identifies a patient as well as the clinical data tied to the patient.

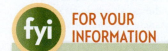 **FOR YOUR INFORMATION**

The entire HIPAA Privacy Rule is located at http://www.hhs.gov/ocr/privacy/hipaa/administrative/privacyrule and is titled 45 CFR Part 160 and Part 164.

Notice of Privacy Practices (NPP) Written notification, which must be signed by the patient/legal representative, that communicates how PHI is used, disclosures made without the need for authorization, the patient's rights regarding PHI, the persons to whom PHI may be released, and the covered entity's legal duties with respect to that information.

The Security Rule

The HIPAA **security rule** speaks directly to the electronic systems used to house, maintain, and transmit health information. It is within the security rule that procedures and methods used to protect electronic health information are addressed. This rule specifically addresses how PHI is stored, accessed, transmitted, and audited.

The security rule addresses *administrative safeguards*, such as the designation of a security team in the organization; *physical safeguards*, such as physically securing computers and creating policies regarding what data can be stored on laptop computers; and *technical safeguards*, including the use of encryption when transmitting data and the means for authenticating the identity of each computer user.

The Code Set Rule

The HIPAA *code set rule* requires healthcare providers and facilities to report diagnosis and procedure codes using the following code sets:

- ICD-9-CM (or ICD-10-CM) for reporting of inpatient and outpatient diagnosis codes and ICD-10-PCS codes for inpatient procedures (at the time of this writing, the effective date is October 1, 2015)
- Healthcare Common Procedure Coding System (HCPCS) level I codes (Current Procedural Terminology, or CPT) for outpatient procedures
- HCPCS level II codes for inpatient and outpatient services
- National Dental Codes (NDC) for dental and oral surgery

The Unique Identifier Rule

The *Unique Identifier Rule* is part of the administrative simplification rule and includes the requirement for a standard unique employer identification number (EIN) code to identify the employer on any HIPAA transactions. In addition, the **National Provider Identifier (NPI)** number, which is a unique 10-digit number identifying each care provider on any administrative or financial transaction. The use of the final standard identification number was to have been required as of November 5, 2014, and is known as the **Health Plan Identifier (HPID)**. An HPID is assigned to all payers (health plans) and will be required on the claim form for Medicare and Medicaid patients. Physicians will be required to include the HPID on all claims as of November 7, 2016.

The Enforcement and Compliance Rule

The *enforcement and compliance rule* contains the provisions that pertain to compliance and investigations of noncompliance, the civil money penalties imposed for violations of the HIPAA Administrative Simplification Rules, and the provision for procedures for hearings.

The entire HIPAA law is lengthy, but all of it pertains in some way to functions carried out by health information staff. It is important to stay abreast of any changes or clarifications in the law. Most state hospital associations and component state associations of AHIMA are excellent resources for updates on regulatory issues. Figure 5.4 recaps the essential rules of HIPAA.

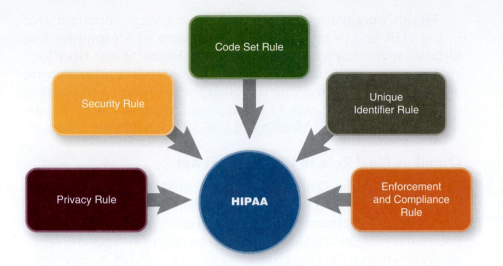

Figure 5.4 The Privacy Rule Is Just One Core Rule of HIPAA

Health Information Technology for Economic and Clinical Health (HITECH) Act

HITECH was initially explained in the chapter covering healthcare in the United States. Briefly, its purpose is to increase the use of EHRs by hospitals and physicians. Funding is available to physicians and hospitals, in the form of incentive grants, for the purchase and Meaningful Use of EHR software. Providers who are already using an EHR are eligible for the grant money if they upgrade to a certified EHR. CMS and the Office of the National Coordinator of Health Information Technology (ONC) have established standards for certified EHRs. Beginning in 2015, most clinics and hospitals that do not have an EHR will be subject to reduced Medicare reimbursement levels.

The intent is that, through the use of an EHR, the quality and efficiency of healthcare will be improved and the disparities often found with paper records will be cut down. Because patients will have easier access to their health information through patient portals, they are more likely to play an active role in their healthcare. The duplication of testing that is frequently seen with the use of paper records should decrease, since providers and hospitals will have access to the records from previous care.

The use of an electronic health record system is key, but just as important is that the data collected and maintained in the EHR are meaningful. The three stages of Meaningful Use started with data capture—pertinent data were collected that would improve patient care and outcomes; the second stage focuses on advancing clinical processes through increased sharing of patients' health information with other healthcare providers who have a need to know—for instance, if a patient is transferred from one hospital to another; and the third and final stage, which has been delayed until 2017 at the time of this writing, focuses on improved patient outcomes through the use of clinical decision support technology, access to self-management tools by patients themselves, and access to comprehensive data, which in turn improves the health of all individuals.

Health information professionals play a very important role in the EHR and in meeting the requirements of Meaningful Use (detailed in the chapter on healthcare in the United States), since they are the experts in the content of health records and the monitoring of documentation in meeting compliance and reporting incomplete or missing documentation to the appropriate providers or departments, so that required Meaningful Use data elements are collected.

Omnibus Final Rule to the HITECH Act

Omnibus Final Rule to the HITECH Act Legislation that updates and clarifies the requirements in the HITECH Act.

In March 2013, the Omnibus Final Rule to the HITECH Act went into effect; compliance was required beginning in September 2013. It includes enhancements to protecting patient privacy, additions to individual patients' rights, and strengthening of the government's ability to enforce the law. HIPAA was also expanded to give more control over any covered entity's business associates—for the HIM professional, these include external coding consultants and software service providers. The Notice of Privacy Practices was expanded and the maximum penalty for violation of the law was increased to $1.5 million per violation. The Omnibus Final Rule to the HITECH Act has enhanced breach notification standards and, by extension, patient rights.

Examples of the enhancement of patient rights include the requirement that providers who utilize electronic health records provide patients with their records in electronic form, when requested. In addition, patients who are paying for their services in cash may instruct the provider not to bill their insurance and not to divulge any information about the services to the patient's health insurance carrier. The intent of both is to ensure that protected health information (PHI) is kept private and secure.

The Final Rule gives patients the right to determine who sees their health information, but it still gives covered entities (a healthcare provider, a clearinghouse, or a health insurance plan) the ability to access necessary PHI to care for patients, collect payment for services rendered, and operate a business (quality review activities, for example).

The Final Rule spells out protected health information as any piece of information that identifies a patient—it includes a patient's name, date of birth, address, email address, and telephone number; a patient's employer; any relatives' names; a patient's Social Security number; his or her medical record number; account numbers tied to the patient's account; the patient's fingerprints; any photographs of the patient; and any characteristics about the patient that would automatically disclose his or her identity (for instance, "the governor of the largest state in the United States"). In addition, PHI includes the medical information that is tied to the person, including diagnosis, test results, treatments, and prognosis; documentation by the care provider and other healthcare professionals; and billing information. HIPAA states (and HITECH enhances) that only persons who have a need to know may have access to a patient's PHI. And to take it a step further, they are entitled to access only the minimum amount of information required to do their jobs.

HIPAA	HITECH	Omnibus Rule
• Privacy • Security • Code sets • Unique identifiers • Enforcement and compliance	• Move from paper health records to an EHR • Requires Meaningful Use of the EHR • Enacts monetary penalties on providers and hospitals who choose not to convert to a certified EHR	• Enhance privacy rules • Expands patients' rights regarding their health information • Increases fines for privacy breaches • Strengthens the government's ability to enforce the law

Figure 5.5 The Key Features of HIPAA, HITECH, and the Omnibus Rule

A thorough knowledge of HIPAA, HITECH, and the Omnibus Final Rule is necessary for HIM practitioners—facility policies must be in line with the requirements and proper procedures followed in order to maintain compliance with the law. Reviewing these three acts against applicable state law should also ensure that policies address the most stringent requirements. Figure 5.5 provides a comparative overview of the key features of the three acts.

5.1 A DAY IN THE LIFE

Eileen is the new Health Records Department director at Memorial Hospital. As she is reviewing health records–related hospital policies, she notices there are no policies for how long health records must be kept; there are no policies or medical staff bylaws stating the time frame within which health records must be completed following discharge or completion of an outpatient encounter; and there is no policy regarding the documentation of operative procedures.

1. Is this a problem? Why or why not?

Penalties for Noncompliance with HIPAA and HITECH

The Office for Civil Rights (OCR) enforces compliance with the privacy, security, and breach notification HIPAA rules (including the HITECH enhancements). Failure to comply with HIPAA rules can result in civil (monetary) and/or criminal penalties. The Omnibus Final Rule enacted the fines found in Table 5.1.

HIPAA and HITECH require that patients be provided with an **accounting of disclosures** upon request. Patients may also request a report of all accesses by internal individuals who had access to their PHI.

Accounting of disclosures A listing of all disclosures of a patient's PHI, including those for treatment, payment, and healthcare operations.

Breach Notification

The US Department of Health and Human Services (HHS) defines a breach as "generally, an impermissible use or disclosure under the

TABLE 5.1	Omnibus Final Rule Fines	
Type of Violation	Fine per Violation	Total Violation When the Breach Involved the Same Provision within the Same Calendar Year
Unintentional breach	$100 to $50,000	$1,500,000
Reasonable cause	$1,000 to $50,000	$1,500,000
Willful neglect (corrected)	$10,000 to $50,000	$1,500,000
Willful neglect (not corrected)	Minimum of $50,000	$1,500,000

Source: American Medical Association. HIPAA Violations and Enforcement.

Privacy Rule that compromises the security or privacy of the protected health information." In the event of an unsecured breach, the affected individual(s), the secretary of HHS, and in certain circumstances the media must be notified. If the breach occurs by a business associate, the covered entity must be notified. Individual notifications must be provided "without unreasonable delay," but no later than 60 days following the discovery of a breach. The breach notification must include, to the extent possible, a brief description of the breach; a description of the types of information involved in the breach; the steps that affected individuals should take to protect themselves from potential harm; a brief description of what the covered entity is doing to investigate the breach, mitigate the harm, and prevent further breaches; and contact information for the covered entity (or business associate, as applicable).

When the breach involves 500 or more residents of a state or jurisdiction, the previously mentioned measures must be taken and the media outlets that serve that area must be notified as well. In the case of breaches affecting fewer than 500 individuals, the secretary of HHS may be notified annually, but no later than 60 days following the end of the calendar year in which the breaches occurred.

5.2   THINKING IT THROUGH

1. What types of facilities need to be aware of the Conditions of Participation?
2. What is HIPAA's security rule? Give one example of how the security rule influences healthcare facilities.
3. Give three nondemographic examples of protected health information.
4. Locate the required Notice of Privacy Practices on the Internet, and write a brief description of its contents.

Voluntary Accrediting Agencies

Unlike licensure and the CoP, accreditation is voluntary. Healthcare is a competitive business; healthcare organizations choose to earn accreditation to gain a competitive edge over those that are not accredited. Also, accreditation shows the community that the organization is committed to providing the highest standard of healthcare. Accreditation standards focus on quality care and safety; thus, they zero in on the management of risk, which may equate to lower liability insurance costs for the facility. Accrediting bodies require continuing education of facility staff, which is helpful in recruiting new staff and retaining current staff. Accrediting bodies advocate an official performance improvement plan as well. In other words, healthcare facilities should have a formal method of identifying areas where improvement is needed, and should improve those areas through a multistep, systematic approach. Depending on the accrediting agency, accreditation may also mean that the facility holds "deemed status," which will be discussed in the next section.

Each accrediting agency has an application process and eligibility requirements. Because accreditation is voluntary, there is a fee involved, which varies by agency.

Accrediting Agencies with Deemed Status

There are many agencies that accredit healthcare institutions. Some agencies hold **deemed status**, which permits the accredited facility to seek reimbursement from Medicare and Medicaid without the need for a separate review process. A facility applies for accreditation and in so doing agrees to comply with a set of standards (as opposed to laws or regulations).

Deemed status By virtue of achieving accreditation status, a facility is also in compliance with the CoP.

CMS-approved accrediting agencies survey healthcare organizations as an agent of CMS. The fact that a healthcare organization holds deemed status does not mean that CMS will never conduct a survey on its own as a result of a specific complaint or as a post-survey visit. CMS surveys are most commonly performed by the department of health in the state where the healthcare organization is located. Also, state departments of health may conduct a survey at any time, and licensure or accreditation surveys may be announced or unannounced. The surveys are conducted on the facility as a whole—not just on Medicare and Medicaid patients—and if the visit is in response to a complaint, all regulations or standards are assessed, not just the one to which the complaint pertains.

Nonaccredited healthcare organizations are surveyed by CMS, usually by the state department of health. Table 5.2 lists the CMS-approved organizations that hold deemed status.

Critical Access Hospital (CAH) A hospital that has no more than 25 inpatient beds; maintains an annual average length of stay of 96 hours or less for acute inpatient care; offers 24-hour, 7-day-a-week emergency care; and is located in a rural area at least 35 miles' drive away from any other hospital or other Critical Access Hospital; the CoP regulations for CAHs differ from those for hospitals that are not CAHs.

Of the accrediting agencies listed in Table 5.2, the most widely known and largest is The Joint Commission. According to The Joint Commission website, 77% of the hospitals in the United States are accredited by The Joint Commission. This includes acute hospitals and **Critical Access Hospitals (CAHs)**. CMS designates which hospitals are CAHs; they are all 25 beds or less, their patients stay 96 hours or less, and they hold critical access status by the state office of rural health. The Joint Commission also accredits ambulatory surgery centers, home health agencies, hospices, behavioral health centers, and psychiatric hospitals. In addition, The Joint Commission accredits clinical laboratories within hospitals and freestanding reference laboratories.

TABLE 5.2	CMS-Approved Organizations Holding Deemed Status	
Organization	**Types of Facilities or Services Accredited**	**Website**
Accreditation Association for Ambulatory Health Care (AAAHC)	Ambulatory surgery center (ASC)	http://www.aaahc.org/
Accreditation Commission for Health Care, Inc. (ACHC)	Home health agency (HHA) Hospices	http://www.achc.org/
American Association for Accreditation of Ambulatory Surgery Facilities (AAAASF)	Ambulatory surgery center (ASC) Outpatient treatment (OPT) Rural health clinic (RHC)	http://www.aaaasf.org/
American Osteopathic Association Healthcare Facilities Accreditation Program (AOA/HFAP)	Ambulatory surgery center (ASC) Critical Access Hospital (CAH) Hospitals	http://www.hfap.org
Center for Improvement in Healthcare Quality (CIHQ)	Hospitals	http://cihq.org/
Community Health Accreditation Program (CHAP)	Home health agency (HHA) Hospice providers Home medical equipment Pharmacies Private duty nursing Infusion therapy Public health Community nursing services Supplemental staffing services	http://www.chapinc.org/
Det Norske Veritas Healthcare (DNV Healthcare)	Hospitals Critical Access Hospital (CAH)	http://www.dnvaccreditation.com/
The Joint Commission	Ambulatory surgery center (ASC) Critical Access Hospital (CAH) Hospitals Home health agency (HHA) Hospices Behavioral health Psychiatric hospitals	http://www.jointcommission.org/
National Committee for Quality Assurance (NCQA)	Health plans	http://www.ncqa.org/tabid/689/default.aspx

Special certifications for certain procedures or services are also available through The Joint Commission. Examples include certification for the treatment of stroke, congestive heart failure, or joint replacement.

One of the hallmark consumer-focused initiatives of The Joint Commission is the QualityCheck® website, which provides consumers with comparative data related to facilities that are accredited by The Joint Commission. Consumers have access to the latest accreditation decision on a facility of interest to them, the effective date of the accreditation, and any certifications that facility holds (see Figure 5.6).

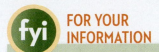
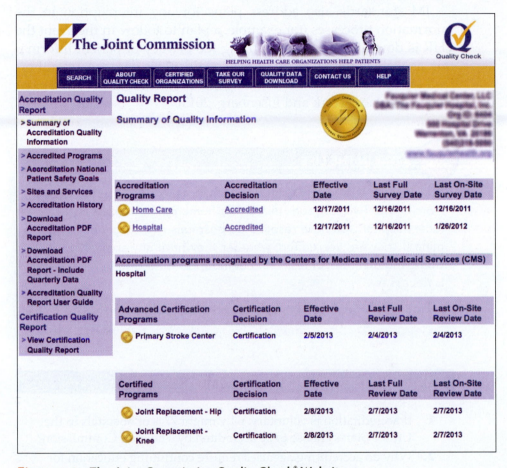

Figure 5.6 The Joint Commission QualityCheck® Website

Though The Joint Commission standards affect all the departments and services in a healthcare facility, the standards directly related to health information include Record of Care, Treatment, and Services (RC), and Information Management (IM) standards. Here is a *sampling* of these standards:

- A medical record must be compiled for every admission/encounter.
- All entries must be dated and timed.
- Nursing assessment must be completed within 24 hours of admission.

- Physician's history and physical exam (H&P) must be completed (or updated, if done within 30 days of admission) within 24 hours of admission and prior to surgery.
- Operative (procedure) notes or reports are to be completed immediately following surgery (before the patient is discharged from the post-procedure care unit [recovery]).
- Medication reconciliation (medications being taken at home) must be done within 24 hours of admission.
- Patient education: documentation of any barriers to communication or patients' needs must be identified and resolved.

IM standards also address plans for any interruption in the information processes (for example, a plan to follow in the event the EHR is down). Policies for ensuring the privacy of patient information as well as the integrity of data against loss damage, unauthorized alteration, unintentional change, or accidental destruction must also be in place (Clark and Eisenberg, 2013).

5.2 A DAY IN THE LIFE

Your neighbor is having gastric bypass surgery at a hospital 60 miles from home. Two surgeons nearer her home perform the surgery at a local hospital. You have researched hospitals and surgeons to determine if they are accredited, whether they have any special certifications, and their outcomes. Your neighbor does not see that any of this is necessary.

1. How would you explain your reasoning to your neighbor?

5.3 THINKING IT THROUGH

1. If accreditation is voluntary, why might 77% of hospitals in the United States choose to be accredited by The Joint Commission?
2. Why do accrediting agencies require continuing education for staff members of accredited facilities?

chapter 5 summary

LEARNING OUTCOMES	CONCEPTS FOR REVIEW
5.1 Differentiate among regulations, standards of documentation, and record-keeping practices. Pages 124–125	• Identify the difference(s) between licensure and accreditation. • Regulations come from two government levels—name both. • Explain how licensure regulations might differ from accreditation standards. • Why do third parties (insurers) have a stake in compliance with licensure regulations or accreditation standards? • Explain HIM's role in compliance.
5.2 Outline the health information regulations of various government agencies. Pages 125–136	• Explain state licensure; what types of medical professionals or facilities must be licensed? Are all state regulations the same? • Differentiate CoP regulations from state regulations. • Explain the typical state and/or CoP regulations that govern documentation and the keeping of health records. • Give examples of CoP regulations. • Name major department- or facility-specific CoP regulations that directly impact health information documentation and the keeping of health records. • Give examples of covered entities. • Explain the HIPAA privacy rule. • Explain the HIPAA security rule. • List the code sets required in the HIPAA code set rule. • Discuss two unique identifiers used on administrative or financial transactions. • Identify the penalties for privacy or security breaches.
5.3 Justify the need for accreditation. Pages 137–140	• What is the focus of accreditation? • Why would a facility choose to seek and maintain accreditation? • Define *deemed status* and give examples of accreditors that hold deemed status. • Define *Critical Access Hospital*. • Explain how consumers can use The Joint Commission's quality initiatives.

MATCHING QUESTIONS

Match each term with its definition.

_____ 1. **[LO 5.3]** accreditation

_____ 2. **[LO 5.2]** Conditions of Participation

_____ 3. **[LO 5.3]** Critical Access Hospital

_____ 4. **[LO 5.2]** Health Insurance Portability and Accountability Act of 1996 (HIPAA)

_____ 5. **[LO 5.2]** protected health information (PHI)

_____ 6. **[LO 5.2]** administrative simplification provisions

_____ 7. **[LO 5.2]** covered entity

_____ 8. **[LO 5.2]** Health Plan Identifier

_____ 9. **[LO 5.1]** licensure

_____ 10. **[LO 5.3]** deemed status

a. Legislation that created rules for the security and transference of health information and insurance

b. Facility or person allowed access to a patient's protected health information

c. Patient-identifying data that must be kept private and secure

d. Designation that shows a facility has gone above and beyond Conditions of Participation regulations

e. Mandatory designation that gives healthcare professionals the ability to practice in their state of residence

f. Regulations that must be followed by any facility that accepts Medicaid or Medicare patients, as well as the payments that accompany such acceptance

g. Voluntary process that a healthcare facility undergoes to prove its maintenance of high standards and quality of care

h. Guidelines that standardized the management of health information

i. Facility characterized by a low bed count and short patient stays

j. Assigned to each health plan as required by ARRA

MULTIPLE CHOICE QUESTIONS

Choose the letter that best completes the statement or answers the question.

11. **[LO 5.1]** Which is true about licensure?
    a. A healthcare professional can be licensed only in a single state.
    b. The licensing process is overseen by federal regulations.
    c. Many healthcare professionals are licensed in multiple states.
    d. Licensing provides a healthcare professional with "specialist" status.

12. **[LO 5.1]** A facility may be awarded "Center of Excellence" status if
    a. it offers competitively priced services.
    b. at least 70% of its physicians are board certified.
    c. it complies with all Conditions of Participation.
    d. it uses electronic health records to prove compliance.

13. **[LO 5.1]** Health records can serve as _____ documents, because they _____.
    a. compliance; must always be correct
    b. narrative; tell the story of patient care
    c. historical; contain a record of every patient encounter
    d. source; can prove what was or was not done for a patient

14. **[LO 5.2]** Which is an example of protected health information?
    a. An unidentified patient is Caucasian.
    b. Joan Philipps is being treated for diabetes.
    c. An identified patient's primary care doctor is Dr. Azore.
    d. An unidentified patient's height is 5'8".

15. **[LO 5.2]** According to most state regulations concerning medical records, a health record should
    a. contain information about appointment-making methods.
    b. be accessible to and editable by all staff of a healthcare facility.
    c. be securely stored in locked cabinets.
    d. reflect each single patient encounter.

16. **[LO 5.2]** How often do healthcare facilities receive licensing review visits?
    a. Annually
    b. Monthly
    c. Depends on state requirements
    d. Only if there are complaints

17. **[LO 5.2]** The Conditions of Participation are
    a. facility-based.
    b. care-based.
    c. provider-based.
    d. treatment-based.

18. **[LO 5.2]** The original intent of HIPAA regulations was to
    a. ensure data integrity.
    b. increase the privacy of health data.
    c. guarantee insurance transference.
    d. assist in electronic record adoption.

19. **[LO 5.3]** Which is a requirement of facilities seeking or maintaining accreditation?
    a. Achieving deemed status
    b. Continuing education for staff
    c. Drafting improvement plans
    d. Retaining staff at least three years

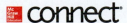 Enhance your learning by completing these exercises and more at http://connect.mheducation.com!

SHORT ANSWER QUESTIONS

20. **[LO 5.1]** Why must facilities that accept Medicare or Medicaid patients follow the Conditions of Participation?

21. **[LO 5.2]** What is the purpose of the *Hospital Interpretive Guidelines of the State Operations Manual?*

22. **[LO 5.2]** Is the information "Patient has quit smoking in the last six months" considered protected health information? Explain.

23. **[LO 5.2]** Discharge planning is one of the major conditions of the CoP. Explain how discharge planning might directly impact health information management.

24. **[LO 5.2]** Summarize the Omnibus Final Rule to the HITECH Act.

25. **[LO 5.3]** What is the benefit to organizations such as state departments of health or accrediting agencies conducting unannounced review visits to a facility?

26. **[LO 5.3]** List three of the Record of Care, Treatment, and Services, and Information Management standards outlined in the text. Discuss how each is relevant to accreditation.

APPLYING YOUR KNOWLEDGE

27. **[LO 5.1, 5.2, 5.3]** Accreditation, even though voluntary, may have stricter requirements than licensure or CoP. Explain why this may be the case, giving specifics as relevant.

28. **[LO 5.2]** Discuss the pros and cons of licensing requirements being variable from state to state. Might this influence the decision of a healthcare provider to obtain licensure in different states? Explain.

29. **[LO 5.2]** Why are HITECH incentive payments earmarked for EHR software purchases or upgrades? Do you think that this earmarking is fair to healthcare facilities? Explain your answer.

30. **[LO 5.2]** How are the privacy and security sections of HIPAA related to the original intent of the law? Give at least two examples of the interrelatedness.

31. **[LO 5.3]** Visit the websites of two accrediting agencies outlined in Table 5.2. Summarize the information you find, and explain its relevance to the field of healthcare.

6

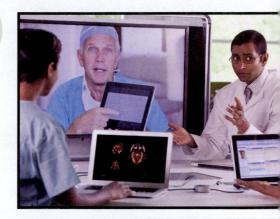

The Active Health Record in Acute Care Settings

Copyright © 2016 by McGraw-Hill Education

Learning Outcomes

When you finish this chapter, you will be able to:

6.1 Describe the flow of health information in an acute care setting.

6.2 Describe electronic tools used by clinicians to document in the health record.

6.3 Contrast electronic tools used in the records management process.

6.4 Classify technologies used in the integration of health information in acute care settings.

Key Terms

Admission, discharge, and transfer (ADT) system
Advance directive
Apgar score
Attending physician
Autopsy
Bar code
Charting by exception
Claims data
Computerized physician order entry (CPOE)
Durable medical equipment (DME)
History of present illness (HPI)
Hospitalist
Interface

Medication Administration Record (MAR)
Nursing assessment
Observation
Pathologist
Patient census
Patient rights acknowledgment
Point of care
Post-anesthesia care unit (PACU)
Property and valuables inventory
Review of systems (ROS)
Template
Verbal order

Introduction

Previous chapters have covered the processes and the staff involved in ensuring accurate, complete documentation of a patient's healthcare. In this chapter, we will look specifically at the documentation itself and how the requirements of external forces affect each piece of this documentation. You will gain an understanding of the flow of information from the time the patient presents for admission or an outpatient encounter to the time he or she leaves the facility. Many of the steps in the process may be repeated several times during the patient's stay. Various electronic systems, such as clinical documentation, laboratory, imaging, and financial systems, interface to tell a seamless story of each patient's encounter with the facility.

6.1 The Flow of Information

Patient Registration

As we saw in the chapter on maintaining health information, the first step of any healthcare encounter is registration of the patient. Recall that registration captures valuable administrative data about the patient and leads staff to the location of any health records from previous encounters, so that they are available to care providers. It is particularly imperative that the records of the *correct* patient are made available. Think of it this way—in any given hospital, there may be 10, 20, 30, or more patients by the name of Mary Smith in that hospital's Master Patient (Person) Index (MPI), the permanent database of all patients who have been treated at that facility. If Mary Smith was a patient there before, her current encounter must be linked with the correct master file for her, which is identified by a unique number for each patient.

Registration may be a multi-part process rather than being completed all at one time. For instance, a patient who is going to have a planned procedure performed at the hospital will begin the registration process when the surgeon's office schedules the surgery date and time. The process will be finalized when she arrives for pre-admission laboratory, radiology, and anesthesiology workup or when she arrives on the day of the surgery.

During the registration process, the patient typically signs many forms, including a consent to treatment, an agreement that he or she is responsible for payment for services, the HIPAA Notice of Privacy Practice (NPP), and the **patient rights acknowledgment**, for instance.

From the registration area, the patient moves on to a nursing unit, as an inpatient, or to the ambulatory surgery area, if the purpose of the encounter is an ambulatory (outpatient) surgical procedure.

Clinical Documentation

From registration, the clinical aspects of care begin. As noted, the health record is the source document that proves everything that was done to or for a patient. Absence of documentation equates to something not being done to or for the patient. For example, if a physician wrote an order for vital signs to be taken on a patient every

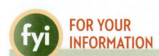
FOR YOUR INFORMATION

The terminology *patient access department* is commonly used to describe registration.

Patient rights acknowledgment A listing of guarantees that a patient should expect, including the right to privacy, the right to make one's own medical decisions, the right to refuse treatment, and the right to be treated fairly.

shift, but there is no documentation of it on the 3-11 shift on May 22, 2014, the conclusion drawn is that the vital signs of the patient were not taken during that shift.

Conditions of Participation Interpretive Guideline §482.24(c) states

The medical record must contain information such as notes, documentation, records, reports, recordings, test results, assessments, etc., to

- justify admission;
- justify continued hospitalization;
- support the diagnosis;
- describe the patient's progress;
- describe the patient's response to medications; and
- describe the patient's response to services such as interventions, care, treatments, etc.

The documentation of physicians and hospital staff must be sufficient to meet this regulation.

Initial Assessment of the Patient

An initial **nursing assessment** is performed after the patient reaches the care unit, or it is updated if started during a pre-admission visit. This assessment consists of a nursing history that includes the reason the patient is being seen or admitted, the course of events that led to the current encounter, the patient's general health status, and his or her past medical, surgical, family, and social histories. Particularly in senior patients, an important part of the social history is the patient's living arrangements, such as whether he or she has a support system to help with activities of daily living (bathing, dressing, getting meals, etc.). Following the history, an initial nursing physical is completed, which includes vital signs (height, weight, respiratory rate and pulse, temperature, blood pressure, blood oxygen level, and in recent years calculation of the patient's body mass index [BMI]). Also, a nursing physical exam may be completed for such issues as pain level, skin condition, and general appearance.

Nursing assessments must be completed within 24 hours of admission, as required by the Conditions of Participation (CoP) and The Joint Commission (TJC). If the health record is electronic, the form is completed using a template on the computer screen. Nurses in facilities using a paper record complete a paper form as the assessment is being performed. This may be the time at which a patient presents his or her completed **advance directive** or is asked whether he or she would like to complete one. A **property and valuables inventory** is also completed and documented during the assessment process.

Nursing and Ancillary Care and Documentation

Throughout a patient's stay, nursing staff enter documentation, including the following:

- Nursing notes: Generally, on each nursing shift there is documentation regarding the patient's status during that time—for instance, "Patient sleeping on rounds," "Patient sitting up in

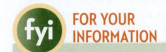

FOR YOUR INFORMATION

Every page in a health record (or on a computer screen) must identify the patient by name and by medical record number. In addition, each entry, whether written or electronic, must be timed, dated, and authenticated. Any written entries must be legible.

Nursing assessment The documentation of a nursing interview and exam performed immediately or shortly after admission that details information such as means of admission (by wheelchair, ambulatory, etc.), reason for admission, events leading to admission, presence of chronic conditions, current medications, drug allergies, person to contact in case of emergency, and whether the patient can perform typical activities of daily living.

Advance directive A document listing a patient's wishes, should he or she be unable to make decisions for him- or herself, or the naming of an individual who is authorized to do so.

Property and valuables inventory A listing of all the personal property (clothing, jewelry, prosthetic devices, wallet, money, etc.) the patient had on his or her person when arriving in the hospital room.

chair, no complaints offered," or "Dressing changed, wound dry." Some facilities use the **charting by exception** method for nursing documentation. The premise is that only unusual, unexpected, or abnormal findings are documented. Though charting by exception does not require as much time documenting, it does represent the patient's progress (or lack thereof) over the course of his or her stay. Nursing notes in an electronic health record (EHR) may be in narrative format, or documentation may be completed using a **template**. Figure 6.1 shows a bedboard based on the documentation entered in nursing templates.

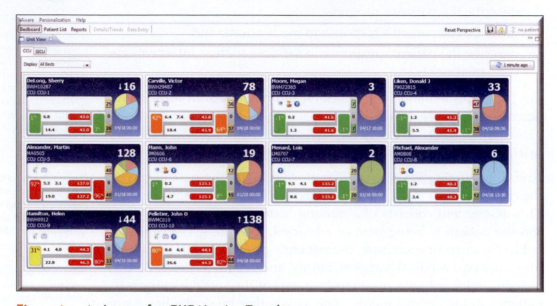

Figure 6.1   An Image of an EHR Nursing Template

- Record of vital signs: Throughout a patient's stay, vital signs are taken per the physician's order. Thus, if vital signs are ordered every four hours, the nurse or patient care technician takes and records the patient's vital signs on that schedule. A particular advantage of an EHR is that vital signs can be shown in graph form (Figure 6.2) to chart each vital sign over time. An impending infection of a patient who has undergone surgery may be readily apparent by a steadily increasing body temperature, as seen on the graph.

- **Medication Administration Record (MAR):** In a paper record, a nurse documents each time a medication is given, including the route of administration (such as orally or by injection, including the site), the time it was given, and the nurse's initials. The name of the medication, the dosage, and the times the medication is to be given are entered on the form as ordered by the physician. In an EHR, the process is much more efficient, because the MAR is a by-product of any medication orders given by the physician, which are entered electronically into the patient's EHR. This flow of data from one part of the EHR to another without human intervention minimizes the possibility of errors.

Other nursing documentation includes treatment records and records of input and output (I&O) as ordered by the physician. Each

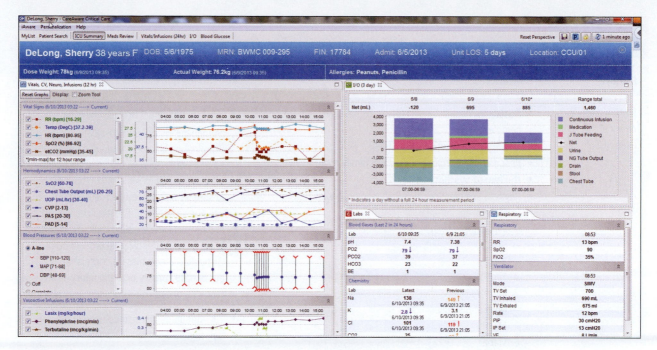

Figure 6.2   An Image of an EHR Screen Showing Graphed Vital Signs

entry must be signed and dated by the nurse (or patient care technician) making the entry. In an electronic system, this is done in real time based on the nurse's log-in credentials (user ID) and the date and time he or she saved the entry.

Physician Documentation

The patient's **attending physician** is ultimately responsible for the care of the patient while hospitalized. The attending physician may also be known as the *physician of record*. Other physicians, such as consultants, surgeons, **hospitalists** (physicians employed by the hospital and based in the hospital), radiologists, and pathologists, may also document in patients' records. In addition, the use of physician extenders, such as physicians' assistants (PAs) or nurse practitioners (NPs), is common. In teaching hospitals, the patient may also be seen by a medical resident or an intern. Regardless, a licensed MD or DO with privileges to practice at that facility must countersign (co-sign) the orders of the physician extender, medical student, resident, or intern.

Nothing can be done to or for a patient without a physician's (or designee's) order, including admission. Before the patient is taken to a hospital bed or a unit of the hospital, either an order is entered (written) by a physician or a **verbal order** is given to a nurse for the status of the patient. Statuses include admission (the patient needs inpatient care of an extended duration), **observation** (the patient needs monitoring and observation of 24–48 hours' duration, though time frames may vary by payer), or ambulatory surgery services. Physicians typically word these orders as "Admit to ICU," "Admit to observation," or "Admit to ambulatory surgery unit." The most common forms of documentation and the required timing are those in Table 6.1.

Attending physician The physician responsible for the care of the patient while hospitalized.

Hospitalist A physician, employed by a hospital and is typically a board-certified internist or family practitioner, responsible for admitting patients, following and assessing patients as needed, and writing orders as necessary.

Verbal order An order given to a nurse either in person or over the phone, then later authenticated by the physician or physician extender.

Observation A patient status used when the patient's condition does not warrant an inpatient level of care but does require observation by medical personnel. Observation typically lasts from 24 hours to no more than 48 hours.

Report	Contents	Specific Requirements
History and physical exam (H&P)	<ul><li>Reason for hospitalization (the patient's chief complaint)</li><li>**History of present illness (HPI)**</li><li>Past medical, surgical, social, and family histories</li><li>**Review of systems (ROS)**</li><li>Physical examination, including (as applicable) – General appearance – Vital signs – Skin – Head – Eyes – Ears – Nose and sinuses – Mouth – Throat – Neck – Chest – Breasts – Lungs – Heart – Abdomen – Genitourinary – Vaginal – Rectal – Musculoskeletal – Lymphatics – Neurologic</li><li>Admitting impression (admitting diagnosis or diagnoses)</li></ul>	<ul><li>The CoP regulation reads as follows: "A medical history and physical examination completed and documented no more than 30 days before or 24 hours after admission or registration, but prior to surgery or a procedure requiring anesthesia services. The medical history and physical examination must be placed in the patient's medical record within 24 hours after admission or registration, but prior to surgery or a procedure requiring anesthesia services."</li><li>TJC standards are in keeping with the CoP regulation.</li></ul>
Operative (procedure) note	<ul><li>Date(s) and time(s) of the surgery</li><li>Name(s) of the surgeon(s) and assistants or other practitioners who performed surgical tasks (even when performing those tasks under supervision)</li><li>Pre-operative and post-operative diagnoses</li><li>Name(s) of the specific surgical procedure(s) performed</li><li>Type of anesthesia administered</li><li>Complications, if any</li><li>A description of techniques, findings, and tissues removed or altered</li><li>Surgeons' or practitioners' names and a description of the specific significant surgical tasks that were conducted by practitioners other than the primary surgeon/practitioner (significant surgical procedures include opening and closing, harvesting grafts, dissecting tissue, removing tissue, implanting devices, and altering tissues)</li><li>Prosthetic devices, grafts, tissues, transplants, or devices implanted, if any</li><li>As with all entries, the time, date, and authentication</li></ul>	<ul><li>CoP: Dictated immediately following surgery</li><li>TJC standards require that the operative report be written or dictated on completion of the procedure and before the patient is transferred to the next level of care, which translates into immediately following the procedure.</li></ul>

Report	Contents	Specific Requirements
Physician's orders	• Orders must be in writing (handwritten or electronic) for admission, transfer, discharge, medications, treatments, diet, ambulation, restraints (including bed rails), and all diagnostic tests. Orders direct the nurses, therapists, and ancillary personnel what they need to do to or for the patient. • Patients may opt to leave the hospital without an order from a physician, which is known as leaving against medical advice (AMA).	• Orders are written (entered) by the physician or physician extender or entered into the patient's EHR. Orders may also be given verbally to a nurse or other staff member who is permitted to do so by hospital policy. • There are specific state licensure and CoP regulations regarding automatic stop orders (for instance, for narcotics) and use of standing orders (a physician's standard orders for certain procedures or diagnoses).
Physician progress notes	• Written (or entered) by physicians to reflect the patient's current status or response to treatment. Progress notes are typically written following a surgical procedure as well as at the time of discharge.	• No specific requirements other than the record must "document the course and results of care, treatment, and services; and promote continuity of care among providers" (Source: CMS), which is the premise of TJC as well.
Consultation reports	• Consultations are ordered by attending physicians when they are seeking an opinion (usually of a specialist) regarding the care and treatment of a patient. • Medical staff bylaws (policies) require the consultant to examine the patient and document his or her findings within a particular period of time. The result of the examination is documented in a consultation report, which must indicate that the patient's health record was reviewed and the patient was examined. The impression and opinion regarding treatment must be documented as well.	• No specific regulations, though the facility's own policies must be followed for timeliness

Discharge summary	• As the name implies, this report summarizes the patient's hospital stay. It is dictated by the attending physician, physician extender, or resident. It includes
	  – Reason for hospitalization
	  – Final diagnoses, including the principal diagnosis, any comorbidities, and/or complications
	  – Significant findings from tests or procedures
	  – Procedures performed
	  – Response to treatment
	  – Condition on discharge
	  – Discharge instructions, including medications, physical activity limitations, diet, and follow-up care
	• A discharge progress note may be substituted for a dictated summary for stays of less than 48 hours or in the case of normal newborns.
		• The CoP require that the medical record, including the final diagnosis, be complete within 30 days of discharge (or in the case of an outpatient, within 30 days of the encounter).
		• TJC standards also state that completion must occur within 30 days of discharge/encounter or in accordance with hospital policy or state licensure requirements, whichever is shorter.

Other Documentation

The documentation and requirements discussed in the previous section are the most common and are found in most health records. The following are required as applicable to individual cases.

Informed Consent

Patients who present to a hospital or other healthcare facility on their own are giving consent to treatment by the very act of presenting

History of present illness (HPI) The symptoms or circumstances leading the patient to seek medical intervention.

Review of systems (ROS) A system-by-system set of questions asked of a patient regarding symptoms he or she may be experiencing.

and requesting care. Still, a general consent to care is required if the patient is able to sign on his or her own. If not, a legal representative of the patient may sign. However, if waiting for someone to give consent for the patient may be detrimental, then care is administered without signed consent. This consent is a general, or blanket, consent form and covers routine care that would be provided to any patient.

An informed consent, on the other hand, is very specific and detailed. Informed consents are necessary when the patient will undergo any procedure that would carry a risk to the patient. In order to be "informed," the patient must be told the name(s) of the procedure(s) to be performed, the risks that may occur as a result of undergoing the procedure(s), any alternatives to having the procedure(s), and the likely outcome. Also, the patient must be informed that the performance of additional procedures may be necessary based on the findings of the original procedure. For instance, a laparoscopic cholecystectomy (removal of the gallbladder through the use of a scope) may need to be converted to an open procedure (through an incision). Another example is removal of a breast lump that is found to be malignant (cancerous)—the patient may have also consented to a lumpectomy or mastectomy.

In the event of a medical emergency (danger to life or limb), a legal representative may give informed consent for the patient.

Both the CoP and TJC address the need for a facility to require informed consent for any surgical procedure or as specified by facility policy.

Pathology

Hospital policy and/or medical staff bylaws identify the tissues or organs removed during a surgical procedure that must be microscopically and/or macroscopically (grossly) examined and diagnosed by a **pathologist**, a physician who examines and diagnoses the tissue or organ specimen. An example of a specimen that may not require pathological examination is a tooth extraction. The pathologist is responsible for providing documentation such as a description of the specimens received and examined and the pathological diagnosis for each.

Pathologists also perform **autopsies** and are responsible for documenting a summary of the events leading to the patient's death, the gross and microscopic findings, and the diagnoses as well as cause of death.

Anesthesia

There are many reports that result when patients undergo any type of anesthesia other than a local anesthetic. Documentation of each event becomes part of the patient's health record.

The pre-anesthesia assessment (see Figure 6.3) is completed by a nurse anesthetist or an anesthesiologist and includes past medical, surgical, family, and social histories; review of laboratory test results, electrocardiogram (EKG or ECG), and chest x-rays; and review of current medications. The patient is asked a series of questions to determine if there are any potential anesthesia risks. The recommended anesthesia method is explained to the patient, who then signs a consent to anesthesia, which becomes part of the health record.

Pathologist A physician whose specialty is dealing with the analysis of a tissue sample to establish a diagnosis.

Autopsy An examination performed after death to examine organs and tissue in order to determine cause of death.

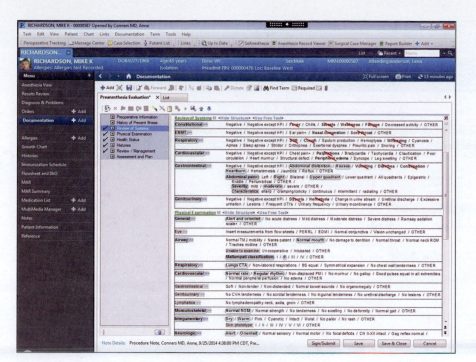

Figure 6.3 A Pre-anesthesia Assessment Screen in an EHR

During anesthesia, the report of anesthesia is compiled by a nurse anesthetist and/or anesthesiologist. It includes documentation of pre-operative medications, the anesthetic agent and dosage used during the procedure, the method used to administer it, and a constant record of the patient's vital signs during the procedure. Any fluid or blood loss during the procedure are documented, as well as the patient's condition during and at the conclusion of the procedure.

The patient is also assessed post-anesthesia before leaving the post-anesthesia care unit.

Post-anesthesia Care Unit

In the **post-anesthesia care unit (PACU)**, also referred to as the recovery room, a nurse oversees a patient as he or she becomes more alert following a procedure and anesthesia. The patient's condition and level of consciousness on arrival and discharge to/from the PACU are documented as is the status of any drains, infusions, or surgical dressings. The patient's vital signs are monitored throughout. Patients can be discharged (or transferred back to the inpatient bed) only upon order of the surgeon.

Imaging (Radiology)

Imaging is more commonly known as radiology. Techniques used to diagnose include plain films (x-rays), computerized axial tomography (CT scans), magnetic resonance imaging (MRI), ultrasound, nuclear medicine scans, and positron emission tomography (PET). Interventional radiology techniques are used to diagnose or treat disease—for example, epidural injections for pain management.

Specialists in this area are known as radiologists. A report (see Figure 6.4) of each procedure must be made a part of the patient's health record. It is dated, timed, and authenticated by the radiologist either electronically or by handwritten signature.

Post-anesthesia care unit (PACU) The unit to which a patient is transferred following surgery for monitoring of vital signs and condition post-surgery.

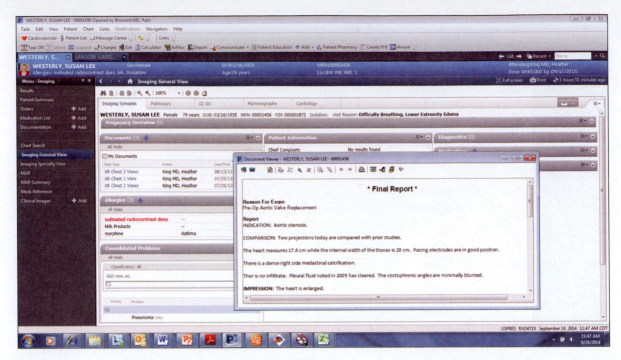

Figure 6.4   An Imaging (Radiology) Report in an EHR

Cardiology Diagnostics

An EKG or ECG is a tracing of the electrical changes in the heart. An EKG technician or nurse places electrodes on various parts of the body, which then provide a tracing of the heart's performance. Figure 6.5 depicts a typical tracing as seen in an EHR. A physician then interprets the tracing for any abnormalities and documents the findings.

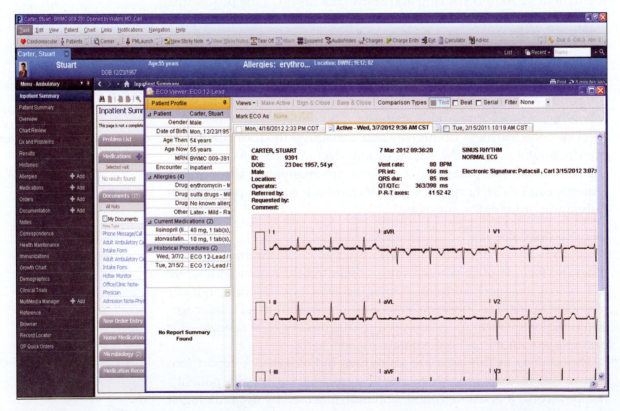

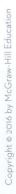

Figure 6.5   An EKG Tracing from an EHR

An echocardiogram is a specialized ultrasound used to diagnose multiple cardiac disorders, including diseases of the heart muscle, heart valves, and coronary arteries. There are different types of echocardiograms, and a physician is present during the procedure, as opposed to only a nurse or technician in the case of an EKG. The physician then writes or dictates a report, which is dated, timed, and authenticated.

Laboratory

Laboratory tests are done on blood and body fluids. Specialized areas include hematology, microbiology, blood chemistry, serology, and blood bank. Laboratory tests must be ordered by a physician; although most results are automated, the tests must be interpreted by a physician as well. Figure 6.6 is an example of a typical laboratory report.

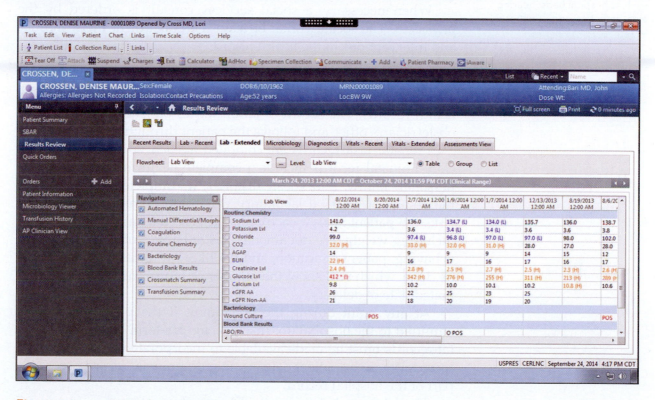

Figure 6.6 **An EHR Laboratory Report**

Rehabilitative Therapy

Rehabilitative medicine takes various forms—physical therapy, occupational therapy, and speech therapy, for example. Though a therapist may recommend the form of therapy, a physician's order is necessary for a patient to be assessed by a rehabilitation service and to begin therapy.

The therapist documents the initial evaluation of the patient, the goals of therapy, the techniques used, the patient's response to the treatment, and progress toward the goals.

Respiratory Therapy

Respiratory therapists analyze pulmonary function tests, administer and monitor oxygen, perform or assist patients with breathing treatments, and start and stop mechanical ventilation. A physician's order is needed before performing any of these tasks. Documentation includes the type, frequency, and duration of treatments; the dose of medication used; oxygen concentration; the time mechanical ventilation was started and stopped, as applicable; and the patient's response to treatment.

Social Services

Social services personnel may have a wide range of responsibilities from assisting the patient and family through personal issues or helping with post-discharge plans (for instance, nursing home placement) to working with an insurance company regarding coverage of **durable medical equipment (DME)** needs at home. These include such equipment as walkers, hospital beds, oxygen, and quad canes.

When necessary, a social services consult is ordered by the physician. The social worker or team then document their findings and interventions in the health record.

Durable medical equipment (DME) Medical equipment meant to be used for long periods, such as hospital beds, hearing aids, orthotics, and prostheses.

Obstetrics

Obstetrics records look very different from general medical/surgical health records. The record of an obstetrics patient is started in the obstetrician's office and follows the patient through the pregnancy.

Prenatal visit records are compiled at each visit to the obstetrician. Prenatal records include a complete health history, including personal, family, and social histories; a complete physical exam; the results of prenatal laboratory work; and an assessment of any risks the patient has. At each prenatal visit, the patient's vital signs, including weight, are documented, as are any problems the patient is having, patient education, and the like. An ultrasound will likely be done, which will show the number of fetuses as well as the estimated date of delivery.

At any point during the pregnancy, if the patient should be admitted to the hospital (for instance, for pre-term labor), the prenatal records must be made available to incorporate with the hospital record. When the patient delivers, the full prenatal record becomes a part of the hospital record.

The labor and delivery (L&D) record, as shown in Figure 6.7, contains very specific documentation from the time the patient is admitted until the completion of the delivery.

Postpartum documentation continues from the time of delivery through the patient's discharge.

Newborn

The newborn record includes the birth history, newborn physical exam, and nursing admission assessment. Often, the labor and delivery summary from the mother's record is made part of the newborn record as well. At one minute and five minutes after birth, the newborn is assessed for heart rate, respiratory rate, muscle tone, reflexes, and skin color—an assessment known as an **Apgar score** (see Figure 6.8). Documentation of any anomalies or medical problems determines the extent of documentation in the newborn's record.

Apgar score A newborn assessment done at one minute and five minutes after birth to assess the newborn's respiratory function, heart rate, muscle tone, reflexes, and skin color.

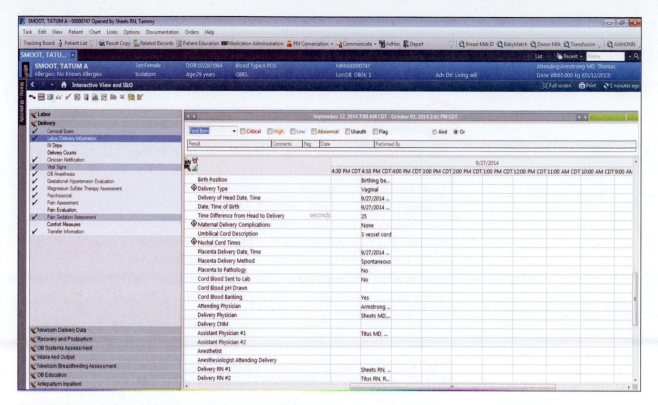

Figure 6.7   A Labor and Delivery Record in an EHR

Sign	0	1	2
Activity (muscle tone)	Absent/limp	Arms, legs flex, show some resistance to extension	Arms and legs actively moving and flexing
Pulse (heart rate)	Absent	Below 100 beats per minute	Above 100 beats per minute
Grimace (response to catheter in nostril after cleared)	No response	Facial grimace	Cough, sneeze, cry, pull away/resist
Appearance (skin color)	Blue, blue-gray, pale	Pink body, blue extremities	Completely pink/normal coloring all over body
Respiratory effort (breathing)	Absent	Slow, irregular, shallow	Good, sustained crying, regular breathing

Figure 6.8   Apgar Score Assessment

Special Care Units

Special care units in a hospital include the intensive care unit (ICU), cardiac care unit (CCU), neonatal intensive care unit (NICU), dialysis unit, hospice unit, and burn unit. Specialty units vary by facility. Each unit may have special documentation requirements as far as timeliness, which is dictated by facility policy.

Outpatient

The documentation described in the previous sections is typically seen in inpatient records. The CoP requirements for a medical record discussed at the beginning of this section also apply to outpatient records. Outpatient care may be an emergency department visit, ambulatory surgery, outpatient diagnostic testing, or outpatient treatment. Outpatient records are typically not as lengthy as inpatient records; however, the documentation in them justifies the reason for the encounter, supports the diagnosis, describes what was done to the patient, and the patient's response.

6.1 A DAY IN THE LIFE

Gerald Shaw has just been admitted for an elective (planned) surgical procedure. He had to go to the hospital a few days ago for lab tests and an x-ray and to meet with the anesthesiologist. He has gone through the admission process, which took about an hour and a half. He is sitting in his chair, shaking his head because it took so long, and now his nurse has entered the room to ask him still more questions. He is irritated and wants the nurse to explain why all these steps and questions are necessary.

1. If you were the nurse, how would you answer Mr. Shaw?

6.1 THINKING IT THROUGH

1. Explain why accuracy is such an important part of the registration process and how an error in the registration process could result in a patient safety issue.
2. For what reason(s) would a history and physical exam need to be completed before surgery begins?
3. Think of the last time you or a family member had been seen by a physician for something minor. Based on that encounter, describe your history of present illness as if you were describing it to a healthcare professional.

6.2 The Use of Clinical Electronic Tools in the Documentation of Healthcare

Computerized Physician Order Entry (CPOE)

Recall that all documentation in a health record must be legible. Handwritten physician orders were often difficult to read, and many phone calls were made to clarify what was actually written. **Computerized physician order entry (CPOE)** enables the physician to place orders electronically; each order is compared against a decision support system to ensure that the order is logical based on other data in the record; then the system sends the order on to the appropriate department (for instance, an order for a urinalysis would be sent to the laboratory). The user's log-in and password result in an automated date and time stamp and authentication. Nurses are able to enter orders on a physician's behalf when verbal orders are given—the order is entered through the nursing system and automatically notifies the ordering physician that verification and authentication are needed.

Computerized physician order entry (CPOE) Electronic means of ordering tests and medications that also provides clinical advice about the drug, the dosage, and any contraindications.

The following are some of the benefits of CPOE:

- At any given time, the status of an order is known to the physician and nursing staff—for instance, "pending physician authentication," "specimen collected," or "results ready."
- Orders do not get lost, which was not true of paper orders.
- Legibility is improved.
- In regard to medication orders, the system automatically checks for drug-to-drug interactions and drug allergies documented in the patient's record.
- Access is provided to clinical decision support systems for clinical guidance.
- Alerts are given for generic equivalents or less costly substitutes for high-cost drugs.

Results Management

Whereas CPOE is automation of the ordering process, results management systems quickly and efficiently provide the healthcare team with online results of diagnostic tests, as in the case of laboratory results. In a paper system, there is a delay in getting the results to the nursing units, because delivery may be made only once a shift. The exception would be for testing that is ordered STAT, which means immediately. Automation of results also includes the capability to flag results that are out of normal range and to display results in a graphic format to see change over time—in the patient's blood glucose level, for example.

Picture Archiving and Communication System (PACS)

The picture archiving and communication system, commonly known as PACS, digitizes radiology film into computer images. X-ray film takes a great deal of valuable floor space for storage, disposal is expensive, and duplication is time-consuming and labor-intensive, should films be needed by another physician or facility. With a PACS, images are stored on an optical disc and easily duplicated or transferred to another provider of care.

Automated Pharmacy Solutions

Gone are the days of counting pills by hand in a hospital pharmacy (or a retail pharmacy, for that matter), since the past two to three decades have seen advances in automated pharmacy systems. The efficiency of filling medication orders has improved through the use of an automated medication dispenser. In an automated system, a robot fills medication orders for each patient through an interface between the CPOE and the bar-coded medication inventory. Dispensing errors are all but eliminated, resulting in improved patient safety. The pharmacist spends less time verifying and approving dispensed drugs. The inventory process is improved, and the costs associated with the pharmacy as a whole are more controllable, because statistics are generated regarding usage, expiration dates, and quantities on hand.

I am Gary, the pharmacy director of a small rural, hospital. I am responsible for the procurement, storage, distribution, administration, and disposal of all medications used within the hospital. Best medication practices that were in their infancy in the early 1990s have been refined and are now commonplace in the hospital setting, regardless of the size of the hospital. Many professional and regulatory drivers have helped improve medication practices within our healthcare system due in part to a 1999 report by the Institute of Medicine, *To Err Is Human*. Practice standards are developed by interdisciplinary professional practice organizations, which define the safe use of medications, both in the community and in the hospital setting. The advances and refinements of technology have made it easier to implement better medication practices.

Automated Dispensing Cabinets, such as Pyxis®, AcuDose, and Omnicell, were initially used in the hospital setting as a way to improve inventory control and recoup lost pharmacy charges. Before that technology was available, pharmacies would have to create medication stock closets or rooms on each nursing unit, which served as the hospital's drug inventory after the pharmacy department had closed for the day. Nursing had to manually record in a log book the medications that were removed to satisfy new medication orders or first doses that were removed for new patient admissions. Nursing's focus has always been on direct patient care, and the pharmacy paperwork didn't always get done. But more importantly, nurses had access to all the medications in the drug closet or med room. There weren't any safety mechanisms in place to help ensure that the right medication was pulled and administered to the patient. Early Automated Dispensing Cabinets limited the nursing staff to the medication they were looking for, plus the other medications that were in the same unlidded, pocketed drawer, referred to as a matrix drawer. These drawers allowed for high capacity but low security. The early cabinets essentially functioned as glorified vending machines. More innovation was needed to improve the medication dispensing process.

Newer versions of the Automated Dispensing Cabinets incorporated additional technology as it became available. Later versions used less of the matrix-style drawers and instead incorporated smaller, pocketed drawers and mini drawers with fewer storage places per drawer. As more hospitals adopted electronic medical records, the cabinets were upgraded with two-way computer interfaces between the cabinet and the hospital's information system software. Through this interface, a patient's drug profile is tracked throughout the patient's admission. As medications are pulled from the Automated Dispensing Cabinet, the removal appears on the electronic medication administration record (eMAR) and allows nursing to chart the dose and route of administration in the medical record. Bar code and

(continued)

scanner capability has been added to the latest versions of the dispensing cabinets. All unit (single) doses of medication now include a bar code. Pharmacy technicians scan the bar code when they are refilling the cabinets, to reduce the possibility of incorrectly filling the pockets with the wrong medication. Nurses now scan the bar code on the patient's wrist band and the bar code on the medication during medication administration. This practice has greatly reduced some types of medication errors.

The very latest software in these cabinets is closely integrated with the hospital's health information system software. Pharmacy has moved from having to manually read and decipher physician orders to verifying medication orders sent through computerized physician order entry (CPOE) systems. Pharmacy reviews the order for contraindications with patient drug allergies and for any dosing adjustments that may be needed based on the patient's age, weight, or renal function. Once the pharmacist verifies the order in the computer system, the drug will appear on the patient's profile of the Automated Dispensing Cabinet closest to the patient's room. Nurses can then go to the dispensing cabinet and remove the medication that is specified in the medication order. After the patient's arm band is scanned and the drug is scanned, the computer system will electronically document the administration of the drug to the patient in his or her eMAR. All these steps are recorded in the patient's electronic health record corresponding to that patient's hospital admission.

Use of technology in documenting and verifying medication orders electronically greatly improves patient safety by making it easier for nurses to follow the seven rights of medication administration: Right Patient, Right Drug Route, Right Drug, Right Amount, Right Time, and Right Documentation, as well as documenting the Right to Refuse Treatment. These advances have also made it possible for pharmacists to become more active in direct patient care through activities such as patient education, medication reconciliation, and interdisciplinary medical team rounding. The increased presence of pharmacists on nursing units has been welcomed by patients, nurses, and the medical staff. The pharmacy department can keep better track of the drug inventory and monitor medication use throughout the hospital. Automated Dispensing Cabinets and the hospital health information computer systems have matured into technologies that have a positive impact on the care given to our patients.

6.2 THINKING IT THROUGH

1. Explain the process of CPOE.
2. Why might a provider like to see a graphic representation of a patient's results or vitals over time? Give an example.

Electronic Admission, Discharge, and Transfer System

Admission, discharge, and transfer (ADT) system
Electronic tracking of the registrations, admissions, discharges, and transfers occurring in a hospital at any given time. It is sometimes referred to as RADT (*R* for "registration").

The **admission, discharge, and transfer (ADT) system** is the electronic system that ties MPI data to the EHR and other systems within and outside the hospital. It is also the system that "admits" the patient, "transfers" the patient to another nursing unit or bed, and "discharges" the patient once the patient has left the nursing unit or other care unit (for outpatients). This is the database that interfaces with the laboratory, radiology, dietary services, or anesthesia documentation system. For instance, if a patient is discharged at 10:02 a.m. on February 7, 2014, the dietary department automatically updates, so that lunch and dinner trays need not be sent to the nursing unit for that patient. Also, housekeeping knows that a bed is empty and needs to be prepared for the next patient; once the bed has been prepared and housekeeping has changed that bed to "ready" status, the bed shows as being empty, and the ADT system can assign a new patient to that bed.

Patient census The number of inpatients occupying beds at any given time.

The ADT system also generates the **patient census** in real time. The census is a count of all patients currently occupying beds. For instance, if the hospital has 210 beds, and 200 patients are currently occupying beds, then the census is 200. The official census is typically taken at midnight but can also be seen whenever needed. For instance, the HIM staff may need to find the location of a patient if records from another facility have arrived and need to be taken to the nursing unit.

ADT reporting plays an important role in Meaningful Use. The automated reports are well standardized, and the files are relatively small and easy to transmit. Most importantly, however, they include timely clinical information. They are commonly exchanged to support transitions in care. For example, when a patient is admitted to or released from a hospital, the patient's status (admitted, transferred from one bed or unit to another, or discharged) is sent to his or her primary care physician and specialists. Alerts are also sent from emergency departments. These alerts keep the medical team in the loop concerning the patient's status.

Medical Transcription and Voice Recognition Technology

Recall that legibility of all documentation is a requirement of the Conditions of Participation and a standard of TJC, and most states' licensure regulations require documentation to be legible. In a paper record, this is often a difficult goal to attain, because much of the record is handwritten. Many reports are dictated by physicians and then transcribed by medical transcriptionists. As discussed in the chapters on the life cycle of health information and maintaining health records, the advent of voice recognition systems has resulted in a much more efficient process, and the medical transcriptionist's role has changed to that of an editor.

The use of an EHR has greatly improved documentation, mainly by standardizing what needs to be documented through prompts or specific templates. A nursing admission assessment template differs from a physical therapist's rehabilitation assessment, because they are different disciplines. Progress notes of any discipline may use a template system as well and improve the efficiency, completeness, and consistency of documentation. Though information is collected in template form, many EHR software systems have the option for the output to be in narrative form, which reads like a traditional note.

Concurrent Documentation Analysis and Improvement

An EHR allows health information staff to monitor the timeliness of required documentation concurrently (during the patient's stay) rather than waiting until discharge to perform quantitative analysis. For instance, at some point during the workday (or more than once) an HIM staff member may review the records of all admissions in the past 24 hours to ensure that a history and physical (H&P) has been dictated and is available on the patient's record. Or the operating room (OR) schedule may be reviewed to ensure that the H&P is a part of the health record before surgery.

The quality of the documentation may be reviewed by a CDI specialist or HIM staff during the stay, as noted in the life cycle of health information chapter.

Bar Coding

In a hybrid records management system, some records are electronic, and some are paper. Stray documents here and there will always be part of a records management system, even in a fully electronic system. The process used to merge the stray document(s) with the remainder of the EHR for a particular patient is called optical scanning, which was discussed in the life cycle of health information chapter. Healthcare facilities may opt to print labels that contain the patient's full name, medical record number, account number, and date of service and that contain a **bar code**, which is scanned using a wand or a gun-style reader like that seen in a grocery store (see Figure 6.9). Bar codes are often used to identify particular report types—H&P, consultation, operative report, discharge summary, nursing assessment, pathology report, and so on. Or as in Figure 6.9, a vial of blood has been bagged for transport and the bar code identifying the patient is being scanned. Placing the label with a bar code identifying the patient and specific encounter increases the likelihood that the document—or report associated with a lab test—is merged with the correct patient's EHR. Bar coding the type of report assists in retrieving the appropriate document when it is needed.

The health information management process for the medical team as well as those who compile and maintain health records has been greatly improved through the use of technology.

Bar code A machine-readable code consisting of vertical parallel bars and white space. Every scanned document contains a bar code identifying the patient and the encounter to which the document belongs. The bar code then matches that document to the correct patient and encounter within the EHR.

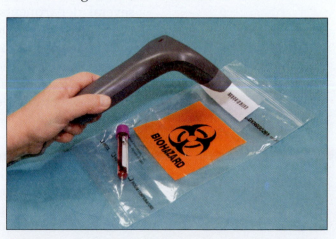

Figure 6.9 **A Bar Code Identifying the Patient to Whom a Blood Sample Belongs**

6.4 Integrating Clinical Systems in Acute Care Settings

Clinical Systems in Point of Care Workflow

Point of care The physical location where a healthcare professional delivers services to a patient.

The **point of care** in an acute setting can occur in a number of locations. An encounter can be in the emergency department, at a patient's bedside, in a clinic for a follow-up appointment, in a radiology clinic, or in any number of other places. The encounter in each of these locations has its own purpose and is supported by special equipment, and typically the services rendered are from specialized healthcare professionals.

This specialization in healthcare has complicated the use and sharing of health information across the delivery system. As described in the previous section, documentation originates from several departments. Historically, each department and specialty has evolved independently, resulting in "silos."

The term *silo* is a metaphor referring to the tendency for departments or groups to not share decision making with other entities and to make decisions based on their self-perceived interests. Silos result in inefficiency and decision making that may not be in the interest of the organization.

Siloed departments present a challenge in acute care settings, because information needs to be shared across departments and locations. Historically, this information was shared as a report in a paper format, as film, or as printed output from lab equipment, which becomes part of the paper record. These transactions often took days to complete and required numerous hand-offs of the patient's chart.

In a paper record system, each department and specialization also tends to develop its own workflow in the patient encounter, the processes for using equipment, and the methods for capturing the information in the medical record. These differences further contribute to the silo effect in acute care settings. Making changes in how health information is captured and shared between departments results in workflow changes. Almost always, these new methods result in resistance from some healthcare professionals and in inefficiencies while the changes are being adopted.

With the advent of HITECH and other healthcare reform initiatives, a major objective has been the introduction of integrated computerized clinical systems using digitized patient records. A standard EHR across all departments is the most important part of this process. While standardized, these EHRs may also provide modules for specializations with unique needs. For example, an obstetrician/gynecologist (OB/GYN) specialist collects different information than a primary care physician does when seeing a patient. EHR creators, therefore, have developed different templates, which appear as screens on the computer for each specialty. The most common specialized templates are for review of systems and care plans.

As depicted in Figure 6.10, all the departments and specialties in an acute care setting must be integrated into a single clinical system. Existing technologies and older (legacy) systems must come together in a single, new system. Integrating the existing and new systems requires customized work and is expensive and time-consuming. But the right information must get to the right place at the right time, and this requires a system developed around and supported by the EHR.

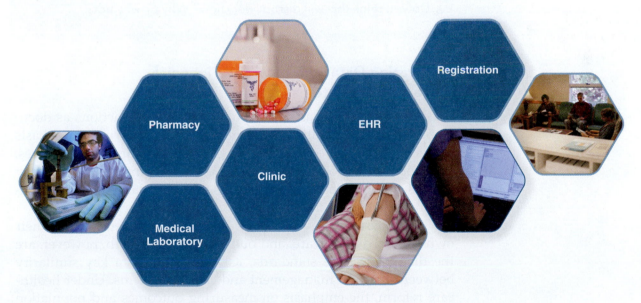

Figure 6.10 **The EHR Is Central to System-Wide Integration**

Standards in Information Flow and Exchange

As described earlier, healthcare has tended to evolve in silos of specialists and departments with their own technologies. As might be expected, the standards for the technologies used in these departments also evolved independently. These separate work spheres now need to be integrated into the larger system and work together. Labs, imaging, medical records, pharmacy, and other departments all use technologies with their own standards and software applications. These standards are detailed in the chapter on EHRs and Meaningful Use. What is important to understand is that the health information collected in these different departments and by different healthcare professionals must be integrated into the larger clinical system in order to support its exchange and use across a hospital setting. Within this process, data integrity must be maintained, security and privacy must be ensured, and data must be made usable across devices. The programs that allow for communication across these devices using different standards are called **interfaces**.

Interface A program that allows two or more similar or different devices to communicate and be interoperable.

6.4 — A DAY IN THE LIFE

Among their responsibilities, chief information officers (CIOs) are responsible for making decisions about the purchase, implementation, and use of information technology to support all the activities in a hospital. Marianne Johnson is the CIO for a large hospital that is implementing a new EHR system. She has to make sure that it can connect all the departments and work with the parts of the existing system that they are going to keep.

1. What makes this process difficult?
2. How should she explain the process to the clinicians and other workers?
3. Do you think this will disrupt workflow? Why or why not?

Integrating Data in Clinical and Financial Management Systems

The medical record has a dual purpose. First, it functions as documentation used for patient's treatment. Second, it serves as the basis for reimbursement for services provided from insurance companies, CMS, or others. Documentation and treatment are encompassed by clinical systems. Reimbursement falls under the larger area of financial management systems.

These systems have also developed independently with their own standards, software, and output. Central to both, however, are the diagnostic code standards, ICD-9/10. This is a key similarity between financial management and clinical systems. Under healthcare reform, the emphasis on measuring outcomes and population health as the basis for reimbursement will require a closer integration between clinical and financial management systems.

Claims data Billing codes that physicians, pharmacies, hospitals, and other healthcare providers submit to payers. These data have the benefit of following a relatively consistent format and of using a standard set of ICD-9/10 codes.

EHRs can allow a provider access to data from financial management systems, or **claims data**. This has jumpstarted the process of bringing these two systems together. When used in conjunction with the clinical data record, claims data can provide a more complete picture of treatment, patient adherence, medicine reconciliation, medical history, and additional information.

In the coming years, there will be movement toward greater integration of claims and clinical data in health information management, driven by changes in reimbursement policies and the additional value added to the patient record by the data. A major step in the integration was slotted under Meaningful Use Stage 2 with the requirement that the clinical diagnosis be input into an EHR using the clinical terminology standard of Systematized Nomenclature of Medicine—Clinical Terms (SNOMED-CT), which will be automatically converted into ICD-10 through translation engines. Although, at the time of this writing, the governmental delay of ICD-10 has put this step on hold, providers are still evolving their systems to allow for the use of a standard clinical terminology. The result will be a rich clinical vocabulary that is used for diagnosis and translated into an equally rich diagnostic code for financial management and analysis.

6.4 THINKING IT THROUGH

1. Why is ICD-9/10 the connecting factor between health records and financial management?
2. Describe the difference between claims data and clinical data. Are there ways that they can be used together?

chapter 6 summary

LEARNING OUTCOMES	CONCEPTS FOR REVIEW
6.1 Describe the flow of health information in an acute care setting. Pages 146–158	<ul><li>The first step of information flow lies with the registration process.</li><li>Accuracy of the MPI and one master file per patient is important in locating the correct patient and providing the past history of the correct patient.</li><li>Clinical documentation is entered by the physicians, nurses, therapists, and other healthcare professionals.</li><li>CoP and TJC have specific requirements for the content and timeliness of each type of documentation.</li><li>Documentation on most records includes<ul><li>Nursing assessment</li><li>Advance directive (optional)</li><li>Property and valuables list</li><li>Nursing notes</li><li>Medication Administration Record (MAR)</li><li>Record of vital signs</li><li>History and physical (H&P)</li><li>Physicians' orders</li><li>Physician progress notes</li><li>Operative note (if applicable)</li><li>Consultation reports (if applicable)</li><li>Discharge summary</li></ul></li><li>Informed consent (if applicable)</li><li>Pathology report (if applicable)</li><li>Anesthesia records (if applicable)</li><li>Imaging reports</li><li>Cardiology diagnostic reports</li><li>Laboratory reports</li><li>Rehabilitative therapy notes (if applicable)</li><li>Respiratory therapy notes (if applicable)</li><li>Social services notes (if applicable)</li><li>Specialty records<ul><li>Obstetrics documentation</li><li>Newborn record</li><li>Special care unit (ICU, CCU, NICU) records</li></ul></li><li>Outpatient (ambulatory) records relate the content and time requirements for each type of document.</li></ul>

LEARNING OUTCOMES	CONCEPTS FOR REVIEW
6.2 Describe electronic tools used by clinicians to document in the health record. Pages 158–161	• Describe computerized physician order entry (CPOE) and how it improves healthcare. • Describe results management software and how it improves healthcare. • The picture archiving communication system (PACS) and its advantages in the imaging department • Automated pharmacy solutions that improve patient care and safety
6.3 Contrast electronic tools used in the records management process. Pages 161–164	• State the purpose of automated admission, discharge, and transfer (ADT) systems. • Describe the patient census. • How does the ADT automated reporting satisfy Meaningful Use and how does it aid in the efficient running of the facility? • Describe how concurrent analysis of documentation improves patient care. • What role does bar coding play in an electronic system?
6.4 Classify technologies used in the integration of health information in acute care settings. Pages 164–167	• Explain what is meant by "point of care." • What is meant by "silos" of documentation? • What is meant by an "interface"? • Why do clinical data need to integrate with financial data?

chapter review

MATCHING QUESTIONS

Match each term with its definition.

_____ 1. **[LO 6.1]** nursing assessment

_____ 2. **[LO 6.1]** Apgar score

_____ 3. **[LO 6.1]** durable medical equipment

_____ 4. **[LO 6.4]** interfaces

_____ 5. **[LO 6.1]** MAR

_____ 6. **[LO 6.3]** patient census

_____ 7. **[LO 6.2]** STAT

_____ 8. **[LO 6.1]** verbal order

_____ 9. **[LO 6.1]** template

_____ 10. **[LO 6.4]** claims data

_____ 11. **[LO 6.1]** charting by exception

_____ 12. **[LO 6.1]** observation

_____ 13. **[LO 6.1]** ROS

_____ 14. **[LO 6.1]** attending physician

_____ 15. **[LO 6.1]** autopsy

a. Postmortem exam conducted to determine a cause of death

b. Doctor on record as being in charge of a patient's in-hospital care

c. Situation in which a patient is in need of monitoring but his or her condition is not critical or severe enough to warrant inpatient hospitalization

d. Roster of all currently occupied beds

e. Documentation format that records only unusual or abnormal findings

f. Data gathered from bills submitted to insurance carriers seeking payment for services rendered

g. Programs that allow two or more devices to communicate with one another

h. Assessment that tracks newborn development in the first minutes after birth.

i. Order that means "immediately"

j. Record of each time a medication was given and by what route

k. General health assessment based on the patient's responses to symptoms he or she experiences by body areas, such as musculoskeletal and respiratory symptoms

l. Items, such as canes or walkers, that make it easier for a patient to function and live at home

m. Preformatted document that identifies where standard information is supposed to go; it makes documentation quicker

n. Preliminary, noncare provider exam done within 24 hours of admission

o. Request given to a nurse without paper documentation

MULTIPLE CHOICE QUESTIONS

Choose the letter that best completes the statement or answers the question.

16. **[LO 6.1]** Who is responsible for performing autopsies and documenting findings regarding a patient's death?
    a. Attending physician
    b. Pathologist
    c. Surgeon
    d. Hospitalist

17. **[LO 6.1]** What is a PACU?
    a. A consent form a patient signs before a surgery
    b. An equipment code used by insurance companies
    c. A room in which patients are allowed to recover after surgery
    d. The room where CTs and MRIs are processed and viewed

18. **[LO 6.1]** Where will a patient's name appear in his or her health record?
    a. On the front page
    b. On every page
    c. On pages that address the patient specifically
    d. On pages that reference the patient's treatments

19. **[LO 6.1]** Which is the best example of charting by exception?
    a. Patient complained of sharp pain at the incision site.
    b. Patient was given 10 mg albuterol as ordered.
    c. Patient was resting comfortably; vitals normal.
    d. Patient indicated no pain or itching near stitches.

20. **[LO 6.1]** Brian Christie is a physician's assistant at County Hospital. Brian would be known as
    a. an attending physician.
    b. a hospitalist.
    c. an intern.
    d. a physician extender.

21. **[LO 6.1]** Which documentation must be completed within 30 days of an occurrence?
    a. Consultation report
    b. Discharge summary
    c. History and physical exam
    d. Physician's order

22. **[LO 6.2]** What is the function of an advance directive?
    a. Tells the nurse which tests to perform
    b. Serves as a listing of patients' wishes if they are unable to communicate them
    c. Details all previous medical physicals
    d. Lists all personal property that the patient took to the hospital

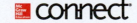 Enhance your learning by completing these exercises and more at http://connect.mheducation.com!

23. **[LO 6.2]** How are pharmacy prescriptions typically filled today?
    a. Hand-counted by the pharmacist
    b. Automatically counted using a robot
    c. Automatically counted with a machine
    d. Scanned and counted via a bar code

24. **[LO 6.2]** A results management system would most likely be used for
    a. viewing lab tests.
    b. filling prescriptions.
    c. reading x-rays.
    d. tracking vital signs.

25. **[LO 6.3]** The _____ system ties MPI data to a patient's EHR.
    a. ADT
    b. bar coding
    c. PACS
    d. medical transcription

26. **[LO 6.3]** An EHR has improved documentation mainly through its
    a. elimination of legibility issues.
    b. quickly downloadable format.
    c. standardization of information.
    d. capability of sending status alerts.

27. **[LO 6.4]** The key to eliminating silos in acute care settings is
    a. adopting an electronic health record system.
    b. hiring a vendor to streamline departments.
    c. moving to a centralized registration process.
    d. taking advantage of HITECH incentive funds.

28. **[LO 6.4]** A program that allows for communication across two or more similar devices is
    a. a template.
    b. a CPOE.
    c. an interface.
    d. a verbal order.

SHORT ANSWER QUESTIONS

29. **[LO 6.1]** What does MPI stand for? What is the MPI's role in registration?

30. **[LO 6.1]** List what each part of a newborn's Apgar score measures.

31. **[LO 6.1]** Why do you think it is necessary to document the items a patient has with him or her on a patient property and valuables form?

32. **[LO 6.2]** What are the benefits of computerized physician order entry (CPOE)?

33. **[LO 6.2]** Besides CPOE, explain at least one other clinical electronic tool used in healthcare.

34. **[LO 6.3]** How do ADT documents influence transition in care?

35. **[LO 6.3]** Explain concurrent documentation, and give at least one of its benefits.

36. **[LO 6.4]** Give an example of the type of encounter that might occur at a patient's bedside.

37. **[LO 6.4]** What is a legacy system?

APPLYING YOUR KNOWLEDGE

38. **[LO 6.1]** Discuss the importance of informed consent. Conduct an Internet search on a recent case involving informed consent regulations, and summarize the outcome of the case.

39. **[LO 6.2]** Of the CPOE benefits listed in the text, which one do you believe serves the greatest purpose in healthcare? Explain, using examples as needed.

40. **[LO 6.2, 6.3]** This chapter discusses some of the tremendous benefits of improving technology in healthcare. However, some feel that there is a "dark side" to this increased reliance on technology. What is your response to that—are they right, or are their concerns unfounded? Explain, giving examples.

41. **[LO 6.4]** This chapter discussed the concept of silos, saying that they result in inefficiency and decision making that may not be in the best interest of the organization. Create a scenario that shows how working in silos is a poor way of operating a hospital. Suggest a way to remove the "silo-ing" and have interhospital departments work together.

42. **[LO 6.1, 6.2, 6.3, 6.4]** Evaluate the reasons for pushback and resistance to EHRs and other healthcare technologies, especially with the knowledge of how many benefits these technologies bring to acute care settings.

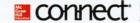

Enhance your learning by completing these exercises and more at http://connect.mheducation.com!

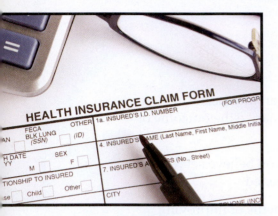

The Post-discharge Health Record

When you finish this chapter, you will be able to:

7.1 Document the elements of the HIPAA designated record set (DRS) and the legal health record.

7.2 Explain required quality assessment activities in healthcare.

7.3 Discuss the role of data in risk management activities.

7.4 Explain payment models used by government and commercial insurance plans.

7.5 Diagram the reimbursement cycle in healthcare.

Key Terms

Accountability measures

Allowed charges

Ambulatory Payment Classifications (APCs)

Benchmarking

Case mix index (CMI)

Copy (cut) and paste

Core measurement system

Designated record set (DRS)

Health plan

Hospital Acquired Conditions (HAC)

Hospital Quality Initiative

Hospital Readmission Reduction Program (HRP)

Hospital Value-Based Purchasing (VBP)

Incident (occurrence) report

Lifetime reserve days

Medicare Severity Diagnosis Related Group (MS-DRG)

Medicare Shared Savings Program (MSSP)

Outlier

Outpatient Prospective Payment System (OPPS)

Peer review

Peer Review Organizations (PROs)

Pioneer ACO Program

Plan, Do, Check, Act (PDCA)

Plan, Do, Study, Act (PDSA)

Pre-authorization

Premium

Present on Admission (POA)

Professional Standards Review Organizations (PSROs)

Provider network
Qualitative analysis
Quality Improvement Organizations (QIOs)
Resource-based relative value scale (RBRVS)
Risk management

Scope of work (SOW)
Six Sigma
Spell of illness
TRICARE
Utilization management

Introduction

The measurement of quality, the prevention and management of risk, and the fiscal success of a healthcare facility are tied to the health record. The health record staff is responsible for ensuring that data, such as coded data, used in quality assessment, risk management, and reimbursement are timely, accurate, complete, and valid. Health information professionals often hold positions in these areas or work closely with those who do.

7.1 The HIPAA Designated Record Set and Legal Health Record

The HIPAA Designated Record Set

As required in the HIPAA privacy rule, patients and/or their authorized designee(s) have a right to access their health information and may request an amendment to their health information. The rule further defines the portions of the patient's health information to which this pertains. This is known as the **designated record set (DRS)** and is defined in the HIPAA regulations:

- Any group of any records maintained by a covered entity including:
  - Patients' medical and billing records as maintained by (or for) the healthcare provider
  - Enrollment, payment, claims adjudication (determination of whether the plan will pay and the amount), and case management or medical management record systems maintained by or for a health plan
  - Medical records that are used in whole or in part by the covered entity to make decisions about individuals.

A covered entity is any **health plan** (insurance or third-party payer), clearinghouse (an entity that verifies that coded diagnoses and procedures are valid and in the proper format), or healthcare provider who stores, processes, and transmits any identifiable health information electronically.

Designated record set (DRS) As defined by HIPAA, any records maintained by a covered entity that are used for patient care or to make payment decisions, such as health records, billing records, insurance enrollment records, insurance claims, and coverage decisions.

Health plan A health insurance company that reimburses for medical care in all or in part.

7.1 A DAY IN THE LIFE

Linda, a HIM release of information coordinator at Memorial Hospital, is helping a former patient, Roberta Lam, who was hospitalized at Memorial Hospital from June 4, 2013, to June 5, 2013. Mrs. Lam tells Linda that her insurance company has denied payment for that stay,

(continued)

and she wants a copy of her record. Linda explains to Mrs. Lam that she may have a copy of her record, and since it is in electronic format, she can have it electronically and/or as a paper copy. Mrs. Lam prefers the paper copy. Linda explains the authorization form to Mrs. Lam, which she signs. The patient shares with Linda that she just does not understand why the insurance company would deny the payment. Linda suggests that she contact her insurance company and informs her that, like her health records, she may also request information from her insurance company, including the coverage decision.

1. What help will Mrs. Lam's health record be in discussing the reason for the denial of payment?

It is necessary to define the designated record set because there are other records maintained by a provider or hospital that contain identifiable patient information to which the patient does not have access and cannot request an amendment. For instance, in the Day in the Life scenario, perhaps the health record of that encounter was selected for an internal audit by the quality assurance department; Mrs. Lam would not have access to the record of the audit. Healthcare organizations must have the definition of their designated record set in health information policies.

The Legal Health Record

The legal health record, which we first discussed in the chapter on maintaining health records, is a bit more complicated than the DRS. It is the information available to physicians, nursing staff, and ancillary staff on which diagnostic and treatment decisions are made, as opposed to what is protected by the HIPAA privacy rule in the case of the DRS. Hospitals and providers must include their definition of the legal health record in facility policy. Whatever the definition, the legal health record must be readily accessible wherever and whenever it is needed, and it must be made available only to the staff and providers needing access. While it stands to reason that the health information compiled by the facility during the patient's encounter would be included in the definition, there are other records that need to be considered as being (or not being) a part of the facility's legal health record, such as all types of media.

When considering the definition of the legal health record, it should be remembered that the legal health record is the official business record of the facility. In addition, the purpose of the health record should be acknowledged. AHIMA, in its practice brief *Fundamentals of Legal Health Record and Designated Record Set*, states

The legal health record serves to:
- *Support the decisions made in a patient's care*
- *Support the revenue sought from third-party payers*
- *Document the services provided as legal testimony regarding the patient's illness or injury, response to treatment, and caregiver decisions*
- *Serve as the organization's business and legal record*

These tenets of a legal health record will influence a facility's definition. A work group or team made up of the HIM director, the IT director, members of the medical staff, the chief nursing officer, and ancillary departments should define the legal health record and need to answer the following questions:

- Are records received from other facilities part of the legal health record?

- Will miscellaneous records that have been presented to the facility become part of the legal record? Examples include patients' Personal Health Records (PHRs) and records that other facilities have sent through a health information exchange (HIE).

- What media types will be included in the legal health record? The inclusion of paper, EHR, images (such as radiology), records maintained in the pharmacy system, tracings, video, and voice recordings all need to be addressed in the definition.

- How will the records of disparate electronic systems, such as the main EHR, laboratory, pathology, anesthesiology, or radiology, be handled?

- How will the facility handle hybrid records (the records of a patient that are still in paper format)?

- How will storage be handled, particularly in an electronic environment? Long-term storage, changes in storage media, and storage costs need to be considered.

In the process, the team must also consider applicable federal and state laws governing health records and privacy. State laws vary regarding the keeping of and access to particularly sensitive information, such as substance abuse and behavioral health records. Also, the retention and destruction policies need to be assessed when the discussion of storage is undertaken.

Information Governance

When defining the legal health record, a facility also needs to consider information governance—who will be responsible for ensuring that only complete information is released or abstracted, and who will track and document the external release of patient information? When statistical reports are required that include diagnostic, procedural, or demographic data, who within the facility will be responsible for providing the reports? Information governance has to do with integrity— the integrity of the documentation itself, how it is stored, how the information is used, by whom, when, and under what circumstances.

The legal health record and designated record set determine how information may be appropriately released. Although it is easy to declare something, such as an EKG WAVE file, as part of the legal health record or designated record set, the organization must consider methods of reproduction; if the file type is not reproducible, consideration should be given to excluding it from the DRS. These decisions are made by a team of individuals who are knowledgeable in technology, legal aspects, compliance, and health record content. Often, this team is led by health information and health IT professionals in the organization.

1. Why might a patient be denied access to documentation that pertains to the him/her, but that is not part of his/her health record?
2. If a healthcare facility has defined the designated record set, why would the facility also need an official definition of the legal health record?

7.2   The Health Record in Assessing Quality

The assessment of quality—whether it is the quality of patient care or the quality of documentation—is of paramount importance in healthcare. As we have seen thus far, the documentation found in a health record is considered proof of the care given to a patient. Quality is assessed internally, through quality assessment and improvement programs, and externally, by outside agencies and auditors. Health information professionals play a key role in the assessment of quality. HIM personnel are responsible for the assignment of coded data in the form of diagnosis and procedure codes using ICD-9 or 10-CM/PCS, CPT, and HCPCS. When quality is assessed, internally or externally, or data are studied, this coded healthcare information is often the starting place. Because of their knowledge of medicine and clinical processes, health information professionals are able to organize data and present them in a way that is meaningful.

Imagine that a surgeon has asked the hospital to spend a million dollars on a new, state-of-the-art piece of equipment for performing cholecystectomies. The hospital's governing board is not going to approve that expenditure without knowing how many patients might benefit from the acquisition of this new equipment and the potential reimbursement for the procedure, which would pay for the equipment in a reasonable period of time. Thus, a staff member in health information may be asked to prepare a presentation showing the number of cholecystectomies (laparoscopic and open) performed for each year over the past five years, sorted by zip code and surgeon, as well as the reimbursement received for each. Health information professionals understand the flow of information throughout the facility, as well as data sources within the facility, and therefore would be able to quickly gather the necessary data to answer the governing board's questions.

Internal Quality Assessment

Quality of Documentation and Health Information Functions

Assessing the quality and completeness of the content in documentation is known as **qualitative analysis**. This type of analysis differs from quantitative analysis, which was covered in the management of health information chapter. Quantitative analysis is a review that ensures that all required reports and signatures are present, whereas qualitative analysis is focused on the content of each report. An operative report that does not contain a patient's

Qualitative analysis A review of documentation to ensure that it is complete, thorough, and accurate.

post-operative diagnosis or the fact that during the procedure the patient's blood pressure rose significantly (as noted in the anesthesia documents) is not quality documentation. Quality analysis may be performed by health information personnel or by personnel in the quality assessment and improvement department. The quality of the documentation—that is, whether the documentation is complete, thorough, and accurate—may be a reflection of the quality of care provided a given patient or patients.

Health information–specific quality assessments occur on a regular basis, particularly in the MPI database. Several examples of common health information quality control measures include the following:

- Looking for duplicate patient entries or incomplete entries
- Ensuring accurate code assignment
- Checking that codes assigned are substantiated by the documentation found in records
- Verifying that records are coded completely

Medical transcription should be an area that is audited for quality on a regular basis. Both means of medical transcription need to be assessed for quality—transcription performed the traditional way, via dictation/transcription, and transcription done via state-of-the-art voice recognition systems in which transcription occurs automatically as a physician dictates a report and the transcriptionist is an editor. Transcriptionists usually monitor their own work as a front-end quality check. An error in dictation or transcription could mean an adverse outcome for the patient.

For example, consider the drugs Actos and Actonel; their names sound similar, but the drugs are very different and might be transcribed incorrectly. Actos is an antidiabetic drug, and Actonel is used to prevent and treat osteoporosis. If a patient is indeed a diabetic taking Actos and the documentation in the history and physical exam reads "Actonel," and is used as the basis for other documentation in the record, that transcription error might lead to a medication error. This type of error can cause the patient harm and lead to legal issues. Should that patient file a lawsuit against the physician or hospital, this documentation error might lead the jury to question the quality of care in general if such an error went unnoticed. Medical errors such as these are known as errors of communication, since the content of the history and physical exam (H&P) was dictated by a physician and, either by human error or computer error, was incorrectly documented in the health record, which, if not caught immediately, is then incorrectly communicated to other members of the healthcare team.

Another example of internal quality review is the review of a filing system. In a manual system, filing quality should be assessed on a regular basis. Hundreds of records may go into and out of file each day, and folders are easily misfiled. Ongoing monitoring and assessment of the files should be a routine task.

The use of electronic health records is changing quality assessment methods. Digital patient records may be reviewed with software programs that identify completeness and accuracy and support in-depth analysis—including factors involving quality of care. A factor that has recently become a focus is so-called copy and paste of patient health information, which is the copying of data into an EHR that were collected in a previous encounter or from an earlier document in the same encounter. Copy and paste can lead to note bloat—documenting more than actually applies to the current encounter, such as past medical problems that no longer exist but are being carried forward to future encounters.

Let's say Jared's record from two years ago reflects a diagnosis of mononucleosis. The physician seeing Jared today copies and pastes mononucleosis into the current problem list in Jared's EHR. The fact that it is documented on the current encounter will result in that condition being coded and thus the claim form will reflect it. Even if no treatment is directed at the mononucleosis on the current encounter, that piece of data is not accurate for *this* encounter; therefore, the integrity of the data as a whole is brought into question. You can imagine the implications for patient care and safety if any information from previous encounters is copied and pasted into current records.

External Quality Assessment Initiatives

Regulatory Requirements

Healthcare facilities must have a formal quality assessment and improvement program (also known as quality assessment) if they are accredited by The Joint Commission. Also, to satisfy CoP regulations, "hospital[s] must develop, implement, and maintain an effective, ongoing, hospital-wide, data-driven quality assessment and performance improvement program."

The federal government's quality initiatives date back to the inception of Medicare (and consequently, the CoP), which requires that any hospital that bills Medicare or Medicaid perform "audits" of care, or quality assessment. A review of the appropriateness of admission and hospital services is also required and is known as **utilization management**. **Professional Standards Review Organizations (PSROs)** contracted with the federal government to perform periodic utilization and quality audits or to do ongoing audits for hospitals that did not adequately do so themselves. The PSROs were replaced with **Peer Review Organizations (PROs)** in the early 1980s as a result of the Tax Equity and Fiscal Responsibility Act of 1982, known more commonly as TEFRA.

In 2002, PROs were renamed **Quality Improvement Organizations (QIOs)**. QIOs, which contract with individual states, are private, not-for-profit entities that employ physicians, nurses, health information professionals, and administrators to focus on improving quality of care and utilization of hospital services for targeted conditions, services or safety issues, or other areas of concern—for instance, coordination of care, as spelled out in what is known as a **scope of work (SOW)**. The SOW changes every three years (the current, tenth SOW went into effect on August 1, 2011), and with each SOW, the projects or targeted areas change. The basis of QIOs is the concept of **peer review**, which takes place when the members

---

Copy (cut) and paste The copying of data from a previous encounter that may or may not be accurate for the current encounter.

Utilization management The review and management of the appropriateness of admissions and facility services.

Professional Standards Review Organizations (PSROs) Organizations charged with monitoring the medical necessity of hospital admissions and the quality of care rendered to Medicare and Medicaid patients.

Peer Review Organizations (PROs) Organizations that replaced PSROs to perform medical necessity and quality of care monitoring.

Quality Improvement Organizations (QIOs) Organizations that replaced PROs to perform monitoring of necessity of services, quality of services, coding of diagnoses and procedures, and adequacy of prospective payments for Medicare and Medicaid patients.

Scope of work (SOW) The work plan for QIOs, which changes every three years, intended to improve the efficiency, effectiveness, economy, and quality of services provided to Medicare and Medicaid patients.

Peer review The review of a professional's work by another in the same profession or specialty. For example, a registered nurse specializing in orthopedic nursing is not a peer of a registered nurse specializing in obstetrics and does not qualify to perform a peer review of the orthopedic nurse's work.

of a profession (in this case, physicians) review and make recommendations or decisions concerning another's work.

An example is the review (by a physician) of a health record to determine if a pacemaker insertion was justified, based on that documentation. If not supported, then the pacemaker insertion was not medically necessary and payment is subsequently denied. The mission of the QIOs as stipulated in legislation is to improve the efficiency, effectiveness, economy, and quality of services provided to Medicare and Medicaid beneficiaries.

Though not regulatory, the CMS **Hospital Quality Initiative** includes Hospital Compare data, which are available to the public online through a website (see Figure 7.1). Reporting in this case is accomplished by surveying discharged patients regarding their experiences in US hospitals. The surveys include questions about the patients' impression such factors as nursing and physician communication, pain control, explanation of ordered medications, facility cleanliness, and the likelihood they would recommend that hospital, among others.

CMS also gathers data to report (by hospital) readmissions, complications, and deaths; the timeliness and effectiveness of care by certain diagnoses; and the use of medical imaging. Also, Hospital Compare includes the ratio of Medicare spending per Medicare patient. For example, if Hospital A's ratio of Medicare spending per Medicare patient is 0.95 and Hospital B's ratio is 0.98, and the national average ratio is 0.97, then Medicare spends less per patient

Hospital Quality Initiative
A program developed by the Department of Health and Human Services to ensure "quality health care for all Americans through accountability and public disclosure."

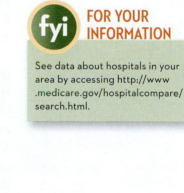

FOR YOUR INFORMATION

See data about hospitals in your area by accessing http://www.medicare.gov/hospitalcompare/search.html.

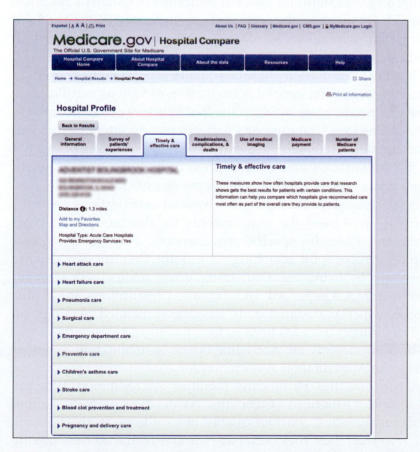

Figure 7.1 Hospital Compare Provides Accessible Quality Information

in Hospital A than it does for patients in Hospital B. This initiative is central to future healthcare reform. The digitization of patient records and the Meaningful Use program are designed to start measuring the value of care delivered by going beyond simply measuring the volume of what is delivered. In the reimbursement section of this chapter, the significance of these data will be further explained.

Accrediting Agency Quality Initiatives

The Joint Commission uses a **core measurement system** to assess quality of care by diagnosis—for instance, myocardial infarction (MI), hip replacement, or congestive heart failure. In addition, The Joint Commission (TJC) process improvement measures include **accountability measures** and non-accountability measures. The accountability measures are based on four criteria, the results of which are used for purposes of proving accountability to external bodies—for example, to prove compliance with accreditation standards, for public reporting, or to insurers that base payment on performance. Non-accountability measures are used within the healthcare organization to assess quality, to provide continuing education of staff, and are a good basis on which to gauge appropriate patient care. (The Joint Commission, 2014). To give one example, three of the seven Joint Commission 2013 accountability measures for the treatment of MI were aspirin given upon arrival, discharged on an aspirin regimen, and prescription of a beta-blocker drug at discharge. For an example of an individual hospital's information measured against state and national indicators in Quality Check, see Figure 7.2. Quality Check is a search engine, powered by The Joint Commission, that allows healthcare consumers to search for TJC-accredited institutions.

The Joint Commission publishes quality reports for its accredited institutions regarding general accreditation as well as certifications in disease-specific areas in which the facility meets certain standards of care or The Joint Commission's national patient safety goals. General accreditation refers to the facility as a whole meeting or exceeding TJC standards. Disease-specific areas include care and treatment of myocardial infarctions or joint replacement, for example. The disease-specific accreditations are advanced certifications awarded to facilities that meet the requirements for disease-specific certification and clinically specific requirements. Anyone can access the quality reports by searching "The Joint Commission Quality Reports" or by using the URL http://www.qualitycheck.org/consumer/searchQCR.aspx. All TJC-accredited institutions are in this database, which is updated daily. The recommended readings list found in Connect contains links to Joint Commission reports.

The Commission on Accreditation of Rehabilitation Facilities (CARF), the Accreditation Association for Ambulatory Health Care (AAAHC), and the Healthcare Facilities Accreditation Program (HFAP) of the American Osteopathic Association, as well as other accrediting agencies, consider quality of care to be in their overall mission as well; thus, they each have standards that address quality assessment and improvement.

Core measurement system
A Joint Commission initiative used to measure the quality and safety of healthcare.

Accountability measures
A Joint Commission system that measures quality and accountability for treatment of certain diagnoses—for instance, myocardial infarction (MI).

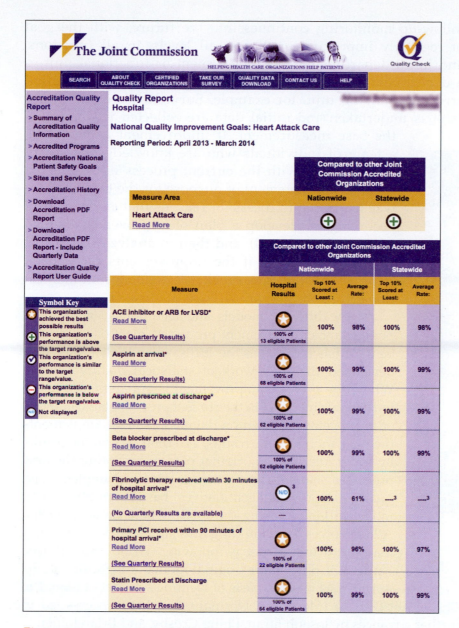

Figure 7.2 Screenshot of a Results Page from The Joint Commission's Quality Check Website

Quality Improvement Models

Quality improvement (QI) activities must be recognized and supported by the facility's governing board and administration. Legislation passed in 1985 requires hospitals to have a written QI plan that includes at least the following:

- A mission statement
- The objectives of the program
- QI values
- The facility's leadership in QI activities
- The organizational structure, methods used, performance measures, communication, and an annual appraisal of the plan

Quality assessment and improvement programs are ongoing, meaning that once improvement is shown in a particular area, follow-up monitoring continues into the future, with the goal of regularly improving quality at all levels, in all functions, and in all departments. Each department or functional unit in a department identifies indicators of quality care—medication errors by nursing unit, for example. Surveillance of that indicator is undertaken and initial data are collected to determine the base measurement. If improvement is indicated, a team of individuals who are knowledgeable about and involved with the current process is established to develop a statement of purpose for the team, to analyze the current process for reasons that errors may be occurring, to develop a plan of improvement (which is then implemented), and then to analyze the results again to determine if the improvements did indeed improve the outcomes (such as a reduction in medication errors on that unit).

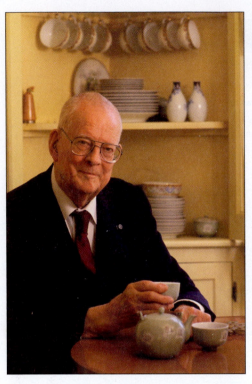

Figure 7.3 W. Edwards Deming, a Leader of the Performance Improvement Movement along with Japanese Business Leaders in 1950s

Plan, Do, Study, Act (PDSA) The statistical model introduced by Walter Shewhart.

Plan, Do, Check, Act (PDCA) The steps of a data-driven quality improvement process to identify reasons for variation, to make plans for improvement, to check results, and to implement the improvements, coined by W. Edwards Deming.

Six Sigma Developed by Motorola in 1986, a data-driven method for improving processes that involves the five-step process define, measure, analyze, improve, and control.

Many different models and techniques are used in performance improvement processes, most of which can be traced as far back as the 1920s, when Walter Shewhart developed the framework of statistical quality control. Where the need for improvement is apparent, a team of individuals involved in the current process plans methods of improvement (based on data assessment), implements the plan, monitors the results, and then acts on the results by either altering the original plan or accepting the new processes. Notably, W. Edwards Deming implemented quality improvement initiatives based on Shewhart's model in Japan during the 1950s, where he assisted the Allied Forces in rebuilding the Japanese economy and manufacturing industry following World War II (see Figure 7.3). Shewhart's original model of Plan, Do, Study, Act (PDSA) was the basis of Deming's model of Plan, Do, Check, Act (PDCA) (Moen and Norman). Deming's success led to further advances by Joseph Juran, Philip Crosby, and Brian Joiner.

Another data-driven method of achieving quality is Six Sigma, which is similar to earlier quality improvement methods in that it, too, is data driven, relies on measurement, and focuses on process improvement. The main process in Six Sigma is to define, measure, analyze, improve, and control (DMAIC); however, there are two Six Sigma subprocesses: the first being define, measure, analyze, improve, and control (DMAIC) and the second being define, measure, analyze, design, and verify (DMADV). The former method is used when improvements to a process need to be made in increments; the latter is used to identify new processes for improvement and for processes that may need a complete reconstruction. Six Sigma requires that the individuals who guide the quality improvement process be specially trained; there are different levels of experts in facilities that adopt the Six Sigma doctrine, such as Champion, Yellow Belt, Green Belt, and Black Belt.

The aim of both the Shewhart model of PDCA and the Six Sigma model of DMAIC is to assess and improve variations in processes.

They are data driven and involve formal steps to assess and solve problems, mistakes, and inefficiencies in procedures or processes. Both require support from the senior leadership of an organization to be effective, and they rely on data as a basis for making decisions or correcting processes rather than on assumptions. The "plan" phase of Shewhart's model is equivalent to the "define, measure, and analyze" steps of Six Sigma; the "do" phase is equivalent to the "improve" step; and "act" is equivalent to "control." Six Sigma also requires specialized training to be Six Sigma certified.

The processes used in any of these models are extensive and are outside the scope of this text. A separate course in quality assessment and improvement is often a part of a health information management educational program at the associate, bachelor's, and master's degree levels.

Quality Initiatives in the Private Sector

Data are reported to the public by private entities such as the Leapfrog Group, which has been reporting hospital quality indicators since 2001. Through reports compiled by the Leapfrog Group based on voluntary self-reporting by hospitals and consumers, hospitals can compare their performance against national quality performance measures, a process also known as **benchmarking**. Benchmarking provides a way for hospitals to identify areas where they need improvement and to then track their progress in reaching their improvement goals.

Healthgrades, Inc. is a private, for-profit entity that provides data on hospitals, nursing homes, and physicians based on patient safety data that are publicly available. Healthgrades provides data and rates hospitals and nursing homes, publishing a "best" and "worst" listing each year. Consumers can search for a facility or physician on the Healthgrades website.

Benchmarking Comparing the performance or outcomes of a provider or facility to that of a similar provider or facility. Examples include infection rate, death rate, and occupancy percentage.

7.2 A DAY IN THE LIFE

Larry is the director of patient access (registration) of Memorial Hospital. He is very frustrated, because Lucinda, the director of nutrition services, has come to him with an issue—patients are no longer taking up a hospital bed because they have been discharged by their attending physicians, but they are not being discharged in the admission, discharge, transfer (ADT) system, so it looks as if the patients are still in a hospital bed, and therefore lunch and dinner trays are being sent to the nursing unit for patients who do not need them. Lucinda says this "always" happens. It also causes a problem for the housekeeping staff, because the room remains empty and could be cleaned in a timely fashion to prepare it for the next patient, but they, too, do not get notified of the discharge. The chief nursing officer, Cassandra, does not think it is a nursing issue, because the nurses "always" discharge a patient in the ADT system as soon as the patient leaves the unit. In order for the ADT system to recognize a discharge,

(continued)

the nursing staff must use the "discharge" application in the system as each patient leaves the nursing unit. Documentation in the nursing notes must show the date and time the patient is discharged, where the patient was discharged to (home, nursing home, expired, etc.), and by whom the patient was accompanied, though that entry does not carry over to the ADT system.

1. Is there variation in the process? What is it?
2. Using what you have learned in this section, what should or could happen to solve the problem?

7.2 THINKING IT THROUGH

1. What is The Joint Commission's core measurement system used for?

2. Explain the significance of the PDCA improvement method.

7.3 The Health Record in Risk Management Processes

Risk management Internal activities performed with the goal of minimizing risk exposure through the identification, evaluation, control of, and response to errors or injuries that could occur or have occurred in order to lessen the facility's liability and to finance incidents for which the facility is found liable.

The management of risk—known as **risk management**—has been a formally recognized discipline in healthcare since the 1970s. As the number of malpractice cases filed against physicians and hospitals increased, so did the need to control risk. Prior to the 1970s, healthcare facilities and providers were seen as being charitable institutions and therefore were not threatened by the possibility of legal actions against them. This status changed, however, with the case of *Darling v. Charleston Community Hospital*. The court's decision set the precedent that patients have the right to compensation when a hospital and/or physician does not perform his or her duties according to professionally acceptable practice or is careless, which is known as negligence. In the event that it is a physician who is accused of negligence, the hospital in which the accusation occurred is also held liable. Because the physician was practicing in that hospital, it has a duty to ensure that anyone practicing or caring for patients inside its walls uses acceptable care in treating its patients.

Through the risk management process, areas of risk are identified—for instance, a high infection rate for a particular nursing unit. Risk is controlled through preventive measures, such as proactive staff education to minimize fall risks. These occurrences that are out of the norm are referred to as *potentially compensable events.* Thus, risk financing—ensuring that funding is available, should an incident occur that results in a financial loss to the organization—is an integral element of a formal risk management plan.

The health record plays a very important role in risk management for obvious reasons. Without the record, there is no proof of what, why, when, or by whom something was done. Health information professionals may work in the risk management field as abstractors of data, as investigators, or as risk managers, who comb through records to glean pieces of data that can lead to the full story surrounding an incident.

Documentation of abnormal incidents (occurrences) is vital in assessing and controlling risk, but documentation of the internal investigation of an occurrence is not part of the patient's health record. The record itself should reflect only the facts, not speculation, hearsay, or history that is unrelated to the occurrence. The findings of an investigation are documented using an **incident (occurrence) report**. Figure 7.4 depicts a typical incident report. Note that this

Incident (occurrence) report Data collected about any abnormal occurrence involving a patient, a visitor, or an employee that detail the circumstances surrounding the incident and are used in the facility's internal investigation.

INCIDENT REPORT

Name of Hospital _____

Address _____ Phone _____ Email _____ Fax _____

Report Prepared By_____ Designation _____

Address _____ Phone _____ Email _____

Incident Report Information

Title of Report _____

Date of Incident ____ / ____ / ____ Duration _____

Location _____

Nature of Incident _____

Brief Description of Incident _____

Persons Involved in Incident _____

Activities of Above Person at the Time of the Incident _____

Any Other Outside Party Involved in Incident _____

Contact Details _____

Witness of Incident, Name and Contact Details _____

Any Injury Taken Place (Provide Details) _____

Any Police Complaint Filed (Provide Details)_____

If Yes, What Corrective Measures Have Been Taken ? _____

Signature _____ Date ___ / ___ / ___

Report Submitted To: Name _____ Designation _____

Figure 7.4   An Example of an Incident Report

image is of an employee incident; facilities may use one form for all incidents or may have separate forms for incidents involving patients, visitors, or staff.

The incident (occurrence) report is never filed as part of the patient's record, nor is the report itself referred to in the record, since its purpose is that of an internal investigation tool. Health information professionals are responsible for reporting inappropriate documentation, as well as documentation that is misleading or accusatory. Facility policy dictates the person or position to which such documentation is reported. It may be to the risk manager, the manager of the department or unit to which the occurrence pertains, or to the health information director.

7.3 A DAY IN THE LIFE

Cassandra is a health record analyst reviewing the record of patient Alicia Powell. A nurse had documented that the patient was very upset because she had overheard a surgical resident, Dr. Lopez, comment to another resident, Dr. Glover, that a mistake must have been made during her surgery. The nurse had documented in the record that "some sort of surgical mishap occurred, and the patient is quite anxious about it." The nurse completed an incident report and documented in the patient's record that the report had been completed and filed with the risk management department.

1. Is any part of this scenario an issue? Why or why not?
2. Is there anything wrong with mentioning the incident report in the patient's record?

7.3 THINKING IT THROUGH

1. What is risk financing?
2. Why is the health record so important in risk management?

7.4 Payment Models

History

Long before the inception of Medicare in 1966, the provision of medical care without regard for ability to pay was taken for granted. Charity care, assistance from religious organizations, philanthropic bequests or grants, and even bartering were used to pay for the services of physicians and hospitals.

Payment was made on a retrospective, fee-for-service basis, which meant that if a physician charged $50 for an office visit, then either the patient (if uninsured) or healthcare insurance (including Medicare or Medicaid) paid the physician $50. The amount charged was typically determined after care had been given (retrospectively), and the amount was not necessarily consistent from patient to patient.

Private healthcare insurance dates back to the late 1920s, when Blue Cross emerged. Blue Shield followed in the 1940s and then the two merged in 1982 to become the Blue Cross Association. Group healthcare coverage through employers then became the norm, and having insurance coverage was the rule rather than the exception.

The Hill-Burton Act, passed in 1946, provided hospitals with funding to construct new buildings or improve facilities to meet the expanding demand for medical care. Up until that time, hospitals did not have sufficient funds to update their facilities. As a result of this legislation, hospitals received funding to improve facilities in return for providing charity care to the needy and un- or underinsured population.

The costs of providing care grew as new, more expensive technologies were introduced. New technologies meant a need for increased training of clinicians, thus increasing salaries. As more and more people were covered by some type of insurance, the demand for services increased. Hospitals and physicians had no incentive to control costs, since they were paid whatever amount they charged. This lack of oversight on the charges for services and no one questioning whether services provided were medically necessary contributed to the out-of-control rise in costs we are still attempting to correct today.

Government Reimbursement Plans

Though employers were providing health insurance at affordable rates or no cost to their employees, the elderly (who were no longer employed) and the poor were without coverage. The federal government then passed Title XVIII of the Social Security Act, which became known simply as Medicare. It was passed into law in 1965 and went into effect in 1966. Medicare covers US citizens and legal residents who are 65 years of age and older or who receive Social Security Disability Insurance (SSDI). Also covered are patients with end-stage renal disease or other conditions, such as amyotrophic lateral sclerosis (ALS). Other qualifications include having paid into the fund through a payroll tax or having paid into the Railroad Retirement fund. Unemployed individuals who have not paid into the Medicare fund are covered if their spouse did pay the payroll tax for at least five years.

Over the years, many changes have been made to the Medicare program, which is administered by the Centers for Medicare and Medicaid Services (CMS). Table 7.1 highlights the major coverage changes in Medicare.

Medicaid (Title XIX of the Social Security Act) is also a federal program, but individual state governments determine eligibility and coverage parameters. However, the minimum coverage stipulated by federal law must be followed in order for states to receive federal monies to help fund the programs. Medicaid assists low-income individuals with the cost of healthcare. Coverage required by the federal government includes inpatient hospital services, outpatient hospital services, diagnostic laboratory and radiology, skilled nursing long-term care, some home health services,

TABLE 7.1   eMedicare Plans

Coverage	Year Implemented	Services Covered	Cost to Individual
Part A	1966	• Inpatient hospital services • Hospice services • Long-term care • Persons with end-stage renal disease (ESRD) • Persons with amyotrophic lateral sclerosis (ALS)	• No monthly **premium** • Responsible for yearly deductible ($1,216 per **spell of illness** for 2014) and a coinsurance applies for days 61–90 of hospitalization for each spell of illness ($304/ day for 2014) • Additional coinsurance charged for **lifetime reserve days**
Part B	1966	• Outpatient physician and nursing services • Outpatient diagnostics, such as x-rays, laboratory and diagnostic tests • Vaccination/immunizations, such as influenza and pneumonia vaccinations • Blood transfusions, renal dialysis, outpatient hospital procedures, limited ambulance transportation, immunosuppressive drugs for organ transplant recipients, chemotherapy, hormonal treatments and other outpatient medical treatments administered in a doctor's office • Durable medical equipment (DME), such as canes, walkers, and wheelchairs • Home oxygen • Prosthetics, such as limbs or breast prostheses	• Monthly premium ($104.90/ month for 2014) • Yearly deductible ($147.00/ year for 2014) • Medicare pays 80% of **allowed charges**. • Individual pays 20% of allowed charges.
Part C Medicare Advantage Plans (formerly known as Medicare + Choice)	1997	• Managed care plans • No traditional Medicare benefits are given up and may have additional coverage. • May include a prescription drug plan	• Medicare Part B premium plus additional, depending on extent of additional coverage
Part D	2006	• Prescription drug plan for Medicare Part A and B beneficiaries	• Out-of-pocket expenses vary, depending on the plan; the drugs covered are determined by the plan chosen.

physicians' office visits, special programs for family planning, the services of a nurse midwife, vaccines for children, rural healthcare, and some periodic screening services (for instance, mammogram or colonoscopy).

Other federal health insurance plans include coverage for active and retired military as well as their dependents. Previously known as the Civilian Health and Medical Program of the Uniformed Services (CHAMPUS), this program has now become one of three major **TRICARE** plans. TRICARE Prime is a managed care plan, TRICARE Standard is a fee-for-service plan in which any physician in the TRICARE network may be seen, and TRICARE For Life supplements Medicare beneficiaries. For a more detailed comparison of the three main TRICARE plans, see Figure 7.5. The TRICARE plans are administered by the Department of Defense rather than CMS. A complete listing of TRICARE plans can be compared and contrasted easily at www.tricare.mil/plans.

As noted earlier, the cost of healthcare had been growing at alarming levels over the past 40 years. However, CMS reports that healthcare's portion of the gross national product (GNP) in 2012 was 17.2%, down from 17.3% percent in 2011. Healthcare spending in 2012 amounted to $2.8 trillion, though healthcare spending in general has been slow since 2009. This slowdown in spending is attributed to the lagging economy but is not expected to last. In fact, healthcare spending is projected to grow as a result of the Affordable Care Act (ACA), as a projected 22 million additional insured individuals are expected to enter the marketplace. The ACA was discussed in the chapter on the evolving healthcare system in the United States.

In the early 1980s, it was more than apparent that the cost of healthcare needed to be contained. The Tax Equity and Fiscal Responsibility Act (TEFRA) marked the first attempt to address the cost issue and resulted in the prospective payment system (PPS); for inpatients, this is known as the Inpatient Prospective Payment System (IPPS). PPS is considered a system of averages—a hospital will make money

Premium The amount paid (typically monthly or quarterly) to an insurer for health insurance, either directly to the insurance carrier for solo coverage or through payroll deductions as part of a group health insurance plan.

Spell of illness A period of consecutive days beginning with the first day on which a Medicare beneficiary begins inpatient hospitalization or extended care (long-term care) services and ending with the close of the first period (up to 90 days) through 60 consecutive days in which the patient is neither a hospital inpatient nor a patient in a skilled nursing facility.

Lifetime reserve days A one-time bank of a maximum of 60 days of inpatient service days after the use of the first 90 benefit days per spell of illness. Lifetime reserve days can be split among more than one inpatient hospitalization.

Allowed charges The maximum amount Medicare (or other third-party payer) will reimburse for services.

TRICARE Prime	TRICARE Standard	TRICARE For Life
• Managed care plan • All active duty military members are covered in one of the Prime plans (Prime or Prime Remote) • Though coverage is automatic, if active duty, enrollment is required • No enrollment fees, no deductibles, and no co-pays for authorized healthcare services or prescriptions	• Fee-for-service, cost-sharing plan • Member pays annual deductible • Member pays 25% of allowed charges • May receive care from any provider who is TRICARE authorized • Includes TRICARE Extra which requires a 20% co-pay and care must be provided by a TRICARE in-network provider	• Supplements Medicare beneficiaries • Medicare pays first; TRICARE For Life is a supplemental policy • Members must participate in Medicare Part B and pay Medicare Part B premiums

Figure 7.5   **Comparison of the Three Major TRICARE Plans**

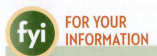

on some patients but will lose money on some; however, in the end, a hospital should at least break even. Its premise is that patients with the same or similar conditions should receive fairly similar care (testing, etc.) and should stay in the hospital about the same length of time; therefore, they should cost about the same to treat. Each patient falls into a diagnosis related group (DRG) based on the patient's principal diagnosis, his or her secondary diagnoses, and the procedure(s) that were performed. The hospital receives the same amount of reimbursement for each patient falling into a particular DRG, but there are exceptions, such as patients who require extra care or who undergo a procedure that is unrelated to their principal diagnosis, for which the hospital would be reimbursed at a higher rate. Some DRGs also take into consideration the patient's discharge disposition—that is, whether the patient expired or was transferred to another hospital. Placing patients into a particular DRG is done with grouper software and cannot be done manually. As of 2007, each case is grouped into a **Medicare Severity Diagnosis Related Group (MS-DRG)**, which takes into consideration the severity of illness and results in a more accurate computation of the costs incurred to care for each patient. Each admission is assigned to only one MS-DRG.

The hospital would be paid the amounts noted in the scenarios regardless of how much it cost to treat the patient. In cases where

7.4 A DAY IN THE LIFE

Scenario 1: Kait, a coder at Memorial Hospital, has just finished coding the record of a 75-year-old woman who was an inpatient from December 22, 2013, to December 24, 2013. Her final diagnosis is documented by the physician as "hypertensive encephalopathy with acute and chronic systolic heart failure, and benign hypertensive heart and chronic kidney disease, stage II." Kait assigns ICD-9-CM codes 437.2, 404.91, 585.2, and 428.23. She runs the MS-DRG grouper software, and MS-DRG 077 is assigned to this case.

Scenario 2: Sandy, also a coder at Memorial Hospital, has just finished coding the record of a 68-year-old man with a final diagnosis documented by the physician as "hypertensive encephalopathy and portal hypertension." The code assignment is 437.2 and 572.3. The MS-DRG grouper software assigns this case to MS-DRG 078.

Figure 7.6 shows an excerpt from the Fiscal Year 2013 Medicare MS-DRG table. The MS-DRGs into which the preceding scenarios fall are MS-DRG 077, hypertensive encephalopathy *with* a major complication or comorbidity, and MS-DRG 078, hypertensive encephalopathy with a complication or comorbidity. Notice the column titled "weights"—the higher the weight, the higher the resources used, therefore resulting in higher reimbursement. Memorial Hospital has a Medicare base payment rate of $3,000.00; thus, the reimbursement for Scenario 1 is $4,887.00 (3,000.00 × 1.6290 = 4,887.00).

Reimbursement for the patient in Scenario 2, for MS-DRG 078, is $2,840.10 (3,000.00 × 0.9467 = 2,840.10).

TABLES—LIST OF MEDICARE SEVERITY DIAGNOSIS RELATED GROUPS (MS-DRGs), RELATIVE WEIGHTING FACTORS, AND GEOMETRIC AND ARITHMETIC MEAN LENGTH OF STAY—FY 2014 Final Rule								
MS-DRG	FY 2014 FR Post-Acute DRG	FY 2014 FR Special Pay DRG	MDC	TYPE	MS-DRG Title	Weights	Geometric mean LOS	Arithmetic mean LOS
077	No	No	01	MED	HYPERTENSIVE ENCEPHALOPATHY W MCC	1.6290	4.6	6.0
078	No	No	01	MED	HYPERTENSIVE ENCEPHALOPATHY W CC	0.9467	3.1	3.9

Figure 7.6 A DRG Table

Source: CMS. FY2014 Final Rules Table.

the costs incurred by the hospital are less than the reimbursement rate, the hospital keeps the difference; if the costs incurred exceed the reimbursement rate, the hospital loses, and the patient cannot be billed for the difference. However, hospitals do receive additional payment when the cost of caring for a patient is extraordinarily high; these cases are known as **outliers**.

Medicare requires the use of MS-DRGs. In addition, many states require them for Medicaid, as do many commercial insurance carriers, though the reimbursement rates differ from the Medicare rates. Assigning every inpatient to an MS-DRG allows the hospital to profile the diagnoses, procedures, and severity of patients treated by computing a **case mix index (CMI)**.

Table 7.2 shows several patients falling into MS-DRGs 100, 121, 175, and 189. Assume these represent one nursing unit for a one-week period. Twelve patients fell into these MS-DRGs, and the relative weight of each MS-DRG is multiplied by the number of patients in each. Adding the total weights for all the patients gives the case mix for that nursing unit, and dividing the total relative weight by the total number of patients results in a case mix index of 1.3797. MS-DRGs with a relative of weight of 1.0000 are considered to have average resource utilization. Therefore, for this nursing unit for this one-week period, the case mix index of patients admitted to that unit was 1.3797, so slightly higher than average.

A similar system for hospital outpatients was implemented in 2000 and resulted in the **Outpatient Prospective Payment System (OPPS)**. This payment methodology was devised to control Medicare spending for outpatients. **Ambulatory Payment Classifications (APCs)**,

Outlier Within the prospective payment system, an inpatient encounter that has an abnormally long length of stay or abnormally high costs associated with it.

Case mix index The average relative weights of all the MS-DRGs representative of the severity of all patients admitted to a facility.

Outpatient Prospective Payment System (OPPS) A system used by Medicare and Medicaid for payment of hospital ambulatory (outpatient) encounters based on an ambulatory (as opposed to inpatient) payment system.

Ambulatory Payment Classifications (APCs) The classification system used by Medicare and Medicaid to calculate payment for hospital ambulatory (outpatient) encounters.

TABLE 7.2	Case Mix Index		
MS-DRG	Relative Weight	No. of Patients in That MS-DRG	Total Weight (Relative Weight × No. of Patients)
100 Seizures with MCC	1.5185	5	7.5925
121 Acute major eye infections with CC/MCC	1.0215	1	1.0215
175 Pulmonary embolism with MCC	1.5346	2	3.0692
189 Pulmonary edema & respiratory failure	1.2184	4	4.8736
TOTAL	—	**12**	**16.5568**
		Case mix index (16.5568/12)	**1.3797**

rather than MS-DRGs, are assigned to certain outpatient encounters (for example, ambulatory surgery, emergency department visits, or blood transfusions) and are based on the CPT codes assigned to each service. More than one APC may be assigned to an outpatient case, though only one is paid at 100%; the others are paid at a lower percentage. Table 7.3 shows an example of three APCs along with the relative weight and payment rate for each.

TABLE 7.3	2014 APC Payment Rate Examples		
APC Description	Relative Weight	Payment Rate
058 Level 1 Cast Application	1.3789	$100.21
100 Cardiac Stress Test	3.3604	$244.21
247 Laser Eye Procedure	5.8928	$428.24

The costs associated with physician services also need to be controlled, and the system used to reimburse for care given to Medicare patients is known as the **resource-based relative value scale (RBRVS)**. CPT and HCPCS codes corresponding to the services rendered to patients are used to determine reimbursement rates.

Linking Quality to Reimbursement: Payment Reform under the ACA

The ACA has a triple aim of improving the quality of care, reducing costs, and improving public health. It includes 14 programs encompassing 8 models that are supported by CMS designed to assist in achieving these aims. These programs center on taking value and quality of care into consideration when providing reimbursement.

Payment reform under the ACA is designed to test various approaches, either individually or in combination. The primary goal is to shift from fee-for-service (FFS) or fee-for-volume reimbursement to fee-for-value (FFV) models. Reimbursement either takes the form of fixed global payments, also called capitated payments, for a population a provider serves or makes fixed payments based on outcome diagnosis and outcome parameters.

Since 2007, hospitals have been required to indicate principal and secondary conditions that were not present on admission as part of the **Hospital Acquired Conditions (HAC)** and **Present on Admission (POA)** reporting provisions of the Deficit Reduction Act of 2005. The indicator is found on the hospital claim form, known as the UB-04. Conditions such as fractures or infections that were not present at the time of admission result in a quality adjustment to what would have been paid for the case. Thus, the hospital is reimbursed less money than what would have been paid for the MS-DRG into which that case fell. This program was expanded under the ACA.

The **Hospital Value-Based Purchasing (VBP)** program, a result of the Affordable Care Act, involves pay-for-performance and applies to inpatient stays. Medicare will adjust a portion of the payments made to hospitals based on (1) how well the hospital performs on each measure as compared to all hospitals or (2) the hospital's level of improvement in each measure as compared to its performance during a previous baseline period. In other words, hospitals will lose money if they are not performing as well as or better than other hospitals in a particular area and/or if they do not show improvement in an area where they were below par. Healthcare consumers can view hospitals' performance by searching Medicare Hospital Compare in an Internet browser.

The **Hospital Readmission Reduction Program (HRP)**, also a result of the Affordable Care Act, has been in effect since fiscal year 2013. Hospitals with high readmission rates for certain high-cost or high-volume conditions—for example, heart attack, heart failure, and pneumonia—receive reduced reimbursement.

Accountable care organizations lead the most recent quality-focused reimbursement initiatives, which were covered in the chapter on new roles in health informatics. ACOs are formal groups of physicians, hospitals, and other healthcare providers who work together to provide high-quality, coordinated care. ACOs receive payments by meeting quality and cost targets based on the characteristics of their patient population. There are two ACO programs: the **Medicare Shared Savings Program (MSSP)** and the **Pioneer ACO Program**.

The following are additional payment reform models supported by CMS under the ACA:

- *Patient-centered medical homes* (*PCMHs*): A model developed by the American Academy of Family Practitioners for patients with chronic conditions to encourage and facilitate involvement by the patient and family in his or her own care
- *Healthcare innovation awards:* $1 billion in funding for organizations that are implementing the most compelling new ideas to delivery better health, improved care, and lower costs to Medicare, Medicaid, and Children's Health Insurance Program (CHIP) enrollees
- *State Innovation Models Initiative:* A CMS program that provides financial support for the development and testing of state-based models for multi-payer payment and healthcare delivery systems for the residents of participating states
- *Pay-for-performance (P4P) programs:* Any of the programs discussed in this section with the purpose of improving the quality, efficiency, and value of healthcare.
- *Bundled Payments for Care Improvement program:* A CMS payment model that includes financial and performance accountability for episodes of care, with the goal of improved quality of care, enhanced coordination of care, and lower costs for Medicare.

Private Health Insurance Plans

The Blue Cross and Blue Shield Association (BCBSA) is an example of a third-party payer, also known as private health insurance. There are 37 individual Blue Cross and Blue Shield companies that are

Hospital Readmission Reduction Program (HRP) Part of the Affordable Care Act (ACA), a program that requires CMS to reduce payments to hospitals with excessive readmission rates.

Medicare Shared Savings Program (MSSP) A CMS program that facilitates coordination and cooperation among providers to improve the quality of care provided to Medicare fee-for-service beneficiaries and to reduce unnecessary cost through participation in an ACO.

Pioneer ACO Program An ACO model for hospitals and care providers who have experience with coordinating care for patients across the continuum of care (across different care settings).

licensees of BCBSA. It is commercial insurance and, according to the BCBSA website, is the third-party payer for more than 100 million people. BCBSA is by far the largest commercial insurance carrier and is accepted by 96% of hospitals and 91% of providers. It is not the only commercial insurance plan, however. Others include Humana, United Healthcare, and Aetna, just to name a few.

As with the government plans, reimbursement was largely fee-for-service, and third-party payers paid the amount charged by the provider. Over the past 30 to 40 years, however, the shift has been made to a managed care system of reimbursement that includes coordination of a patient's plan of care, a focus on wellness, the education of patients, quality care, and the control of costs. In a managed care plan, patients may have to name a primary care provider, and some plans require enrolled individuals to see only providers within a **provider network**.

Provider network A network of hospitals, physicians, ambulatory clinics, and so forth with which a managed care insurance plan contracts to provide services to enrollees at an agreed-upon reduced rate, saving the enrollee out-of-pocket expenses for medical care; often referred to as "in network."

Common types of managed care include health maintenance organizations (HMOs), preferred provider organizations (PPOs), exclusive provider organizations (EPOs), and point of service (POS) plans. The following are some of the benefits of managed care:

- Coordinated care through a primary care physician (also known as a gatekeeper)
- Focus on preventive care (wellness)
- Use of disease management tools (evidence-based or clinical practice guidelines)
- Case management
- Cost controls

The negative aspects of managed care include the following:

- Time spent and work involved in seeking pre-approval of services
- Requirement to see in-network providers
- Physicians feeling that they are told how to treat their patients and cannot make decisions without approval of the managed care plan
- Fear that quality will be sacrificed to save money

The negative aspects may be perceived or real, depending on the perspective of the person with the opinion. A physician caring for a patient does not want to stop the process, or await approvals, yet the patient wants high-quality, cost-effective care.

7.4	THINKING IT THROUGH

1. How did the advent of private insurance change the field of healthcare?
2. Why has managed care basically replaced the fee-for-service model?
3. Esther Oakes uses her Medicare to pay for monthly prescription refills. Which part of Medicare does Mrs. Oakes use for this purpose?

Prior to prospective payment and managed care, the reimbursement cycle started when the patient was admitted for an outpatient encounter, the medical record was compiled, diagnosis and procedure codes were assigned, and the claim form was manually or electronically submitted to the insurance company. Then, the hospital or office simply awaited payment. Seeking reimbursement has now become much more labor-intensive, and there are many more variables, so this cycle is no longer the norm.

Instead, there is more "front-end" work to be done, particularly for ambulatory surgery or expensive diagnostic tests. A patient whose physician has recommended a tonsillectomy, whether he or she is covered by Medicaid or private insurance, may need **pre-authorization** from Medicaid or the insurance company before the procedure can even be scheduled. Some third-party payers today will pay for an MRI just on the basis of a physician's order (and medical necessity); others require pre-authorization before the test can be done.

Some managed care plans require authorization of inpatient stays that follow emergency department visits or direct admits from a physician's office. This authorization is required often within 24 to 48 hours of admission and is generally the responsibility of the utilization management department.

Throughout the stay, particularly for patients who may require a lower level of post-discharge care (a nursing home, for example), case managers work with the physician, patient, and/or family to ensure that the discharge plan is ready when the patient can be discharged.

The coding of diagnoses and procedures is also anticipated to become much more challenging once ICD-10-CM/PCS is implemented, and the quality of health record documentation will need to very clearly support the diagnosis and procedure codes assigned. Diagnosis and procedure codes are required on every claim submitted to Medicare, Medicaid, TRICARE, and commercial insurance plans. Not only is this a requirement of the HIPAA code set and electronic transactions rule, but it is also a requirement of all third-party payers. Incorrect or incomplete coding (or any incomplete claims data) delays payment of the bill, thus slowing cash flow into the organization.

The business office or billing department must have policies and procedures in place to quickly yet accurately submit claims to third-party payers. The longer it takes to file a claim, the longer it takes to receive reimbursement. Sloppy coding and or billing practices can significantly affect a facility's financial bottom line.

Figure 7.7 illustrates a typical reimbursement cycle. Many of these steps may be repeated throughout the patient's episode of care. For instance, pre-authorization may not be approved the first time it is requested; the physician may need to be clearer or more detailed in his or her documentation first. Or a claim may be submitted but initially denied because of an error or a question about medical necessity and must be resubmitted. Even when the steps do need to be repeated, they should be done with efficiency and in a timely manner.

Pre-authorization The requirement of some managed care plans that patients seek authorization (approval) for testing or admission in order for the insurance to pay for the services (providing that other requirements, such as medical necessity, are met).

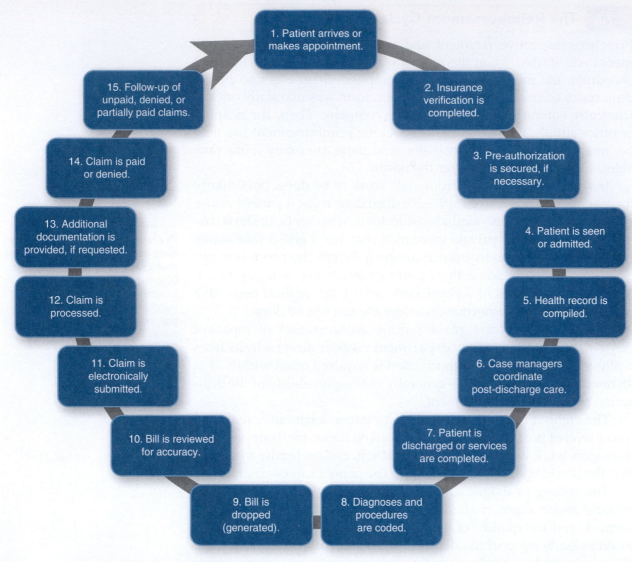

Figure 7.7   A Typical Reimbursement Cycle

The boxes in the cycle read:

1. Patient arrives or makes appointment.
2. Insurance verification is completed.
3. Pre-authorization is secured, if necessary.
4. Patient is seen or admitted.
5. Health record is compiled.
6. Case managers coordinate post-discharge care.
7. Patient is discharged or services are completed.
8. Diagnoses and procedures are coded.
9. Bill is dropped (generated).
10. Bill is reviewed for accuracy.
11. Claim is electronically submitted.
12. Claim is processed.
13. Additional documentation is provided, if requested.
14. Claim is paid or denied.
15. Follow-up of unpaid, denied, or partially paid claims.

7.5   THINKING IT THROUGH

1. Why are there so many steps in the reimbursement cycle?
2. Why might some insurers require pre-authorization for procedures?

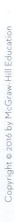

Chapter 7 **summary**

LEARNING OUTCOMES	CONCEPTS FOR REVIEW
7.1 Document the elements of the HIPAA designated record set (DRS) and the legal health record. Pages 175–178	• DRS is required as part of the HIPAA privacy rule. • What patients' rights are afforded as a result of HIPAA? • What must be considered when developing the definition of the DRS? • What is the relationship among a facility, a clearinghouse, and a health plan? • Differentiate between the DRS and the legal health record. Why might they differ in health facilities? • What should be taken into consideration when a facility is defining its DRS and legal health record? • Explain information governance. Why is it an emerging specialty area in HIM?
7.2 Explain required quality assessment activities in healthcare. Pages 178–186	• Discuss the internal and external needs for quality assessment activities. • What role do coded data play in the monitoring of quality? • What are the current concerns for copying (or cutting) and pasting documentation from one record to another? • Why would external agencies require internal quality assessment activities in healthcare organizations? • Discuss the history of quality initiatives in healthcare. • What is the purpose of a QIO? • Why is peer review an important component of quality assessment? • Explain various quality initiatives currently in place by TJC and CMS. • What options do healthcare consumers have to view quality of care data on individual facilities? • Discuss the history of quality assessment models. • How does benchmarking improve the measurement of quality?
7.3 Discuss the role of data in risk management activities. Pages 186–188	• List the typical elements of a risk management program. • What led to the risk management movement? • Give examples of how data impact risk management activities. • Define *occurrence*. • What are the documentation rules when documenting internal investigations of occurrences?
7.4 Explain payment models used by government and commercial insurance plans. Pages 188–196	• Outline the history of federal and state reimbursement plans. • Discuss the various options for Medicare coverage. • Explain what is meant by a managed care plan. • Given applicable figures, calculate MS-DRG payments. • Given applicable figures, determine the case mix index (CMI) for a hospital.

(continued)

LEARNING OUTCOMES	CONCEPTS FOR REVIEW
	• Differentiate between the IPPS and the OPPS. • Explain various payment models that link quality to reimbursement. • How do Hospital Acquired Conditions affect reimbursement in a pay-for-performance model? • Discuss common managed care models: HMO, PPO, EPO, POS.
7.5 Diagram the reimbursement cycle in healthcare. Pages 197–198	• At what point does reimbursement begin? • At what point does the reimbursement cycle end? • How does pre-authorization affect reimbursement? • Place the steps of a typical reimbursement model in order from start to finish.

chapter review

MATCHING QUESTIONS

Match each term with its definition.

_____ 1. **[LO 7.2]** Six Sigma

_____ 2. **[LO 7.3]** incident report

_____ 3. **[LO 7.5]** pre-authorization

_____ 4. **[LO 7.1]** information government

_____ 5. **[LO 7.4]** HAC

_____ 6. **[LO 7.4]** spell of illness

_____ 7. **[LO 7.4]** RBRVS

_____ 8. **[LO 7.5]** utilization management

_____ 9. **[LO 7.4]** TRICARE

_____ 10. **[LO 7.2]** scope of work

_____ 11. **[LO 7.4]** managed care

_____ 12. **[LO 7.4]** Hill-Burton Act

_____ 13. **[LO 7.4]** outlier

_____ 14. **[LO 7.4]** prospective payment system

_____ 15. **[LO 7.4]** lifetime reserve days

a. Legislation that provided hospitals with expansion and improvement funding

b. A Medicare definition of coverage based on the consecutive days a patient is receiving care

c. Case in which the cost of patient treatment is unusually and extremely high compared to other patients with similar conditions and treatment

d. Ailments or injuries sustained by a patient during his or her hospital stay

e. Medicare system used to reimburse physicians

f. Data-driven quality improvement process

g. Plan for targeting and implementing quality improvements

h. Method of estimating patient care costs; effort to reduce healthcare spending

i. Insurance plans that focus on coordinating care, preventive care, and patient education

j. Obtaining permission from an insurance company prior to treatments or procedures being performed

k. The functions that ensure the appropriateness of admission, the medical necessity of planned hospital services and the securing pre-authorization from third-party payers to perform services

l. Determining who will be responsible for the release and tracking of patient data

m. Documentation of unusual or abnormal situations

n. Inpatient days that are paid by Medicare when a patient has exceeded 90 days of admission

o. Federal health insurance coverage for active and retired military service members

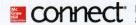
Enhance your learning by completing these exercises and more at http://connect.mheducation.com!

MULTIPLE CHOICE QUESTIONS

Choose the letter that best completes the statement or answers the question.

16. **[LO 7.1]** Which of the following staff members would most likely be asked to join the team responsible for managing questions about the legal health record?
    a. Compliance coordinator
    b. IT analyst
    c. Medical assistant
    d. Office manager

17. **[LO 7.1]** Blue Cross/Blue Shield Insurance Company is considered a
    a. clearinghouse.
    b. covered entity.
    c. designated record set.
    d. provider.

18. **[LO 7.2]** Which regulatory agency maintains a database of its institutions' quality reports?
    a. AAAHC
    b. AHIMA
    c. Centers for Medicare and Medicaid Services
    d. The Joint Commission

19. **[LO 7.2]** Health information–specific quality assurance checks regularly occur with
    a. drug inventories.
    b. equipment purchases.
    c. the MPI.
    d. transcription.

20. **[LO 7.2]** Meeting regulatory standards is part of a hospital's fulfillment of _____ quality assessment initiatives.
    a. external
    b. internal
    c. important
    d. voluntary

21. **[LO 7.3]** Risk management has been a recognized discipline only since the 1970s because
    a. lawsuits were not as prevalent prior to 1970.
    b. hospitals did not accept insurance before then.
    c. malpractice was not an acceptable legal action until 1974.
    d. hospitals were previously viewed as charitable organizations.

22. **[LO 7.3]** A risk manager is reviewing the health record documentation of Nurse Davis for an ongoing legal case. Which piece of information would need to be reported as inappropriate?
    a. "Patient received her 7 p.m. dose of acetaminophen 15 minutes late."
    b. "Nurse Smith took too long taking patient's vitals."
    c. "Patient slept 9 hours through the night without waking."
    d. "Patient complained of a headache."

23. **[LO 7.3]** Making all nursing assistants go through training on bedside manner is an example of risk
    a. financing.
    b. identification.
    c. prevention.
    d. termination.

24. **[LO 7.4]** Prior to 1966, elderly people
    a. could get coverage only under Medicaid.
    b. did not have to pay for healthcare.
    c. were charged only for preventive care.
    d. may not have had access to healthcare coverage.

25. **[LO 7.4]** Which of the following ties reimbursement to quality of care?
    a. APC
    b. DRG
    c. POA
    d. PPS

26. **[LO 7.4]** Requiring a patient to select a primary care physician is a typical practice for which type of healthcare plan?
    a. Managed care
    b. Fee-for-service
    c. Government
    d. Third-party

27. **[LO 7.5]** Which is true of the reimbursement cycle?
    a. Each step is done one time.
    b. Each step is done every time.
    c. Some steps are repeated.
    d. Some steps are optional.

SHORT ANSWER QUESTIONS

28. **[LO 7.1]** List the four main roles of the legal health record.

29. **[LO 7.1]** What is a clearinghouse?

30. **[LO 7.2]** Define *DMAIC*.

31. **[LO 7.2]** What is benchmarking?

32. **[LO 7.3]** Describe the significance of the *Darling v. Charleston Community Hospital* case.

33. **[LO 7.4]** What is a fee-for-service model of healthcare?

34. **[LO 7.4]** How do Ambulatory Payment Classifications differ from diagnosis related groups?

35. **[LO 7.5]** Why is it best practice for a healthcare facility to submit claims in a timely manner?

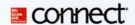 Enhance your learning by completing these exercises and more at http://connect.mheducation.com!

APPLYING YOUR KNOWLEDGE

36. **[LO 7.2]** Search the Internet for a case in which transcription errors caused an adverse medical/patient scenario. Discuss how the errors could have been avoided.

37. **[LO 7.2]** What are your thoughts about the process of peer review? Are there any drawbacks to this initiative? Explain your reasoning, using examples as needed.

38. **[LO 7.1, 7.3]** Why is risk management such an important function for hospitals? Citing your source, summarize at least one recent incident in which a hospital was involved in malpractice or liability proceedings.

39. **[LO 7.4]** Section 7.4 of the text focused in large part on the extreme cost of healthcare. Imagine that you work at Central Hospital, which is sponsoring a contest to generate cost-saving ideas. Create a plan of at least four points—three that address facility-specific cost reductions and at least one point that suggests how national healthcare costs can be controlled or reduced. Give examples as needed.

40. **[LO 7.4]** Do you believe that the negatives surrounding managed care programs are valid? Explain your answer.

41. **[LO 7.4, 7.5]** Which sections of the reimbursement cycle would be most affected by hospital/care quality? Explain.

chapter **eight**

8

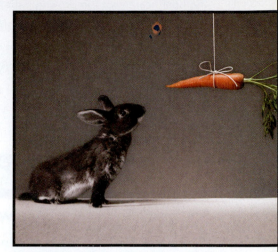

The Electronic Health Record: *Meaningful Use of*

Patient Records

Learning Outcomes

When you finish this chapter, you will be able to:

8.1 Define Meaningful Use and the goals for each stage of Meaningful Use.

8.2 Explain technologies used to process health information.

8.3 Describe the principal standards used for the digitization and exchange of patient records.

8.4 Evaluate the concept of health information exchange, especially in terms of Meaningful Use.

8.5 Analyze the technologies required to support Meaningful Use.

Key Terms

Clinical Document Architecture (CDA)
Continuity of Care Document (CCD)
Continuity of Care Record (CCR)
Direct Messaging
Healtheway
Health Information Organization (HIO)
Health Level Seven (HL-7)
Logical Observation Identifiers Names and Codes (LOINC)

Natural language processing (NLP)
Payer
RxNorm
Standards
Systemized Nomenclature of Medicine—Clinical Terms (SNOMED–CT)
Vaccine Administered (CVX)

The federal government's initiative to modernize the healthcare system is built on the core policy goals of lowering healthcare costs, improving patient outcomes, and having a healthy population. The use of electronic health records (EHRs) in specific, "meaningful" ways determined by the federal government serves as the cornerstone initiative, as well as a key line item of the $32 billion being spent for accomplishing these goals. This chapter examines the use of EHRs to achieve policy directives by detailing the elements of Meaningful Use, electronic health information processes, key technical standards that support these processes, and health information exchange.

8.1 The Electronic Health Record: Meaningful Use of Patient Information

What Is Meaningful Use?

In the face of unsustainably high healthcare costs combined with comparatively poor patient outcomes, the United States has undertaken numerous policy changes during the past decade. These include a number of new laws and regulations, changes in Medicare and Medicaid reimbursement rules, and a variety of policies designed to support reform. The greatest changes occurred in 2009 with the passage of the Affordable Care Act (ACA) and the American Recovery and Reinvestment Act, which included Health Information Technology for Economic and Clinical Health Act (HITECH). All of these measures were designed to change both healthcare delivery and payment models.

Several agencies, primarily in the Department of Health and Human Services (HHS), are spearheading the implementation of HITECH and ACA. Of these agencies, the two most prominent are the Office of the National Coordinator for Health Information Technology (ONC) and the Centers for Medicare and Medicaid Services (CMS).

The HITECH Act is centered on the digital capture, exchange, and analysis of clinical and financial patient records and the efficient use of these records. Its goals are to achieve improved patient outcomes and lower healthcare costs. Under HITECH, $32 billion of federal funds were spent to subsidize healthcare providers, allowing them to purchase electronic health record (EHR) systems, to develop health information exchanges to share data, to support education and training programs for workers, and to sustain various pilot projects.

The programs funded by HITECH are administered by both ONC and CMS. They ensure that tax dollars are being well spent and that resulting systems support *interoperability*.

In order to receive more than $44,000 in incentive payments per doctor to help pay for EHRs, healthcare providers and hospitals must show that they are using a government-certified EHR and that the digital health information captured by the EHR is being used in a "meaningful" way. There are three stages to Meaningful Use spread over a period of six years. The requirements under Meaningful Use increase at each stage. Providers and hospitals must demonstrate that they have achieved the new requirements at each point in time.

FOR YOUR INFORMATION

The Office of the National Coordinator for Health Information Technology (ONC) is part of the Department of Health and Human Services. It leads the charge to integrate advanced health information technology and the electronic exchange of health information into our healthcare system.

FOR YOUR INFORMATION

The Centers for Medicare and Medicaid Services (CMS) covers insurance and other health-related benefits for more than 100 million Americans. CMS is developing programs to support the ACA in a variety of areas, including care coordination, changes in provider reimbursement models, simplification of paperwork, and support of electronic health records and health information exchange.

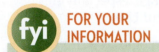

What happens if a provider decides to "stay with paper" and not to adopt an EHR? That is an option, although probably not one that will be very common. If providers and hospitals do not qualify under Meaningful Use, they will begin to have a reduction in the payments they receive for Medicare patients. More than 94% of hospitals have installed a basic EHR system and are in the process of "going digital." About 78% of office-based physicians use EHRs. Once most of healthcare data are being used electronically, there are more reasons to go electronic. Banks were paper-based in the 1980s; today, are there any banks without an ATM?

The Stages of Meaningful Use

In 2009, fewer than 20% of all healthcare providers used an EHR and the exchange of digital patient records between providers was extremely limited. The purpose of HITECH funding was to jump-start the digitization of patient records, the use of EHRs in patient care, and the exchange of the records by computerized systems. Also, policymakers wanted to use the Meaningful Use requirements to support some of the changes required by the ACA. As these changes would clearly take time, policymakers decided to spread out incentive payments over three points in time and to develop rules for implementing Meaningful Use over six years.

Table 8.1 summarizes the stages and focus of Meaningful Use. The requirements and their deadlines are established by the ONC, with public and industry feedback. Two years after attesting to Stage 1 Meaningful Use, a provider moves to Stage 2. Due to technological problems, some providers have been allowed three years at this Stage 1 level instead of automatically advancing to Stage 2. The start date for Stage 3 is still subject to final agreement, but it is scheduled to begin two years after Stage 2. Meaningful Use rules continue to change, but the objectives of the program remain consistent.

By staging the Meaningful Use requirements, the later objectives are built upon the earlier ones. Also, the objectives can be refined as more is learned about how to implement healthcare reform. ONC describes the stages of Meaningful Use as consisting of

1. Stage 1: The capture and sharing of data by EHRs and health information exchange
2. Stage 2: Advancing clinical outcomes through improved measurement and patient-directed exchange
3. Stage 3: Improved outcomes through coordination of the elements built under the earlier stages

Meaningful Use involves demonstrating the achievement of very specific objectives linked to these larger goals. This consists of meeting core objectives and selecting additional objectives from a menu of alternatives. For example, under Meaningful Use Stage 2, office-based providers must meet 17 core objectives and 3 menu objectives from a list of 6 alternatives. The result is 20 requirement objectives for Stage 2.

Hospitals have a separate set of core and menu objectives and a requirement consisting of 19 in total. Figure 8.1 provides a summary of Stage 1 core and menu objectives as well as the percentage of non-federal acute care hospitals.

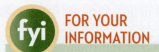

FOR YOUR INFORMATION

Interoperability and Meaningful Use are key ideas that were covered in the introductory chapter and the chapter on health information. Remember, interoperability is the ability of two or more systems to exchange data and use the information once it has been received. It is one of the most important requirements of Meaningful Use, which sets specific objectives that eligible professionals and hospitals must achieve to qualify for Centers for Medicare and Medicaid (CMS) incentive payment programs.

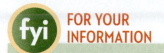

FOR YOUR INFORMATION

HealthIT.gov

The Objectives of Meaningful Use: (1) Improve quality, safety, and efficiency, (2) reduce health disparities, (3) engage patients and families, (4) improve care coordination and population/public health, (5) maintain privacy and security of patient health information.
Ultimately, it is hoped that Meaningful Use compliance will result in (1) better clinical outcomes, (2) improved population health outcomes, (3) increased transparency and efficiency, (4) empowered individuals, and (5) more robust research data on healthy systems.

TABLE 8.1 — The Stages and Goals of Meaningful Use

STAGE 1: 2011–2012	STAGE 2: 2014–2015	STAGE 3: 2017
Meaningful Use Criteria Focus On	**Meaningful Use Criteria Focus On**	**Meaningful Use Criteria Focus On**
• Electronically capturing health information in a standardized format • Using that information to track key clinical conditions • Communicating that information for care coordination processes • Initiating the reporting of clinical quality measures and public health information • Using information to engage patients and their families in their care	• More rigorous health information exchange (HIE) • Increased requirements for e-prescribing and incorporating lab results • Electronic transmission of patient care summaries across multiple settings • More patient-controlled data	• Improving quality, safety, and efficiency, leading to improved health outcomes • Decision support for national high-priority conditions • Patient access to self-management tools • Access to comprehensive patient data through patient-centered HIE • Improving population health

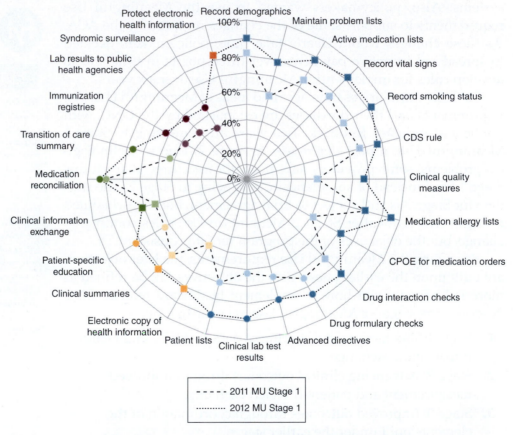

Figure 8.1   Nonfederal Acute Care Hospitals and Meaningful Use Stage 1

Squares (ν) represent Stage 1 core objectives. **Circles(λ)** represent Stage 1 menu objectives.
Blue = Objectives to improve quality, safety, and efficiency. This includes the right side of the chart (12 to 6 o'clock.) Record Demographics through Patient Lists are blue.
Orange = Objectives to engage patients and families, including Patient-specific Education, Clinical Summaries, and Electronic Copy of Health Information.
Green = Objectives to improve care coordination, including Transition of Care Summary, Medication Reconciliation, and Clinical Information Exchange.
Purple = Objectives to improve public and population health, including Syndromic Surveillance, Lab Results to Public Health Agencies, and Immunization Registries.
Red = Objective to ensure privacy and security for personal health information.

Source: Office of the National Coordinator for Health Information Technology.

The Meaningful Use Stage 1 objectives depicted in Figure 8.1 were carefully designed, based on lengthy negotiation and analysis, to be achievable. All of the objectives are measurable and auditable. They have been derived from the criteria in Table 8.1.

Meaningful Use and HIM

From the health information management perspective, the implementation of and adherence to the requirements and progression of Meaningful Use means that patient data are going to be used in more places and for new uses. As such, the responsibilities of health information management will increase and more healthcare workers with a wide variety of job responsibilities will need to understand HIM principles and guidelines.

8.1 A DAY IN THE LIFE

Adam Wagner is the CEO of a regional stand-alone hospital in the Midwest. The hospital has reached the requirements for Meaningful Use Stage 1 and is now required to meet Stage 2 requirements in two years. He is developing a strategy to meet that new goal.

1. How should he approach developing this strategy by building upon Stage 1?
2. What major challenges could the hospital face in meeting Stage 2 requirements, and what can Adam do to prepare?

8.1 THINKING IT THROUGH

1. Examine the Meaningful Use Stage 3 criteria outlined in Table 8.1. How can they directly result in improved efficiency and improved patient outcomes?
2. Describe how Meaningful Use can lead to higher levels of patient engagement.

8.2 Electronic HIM Processes

The Computerization of Health Information Functions

The maintenance of health records, even in a paper world, has for the most part been computerized for more than 25 years. The first computerized functions included tracking admissions, discharges, and transfers (ADTs) and, consequently, the Master Patient Index (MPI), which houses the demographic and administrative data (such as admission and discharge date or date of encounter), attending physician, and basic insurance data.

The advent of a computerized MPI significantly reduced duplicate master files, increased efficiency for health information staff, and allowed for the collection and maintenance of vast amounts of data. It is from the MPI that all other electronic functions flow.

Chart Tracking

Electronic tracking of health records is integral in a paper environment. It is not unusual for paper records to be moved 10 or 20 times a day. Unfortunately, the original location to which a paper record is "signed out" and the return of the record to the health information department are the only times that the true location of a record is known. Take, for instance, the record of a patient named Sally Stone, who is being seen in the emergency department (ED). The patient's old records are pulled by health information staff and taken to the ED. The record is signed out to the ED in the chart tracking system. Sally is then admitted to nursing unit 4F. The day after Sally is admitted to 4F she moves to surgery; her current record accompanies her, but her old records remain on 4F. After surgery, she is sent to the post-anesthesia care unit (PACU), then is transferred to 5E; her old records are sent to 5E by the unit coordinator on 4F. Sally remains in 5E for three days and is then transferred to the rehabilitation unit of the hospital. She acquires a new attending physician in the rehabilitation unit. The new physician needs to read her past history, which is found in the old records, but because the location of the old records was not tracked, it takes over an hour to locate them.

Had Sally's records been tracked, for instance, through a system that interfaces with the MPI, they would have been located easily and quickly. A bar coded system is often used to identify a record, particularly if the chart tracking technology does interface with the MPI. The bar code contains the patient's medical record number and the patient's name, requiring only the verification of the correct patient's record by the individual scanning the bar code.

The use of chart tracking software is unnecessary when the EHR is used, since a record is always accessible to more than one individual at a time, as long as the patient's name is spelled correctly or the correct medical record number is entered in the search field.

Record Completion

In manual (paper) systems, retrospective review of health records is performed to ensure the completeness of documentation. Discharge analysts review the discharged records and use an "incomplete record slip" to alert each physician of missing documentation (history and physical or discharge summary, for example) and any missing signatures. Incomplete records are sent to the "incomplete record room," where they sit, waiting for physicians to complete their records. Any records that remain incomplete for 30 days (or, in some cases, less) are considered delinquent. Some hospitals suspend physicians' admitting privileges or elective surgeries until delinquent records are complete, whereas others fine physicians a certain amount per day until the records are complete. Needless to say, this is a long process, and it can often take months for a record to be truly complete and permanently filed.

In an electronic system, there are still HIM professionals who review each record, but it is done electronically and often concurrently (while the patient is still in the hospital). Physicians are notified of their incomplete records by HIM professionals, who place them in the individual physician's queue.

Complete, accurate health records are necessary in order to satisfy CoP and accreditation requirements and standards, to ensure a smooth coding and billing process, and most importantly to achieve quality patient care. Allowing a record to sit incomplete for a month or more after discharge casts doubts on its validity. The longer the time that elapses between the time of the encounter and the documentation of that encounter, the greater the probability that important clinical information will be forgotten or misrepresented. In addition, should there be an accusation of negligence or malpractice if the record is called into court proceedings, the plaintiff's attorney will surely use that lapse in time to build the case.

In order to satisfy accreditation standards, hospitals must report the average number of incomplete and delinquent records to the Medical Records Committee (a standing committee of the medical staff). Hospitals with a delinquent record rate of 50% or greater of the average monthly discharges will likely receive a citation from the accrediting body. The HIM staff is responsible for reporting deficiencies by physician, by medical department, and in total. With an electronic system, reports are automatically generated and can be presented in multiple ways. Figure 8.2 is an image of deficiencies by a particular physician.

Memorial Hospital
Deficient Records Report by Physician

Delinquencies for: Robert K. Reynolds, MD

Patient Name	MR Number	Reason	Due Date
Robertson, Kyle	12-12-45	Op note	03/25/2014
Olensky, Hannah	11-24-45	Final Dx	03/25/2014
		E-sig orders	03/25/2014
Colburn, Rudolph	14-18-48	E-sig H&P	04/05/2014
		E-sig orders	04/05/2014
		E-sig prog notes	04/05/2014

Report run date: 03/20/2014 by MBS

Figure 8.2 **A Deficiency Report by Physician**

Through use of an electronic record completion system, a summary of deficiencies is run on demand to determine, at any point in time, the number of incomplete and delinquent records. Figure 8.3 demonstrates a summary report.

Electronic Signature

Electronic signature capability has been in use for many years, in both paper and electronic systems. This is particularly true in hospitals that utilize a hybrid system, in which a portion of their health records are

Memorial Hospital
Record Deficiency Summary

Date: 03/20/2014

Days Deficient	Number of Records Deficient
1–10 days	310 records
11–15 days	200 records
16–30 days	100 records
>30 days	85 records

Figure 8.3   A Summary of Record Deficiencies

paper and a portion are electronic. Physicians' orders, dictated reports, and even progress notes are often electronically signed in a hybrid system. A full description of eSignatures is given in the life cycle of health information chapter. From an HIM perspective, the use of eSignatures further streamlines the record deficiency tracking process.

Coding

Coding diagnoses and procedures begins with the documentation found in a health record. The diagnoses and procedures in the record are converted to numeric or alphanumeric format. Diagnoses are coded using ICD-9/10-CM; for inpatients only, procedures are converted to ICD-10-CM/ICD-10-PCS codes. Outpatient procedure and service codes are converted to Current Procedural Terminology (CPT) codes. Coders read the health record, ensure the specificity necessary to code the case completely and accurately (or query the physician if additional specificity is needed), and assign the numeric or alphanumeric code. Coding software, known as encoder software, is used in conjunction with code books to assign the codes. Encoder software is based on algorithms that convert the written format of a diagnosis or procedure into coded data. Without this transformation, filing of insurance claims and statistical reporting and analysis would be impossible.

Encoders may be logic based (Figure 8.4), where the coder answers a series of prompts that appear based on previous responses, to assign diagnosis or procedure codes, or they may be book based (Figure 8.5), in which the screens look much like paper coding manuals.

ENTER DIAGNOSIS ASTHMA

ASTHMA/ASTHMATIC

- With chronic obstructive pulmonary (lung) disease
  - With acute bronchitis
  - Unspecified
- With hay fever
  - With (acute) exacerbation
  - With status asthmaticus
  - Unspecified
- With allergic rhinitis
  - With (acute) exacerbation
  - With status asthmaticus
  - Unspecified

Figure 8.4   A Logic-Based Encoder

Asthma, asthmatic (bronchial) (catarrh) (spasmodic) 493.9
with
    chronic obstructive pulmonary disease (COPD) 493.2
    hay fever 493.0
    rhinitis, allergic 493.0

Figure 8.5   A Book-Based Encoder

Computer-assisted coding (CAC) is the latest technology to assist coders in capturing all pertinent information to assign correct and specific codes in a timely manner. Once in effect, due to a learning curve, the use of ICD-10-CM is expected to cut coder productivity, and CAC may make up for some of the loss of productivity because codes are suggested based on documentation in the record. CAC software utilizes **natural language processing (NLP)** to "read" the health record and suggest codes. The coder then uses encoder software and CAC (which may be interoperable) to verify the suggested coding. Computer-assisted coding (CAC) is not a substitute for a human being and neither is an encoder, but they are tools to enhance productivity, efficiency, and accuracy.

The abstracting process was discussed in the management of health information chapter. The collection of data to satisfy the Uniform Hospital Discharge Data Set (UHDDS) is now accomplished through the registration and coding processes. The data gathered through abstracting are used to provide statistics internally, for purposes such as strategic planning, quality assessment and improvement activities, and medical staff credentialing, as well as externally, in response to queries from public health agencies, media outlets, state and federal government agencies, and third-party **payers**, just to name a few.

Release of Information (ROI)

The release of health information has changed greatly over the past 20 or so years. Manual systems of opening and logging requests for health information, copying the record, and mailing the requested documents were laborious and inefficient. With the EHR or even a hybrid health record and the use of release of information software, this process has become streamlined and efficient. Patient portals, now a Meaningful Use requirement, further add to the efficiency release of information (ROI) software brings to the process. In the near future, a patient or designated caregiver will be able to request health information and receive it electronically through a patient portal. HIM staff, however, must still ensure that the record is complete and that the correct patient's records are authorized to be sent through the portal.

Though facilities still receive paper requests, ROI software that is interoperable with the facility's MPI makes logging the request much faster and most likely more thorough and accurate. In many cases, an EHR or even scanned images enable staff to electronically fulfill the request rather than mailing paper copies.

A log of requests generally includes the following:

- Patient's name, date of birth, medical record number, and date(s) of service or time frame of encounter
- Type of request (e.g., other physician or hospital, patient, attorney, or disability determination)
- Status of the request (e.g., incomplete record, pending authorization, open, or closed)
- Purpose of request (per the requestor)

Natural language processing (NLP) The ability of a computer to understand what is written in an EHR or to understand human speech.

Payer An entity other than the patient who pays for or finances healthcare services. These include insurance companies, the Centers for Medicare and Medicaid Services, and self-insured employers.

- Invoice generation
- Cover letter generation
- Date the request was answered (closed)
- Documentation supplied to the requestor
- Documentation mailed, sent electronically, faxed, through patient portal, and so on
- Identification of the staff member who answered the request

Reporting capability generally includes the following:

- Income for a particular time period
- Profit/loss for a particular time period
- Outstanding invoices by time frame
- By patient, the requestors, records requested, date requested, and so on
- Accounting of disclosures, as required by HIPAA

ROI software has become a staple of most health information departments, particularly since the passage of the HIPAA privacy rule. The software's ability to track and report who requested health information, what was sent in response, when, by whom, and in what form makes it a particularly important tool for ensuring compliance. Patients can request an accounting of disclosure at any time, and the hospital or healthcare facility must be able to provide that information when requested. Not only valid requests and fulfillment of the requests but also any breaches in disclosure need to be reported upon request.

Consider, for example, a request for the records of William I. Withers by a local attorney. William's date of birth (DOB) is July 8, 1955. It just so happens that there is also a William J. Withers, DOB July 8, 1955, in the hospital's MPI and the staff member releases William J. Withers's records rather than William I. Withers's. An incident (occurrence) report would be necessary in this case, and William J. Withers would need to be notified of the breach of confidentiality. Though the release of the wrong record was unintentional, it still constitutes a breach.

8.2 THINKING IT THROUGH

1. Some hospitals concurrently review records for deficiencies; others review retrospectively. Which is the best practice, and why?

2. Mr. Matthews, the administrator of Memorial Hospital, is preparing for a board meeting that begins in three hours. He needs to provide the board with statistics on the number of laparoscopic cholecystectomies performed over the past three years, by physician, and by age of patient. He calls you, the director of HIM, to get these statistics for him within the hour. Is that possible? If it is possible, of the computerized processes covered in this section, which will be used to fill this request?

8.3 Standards and Interoperability for Digitized Records

The Meaningful Use of patient data requires interoperability, the foundation of which is **standards**. Standards allow various technologies to work together. Like other businesses, healthcare has had specific standards that have developed for their software and hardware.

The healthcare industry has always been fragmented by both region and specialization. There is no national healthcare system and, historically, federally mandated standards were primarily concerned with reporting requirements for Medicare and Medicaid patient reimbursement. Vendors of HIT products and services independently developed their own products, with limited focus on connecting with others. Providers added to the problem by independently deciding what data to collect, how to encode and store the data, and how to define what the data meant by creating their own local data dictionaries. Some standards began to evolve, but they were not sufficient to meet the needs of expanding technology under the HITECH Act.

The Office of the National Coordinator for Health Information Technology (ONC) is responsible for coordinating the activities that establish standards for health IT and has created standard-making bodies for HIT. The ONC assists in organizing the activities of numerous stakeholders, including vendors, providers, government agencies, and the standard creating bodies. Most of the work in establishing the standards to support Meaningful Use is being done by the Health IT Standards and Health IT Policy Committees, which is responsible for making recommendations to ONC. As standards are established, they go through a federal rulemaking process that includes a public comment and response period. This process allows for the consideration of the definition of the standards as well as how they are implemented and how vendors can be certified to use them.

The ONC Health IT Standards Committee has identified five elements, or outcomes, for interoperability that need to be supported by standards. Each of these elements and their implications for HIM are described in Table 8.2.

Standards A prescribed set of rules or formats for how technologies operate and interact. Standards are approved by recognized industry bodies or can evolve *de facto*. In healthcare, standards exist for programming languages, operating systems, data formats, communication protocols, and electrical interfaces.

TABLE 8.2	Interoperability and HIM
Element of Interoperability	**Implications for HIM**
1. Adoption and optimization of EHR and HIE services	Capturing patient data, accuracy, relevance, and exchange in an interoperable manner
2. Standards to support implementation and certification	Supports the validity, reliability, and usability of health information
3. Financial and clinical incentives	Value propositions lowering costs and improving measurable patient outcomes
4. Privacy and security	HIM management, HIPAA compliance, trust
5. Rules of engagement or governance	Agreements between nonaffiliates on how health information is collected, exchanged, and used

Standards for Digital Records

There are dozens of technical standards used in HIT that impact patients' digital records. They can be organized by healthcare delivery functions, such as laboratory, imaging, pharmacy, clinical, or financial and administration. Alternatively, the ONC Health IT Standards Committee organizes its work within three very broad areas:

- Clinical operations
- Clinical quality
- Privacy and security

Other approaches organize standards by functionality, such as disease surveillance, database registries, or medication management or by educational domains, such as public health, clinical outcomes, or consumer health.

However, HIM professionals should be aware of key standards and their definitions. Table 8.3 provides a summary of important standards under Meaningful Use requirements.

TABLE 8.3	Key Standards for Meaningful Use
Standard	**Application**
Health Level Seven (HL-7)	HL-7 international is a standards body focused on the exchange, integration, sharing, and retrieval of electronic health information that supports clinical practice and management. HL-7 programming is critical to interfaces between systems to allow interoperability. HL-7 is an exchange format.
Clinical Document Architecture (CDA)	CDA is a standard from HL-7 to support interoperability and exchange. CDA defines the characteristics of a clinical document, including semantics, encoding, and structure.
Continuity of Care Document (CCD)	Based on the CDA standard, the CCD is the standard for the actual health record. It is an XML-based document and has been selected as one of two formats (the other being CCR) accepted under Meaningful Use. The CCD is more commonly used than the CCR standard and has greater traction with vendors and providers because it supports more applications.
Continuity of Care Record (CCR)	Developed by medical practitioners through the American Society for Testing Materials (ASTM), the CCR consists of a patient care summary with defined elements. CCR is XML-based and designed to be exchanged and easily usable by providers and patients. It is one of two health record standards (the other being the CCD) that is acceptable under Meaningful Use.
Systemized Nomenclature of Medicine—Clinical Terms (SNOMED–CT) but commonly referred to as SNOMED)	SNOMED is an established international standard for clinical medical terms to allow for common definitions in electronic data. This standard is part of EHR requirements under Meaningful Use Stage 2. SNOMED must be used for coding the data input from the medical encounter. It is a terminology that contains more than 300,000 medical term concepts to accurately record an encounter or care episode.
International Statistical Classification of Diseases and Related Health Problems, 10th Revision (ICD-10)	ICD-10 is a classification system published by the World Health Organization. It is a diagnostic tool for epidemiology, health management, clinical purposes, and reimbursement. CMS has mandated a conversion to ICD-10 from ICD-9 on October 1, 2014. ICD-10 provides greater detail than ICD-9, with 68,000 diagnostic codes and 72,000 procedural codes. As a classification system, ICD-10 represents a way to organize the output from a database.

(continued)

Standard	Application
Logical Observation Identifiers Names and Codes (LOINC)	LOINC is a standard required under all stages of Meaningful Use. LOINC is used to identify and code laboratory observations (e.g., test results) to be exchanged between labs, providers, and other stakeholders.
Vaccine Administered (CVX)	CVX is the standard used for immunization messages. The Centers for Disease Control and Prevention (CDC) develops and maintains CVX codes under HL-7. The use of CVX standards is required for the immunization objectives encompassed under Meaningful Use.
RxNorm	RxNorm provides for the normalization of names for clinical drugs used in pharmacy management and drug interaction software. RxNorm is required for pharmacy databases and messaging under Meaningful Use. RxNorm was developed and maintained by the US National Library of Medicine.

While these standards are very complex to implement, conceptually they are relatively straightforward. HL-7 is used for exchange and interfaces between devices. Clinical Document Architecture (CDA) defines what a patient summary record contains and is exchanged as a Continuity of Care Document (CCD). Logical Observation Identifiers Names and Codes (LOINC) is the standard for labs. RxNorm is the standard for pharmacies, and Vaccine Administered (CVX) is the standard for vaccinations.

Systemized Nomenclature of Medicine (SNOMED) and IDC-10 require special consideration. It is easy to confuse the roles of these standards. In fact, Meaningful Use Stage 1 allowed certified EHRs to store patient data through either ICD-9 (then the standard) or SNOMED. Meaningful Use Stage 2 requires the use of SNOMED for capturing patient problems in a summary of care record and the use of ICD-9 or 10 for billing. The reason for this is that SNOMED provides more detailed information about the encounter. SNOMED is far more granular than ICD-10. Since ICD-codes have been primarily used for data collection and billing, they do not necessarily correspond to the language and organization used by clinicians. Clinicians developed SNOMED for the purpose of succinctly capturing clinical encounters and procedures. Also, SNOMED excludes extraneous information used for billing or other purposes, which is often included in ICD-10.

SNOMED does not replace ICD-10. In fact, they have different functions and are complementary. As a terminology, SNOMED represents input into a database. As a classification system, ICD-10 represents a way to organize the output of a database for analysis. The use of SNOMED will help the conversion to ICD-10. Numerous products are being developed that automatically map SNOMED to ICD-10.

8.3   THINKING IT THROUGH

1. Describe the role of the ONC in setting standards.
2. How do the Meaningful Use standards improve the quality of information used in patient care?

In order to change both healthcare delivery and payment models, patient data must be at the right place at the right time. This requires the exchange of data among hospitals, clinics, payers, patients, and other stakeholders, a process called health information exchange. The term can be somewhat confusing, because it is used as a verb, to exchange information, and as a noun, an organization that provides the electronic exchange of data between stakeholders.

Health Information Exchange: The Verb

In order to achieve Meaningful Use and be eligible for incentive payments, providers must electronically exchange data with labs, public health departments, patients, and nonaffiliated providers. The Meaningful Use rules do not state how this should be accomplished, only that electronic exchange must occur (fax machines and physical media, such as flash drives, are not considered electronic exchange). The ONC encourages the maximum amount of health information exchange and does not define who provides the exchange infrastructure. By using such a policy, ONC is supporting the process of "health information exchange," as opposed to the organization (the noun) operating the technology to accomplish the process of exchange.

The ONC's approach allows the market for health information exchange to evolve based on local and regional needs. It also means the government does not have to "pick winners and losers" by defining the type of health information exchange organization providers must use. The market for health information exchange is still very young, and it is impossible to know the best structure or which types of organizations will ultimately succeed.

In sum, federal policy is to encourage the greatest amount of health information exchange through any organizations that providers choose. These can be public or private organizations. The stated policy is to support health information exchange, "the verb."

Health Information Exchange: The Noun

In order to accomplish health information exchange, there must be organizations that run the technologies, establish participation agreements between parties for the exchange, and meet all privacy and security requirements. These organizations are called health information exchanges, typically referred to as HIEs.

HIEs can be public, nonprofit community or government-owned organizations, or they can be privately owned, such as those run by large hospital systems. There continues to be great debate about whether public or private HIEs will prove to be the ultimate sustainable survivors. The financial track record for public HIE organizations has been bad. The earliest HIEs in the 1990s were called Clinical Health Information Networks (CHINs), and all were unsuccessful. A second attempt at regional HIEs occurred in the mid-2000s, with **Health Information Organizations (HIOs)**, and all but a very few failed.

Health Information Organization (HIO) A health information exchange organization that provides services only in a smaller region, usually a metropolitan area.

As part of the HITECH Act, ONC provided grants to all states for a period of five years to support the development of health information exchange under Cooperative Agreement Grants. The idea behind the grants was that states were closer to the stakeholders, consumers, providers, and payers and therefore would have the information necessary to make better decisions in spending the money. Each state developed its own strategic plan and decisions on funding allocation. In some states, the funds were used to support several regional HIOs. In others, all the funding was spent to develop statewide networks. There is no consistency from state to state. The end result is that in most states there are several public HIOs competing with each other and, in some cases, competing with statewide networks, all with no clear sustainability model. Figure 8.6 identifies the various types of HIE organizations.

Large hospital systems, payers, and vendors have launched private HIEs. Many of these large hospital systems are known as integrated delivery networks (IDNs), which are hospitals that own or operate ambulatory clinics, long-term care, wellness centers, and other facilities. Most IDNs have developed large networks that support health information exchange among their facilities. They can also extend these networks to nonaffiliates, thereby competing with HIEs.

Payers have had robust networks to support claims and payments, but not clinical data. They are now beginning to get involved in more robust health information exchange, often in partnership with large hospital systems, typically organized as accountable care organizations (ACOs). ACOs are data and analytics driven, because they are paid based on the health of their patient population as opposed to a fee-for-service model. ACOs are described in greater detail in the chapter discussing healthcare reform.

Vendors of EHRs have also developed private HIEs. These are a logical extension of an EHR. Vendors provide connection within a hospital or system or can even interconnect with other hospitals using the same EHR. An example of this is the "Care Everywhere" service provided by one of the largest vendors, Epic Healthcare.

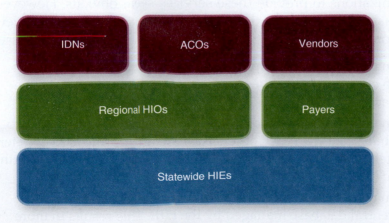

Figure 8.6 **The Types of HIE Organizations**

How HIEs Improve Care and Lower Costs

The premise behind spending on EHRs and ensuring that they are used in a meaningful way is that by getting data to the right place at the right time and by allowing all stakeholders to participate in generating and sharing data, better healthcare decisions will be made. The goal is to make healthcare more patient-centric, to encourage delivery based on a team approach, and to have patients take an active role in decision making. Central to this model are HIE organizations that facilitate the exchange of health information and are trusted parties.

Key ways health information exchange can improve care include the following:

1. Accurate and timely Continuity of Care Document (CCD)
2. Standards-based exchange for labs, diagnostic tests, pharmacy, and other data
3. Medicine reconciliation at all points of care
4. Clinical decision support, such as allergies and drug interaction notifications
5. Reduction in redundant tests
6. Admission, discharge, transfer (ADT) alerts to stakeholders
7. Continuity of care between hospitals and primary care providers after patient discharge
8. Engagement of patients and their caregivers
9. Patient-generated data
10. Public health, including electronic disease surveillance
11. Disease registries, such as those for cancer and diabetes
12. Chronic disease management and real-time monitoring

This is a partial list. Health information exchange enables the changing of the paradigm for healthcare delivery by giving all stakeholders access to the health information, particularly the most important stakeholder, the patient.

The Challenges Facing Health Information Exchange

The need for and value of health information exchange and for HIE organizations to provide these services seem obvious. However, as discussed, HIE organizations have had great difficulty in achieving economic sustainability. Several factors are at the root of this issue:

- In most regions, competing HIE organizations are trying to establish themselves as the principal source of exchange services.
- In many cases, competing hospital systems are unwilling to share data with each other. They are attempting to keep referral networks intact, since most healthcare reimbursement continues to be fee-for-service based.
- In most cases, providers do not want patient data kept in a central database managed by the HIE. This results in more expensive and cumbersome database systems.

- The technologies for health information exchange continue to evolve and are expensive. Particular problems are the interfaces between EHRs and HIEs. Each time services are added to an HIE, interfaces must be modified, adding significant expense and complexity.
- Privacy and security standards are evolving. Some state laws require patients to opt-in (as opposed to opt-out) to allowing their records to be part of an HIE. Opt-ins are challenging to organize and result in lower patient participation in the HIE.

With these issues as context, the single greatest issue facing HIE organizations is economic sustainability. Various models are being tried. The problem is establishing the value propositions in the current fee-for-service healthcare system to justify charging providers to use the HIE. Until more providers are willing to share their data through HIEs, there is a "chicken and egg" problem in attracting providers to the service.

The HIE sustainability problem will diminish as payment reform takes effect, with the resulting movement toward population management using a fee-for-value approach instead of a fee-for-service model. Providers will want to get as much information as possible on a patient, and there will be no competitive incentive to withhold patient information. HIEs will take the form of a "network of networks" much like how the Internet evolved to be what it is today.

8.2 A DAY IN THE LIFE

In planning to meet Meaningful Use Stage 2 requirements, Adam Wagner, the CEO for a regional hospital, has decided to suggest to his board that the hospital join the statewide HIE. This will require paying an annual subscription of about $100,000. Adam needs to get hospital board approval for the expenditure.

1. How can he describe the advantages of joining the HIE to the board? In what ways can joining an HIE improve care?
2. If the board asks him about problems facing HIEs, how should he describe them?

8.4 THINKING IT THROUGH

1. Describe the role that health information exchange plays in Meaningful Use.
2. Evaluate the reasons HIEs have not been sustainable.

8.5 The Infrastructure Supporting Meaningful Use

In order to make Meaningful Use work, a complex infrastructure is required. Figure 8.7 depicts various components of this infrastructure and how they fit together. At the basic level, there is a certified

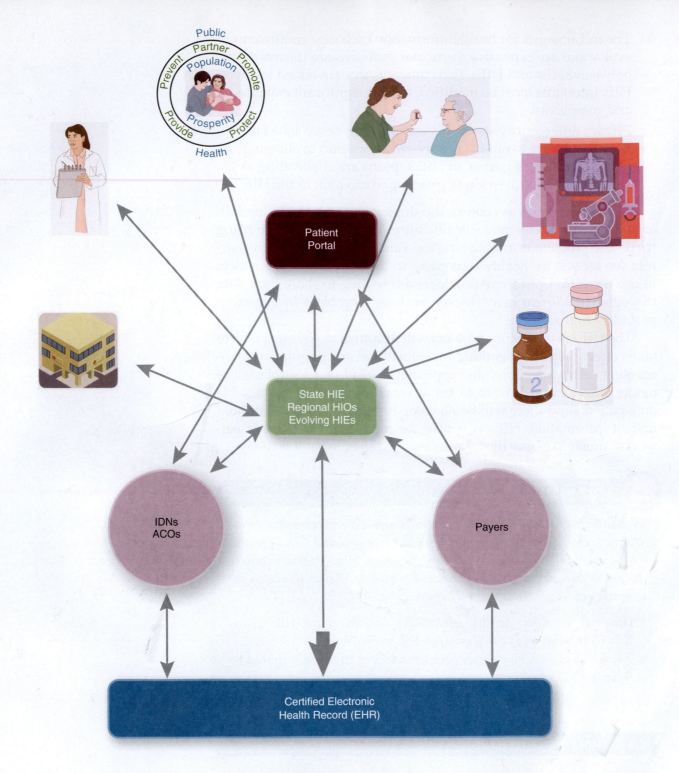

Figure 8.7 The Infrastructure of Meaningful Use

EHR that links information not only within an organization but also with external HIEs. Being certified, the EHR will use the various required standards and have required components, such as computerized physician order entry (CPOE). Interfaces will be used to support interoperability and will be based in HL-7 standards.

At the next level are private HIEs, often the location where the clinician works and the owner of the EHR. These may be the networks of large hospitals, such IDNs, or may interconnect the hospitals or payers that have formed an accountable care organization. Under

Meaningful Use requirements, these private HIEs connect with larger public HIEs, which represent the next level in the infrastructure. The degree to which private HIEs share data and fully engage in exchange beyond the requirements of Meaningful Use remains a key issue.

The third level from the foundation consists of regional HIOs and statewide HIEs. This is where a connection among nonaffiliated providers, pharmacies, labs, public health, case workers, and other caregivers occurs. This third level is critical to continuity of care, building a care team, and achieving larger goals of reducing costs and improving patient outcomes.

If there is no entity for health information exchange at the regional or state basis, or an HIO/HIE lacks the needed infrastructure, providers may meet the Meaningful Use requirements by using either of the two national-level health information network initiatives. One of these is **Direct Messaging**, an ONC-sponsored service. This service allows two clinicians to send patient data through HIPAA-compliant communications (similar to email) as an attached document. Provider organizations and clinicians must register for Direct Messaging and obtain a unique address and identification number. Direct Messaging has had varying levels of success, but it is an important alternative in regions where health information exchange has not developed. Direct Messaging is viewed as a transition technology to full health information exchange.

The second is a national network initiative designed as a "network of networks." The original effort was known as the Nationwide Health Information Network (NHIN or NWHIN) and has now evolved into **Healtheway**, a nonprofit private public partnership with the goal of nationwide interoperability of health information exchange. Ultimately, Healtheway depends on the success of regional and state-level exchanges, with which it will then interconnect as a network or networks.

Finally, Meaningful Use has patient engagement requirements. For example, under Stage 2, providers must demonstrate that at least 5% of their patients are accessing their records online and viewing, downloading, or transmitting them. The infrastructure for this is a patient portal. Patient portals are described in detail in the chapter on the patient's role in healthcare.

Portals also offer a way for patients and their caregivers to contribute information they believe relevant to their healthcare. Patient-sourced data in a portal may include data from remote monitoring devices, such as smartphones or wireless blood pressure or glucose monitors.

Direct Messaging Formally known as Directed Exchange or Direct Secure Messaging, a health information network initiative used by providers to easily and securely send patient information—such as laboratory orders and results, patient referrals, or discharge summaries—directly to another healthcare professional. This information is sent over the Internet in an encrypted, secure, and reliable way among health-care professionals who already know and trust each other, and is commonly compared to sending a secured email.

Healtheway The successor to the Nationwide Health Information Network, a nonprofit organization chartered to operationally support the eHealth Exchange, a rapidly growing community of exchange partners who share information under a common trust framework and a common set of rules. Healtheway leads in the development and implementation of strategies that enable secure, interoperable nationwide exchange of health information.

| 8.5 | THINKING IT THROUGH |

1. Why might Meaningful Use mandate that at least 5% of patients actively use a patient portal?
2. Direct Messaging has been criticized as "being secure email with a pdf attachment." Why is this inferior to the exchange of a full summary of care document through a health information exchange?

chapter 8 summary

LEARNING OUTCOMES	CONCEPTS FOR REVIEW

8.1 Define Meaningful Use and the goals for each stage of Meaningful Use. Pages 206–209

- Meaningful Use is a program administered by ONC and CMS that establishes specific objectives that providers must reach in order to qualify for incentives to help pay for the adoption, implementation, and upgrading of certified EHRs.
- Based on the long-term goals and complexity of achieving Meaningful Use, the program is being phased in through three stages over six years.
- The first stage was from 2011 to 2012, with a focus on capturing data by EHRs and using health information exchange, specifically
  1. Electronically capturing health information in a standardized format
  2. Using that information to track key clinical conditions
  3. Communicating that information for care coordination processes
  4. Reporting specific clinical quality measures and public health information
  5. Using information to engage patients and their families in their care
- The second stage began in 2014 and is focused on advancing clinical outcomes through improved measurement and patient-directed exchange, specifically
  1. More rigorous health information exchange
  2. Increased requirements for e-prescribing and incorporating lab results
  3. Electronic transmission of patient care summaries across multiple settings
  4. More patient-controlled data
- The third stage is scheduled to begin in 2016 with a focus on improved outcomes through coordination of the elements built under the earlier stages, specifically.
  1. Improved quality, safety, and efficiency, leading to improved health outcomes
  2. Decision support for national high-priority conditions
  3. Patient access to self-management tools
  4. Access to comprehensive patient data through patient-centered health information exchange
  5. Improved population health

8.2 Explain technologies used to process health information. Pages 209–214

- Early computerized functions: tracking admissions, discharges, and transfers (ADTs) and the Master Patient Index (MPI)
- Chart location software: useful in a manual record system but not necessary in an electronic system
- Record completion software: used by discharge analysts to notify physicians of missing or unsigned documentation
- Electronic signature: used to authenticate electronic entries
- Encoder software: assist coders in locating correct codes
- Computer-assisted coding: utilizes natural language processing to assign codes, which are later verified by coders
- Release of information: logs, tracks, documents health information released to external entities

LEARNING OUTCOMES	CONCEPTS FOR REVIEW

8.3 Describe the principal standards used for the digitization of patient records. Pages 215–217	• A standard is a prescribed set of rules or formats for how technologies operate and interact.
	• There are a variety of ways to organize the standards used in EHRs. ONC organizes them by clinical operations, clinical quality, and privacy and security.
	• There are key standards used in Meaningful Use.
	  1. HL-7 for exchange of data
	  2. Clinical Document Architecture for defining the characteristics of a health record in the form of a CCD or CCR
	  3. LOINC for laboratory data
	  4. RxNorm for pharmacy data
	  5. CVX for vaccination
	  6. SNOMED for clinical information input
	  7. ICD-10 for some types of clinical information output

8.4 Evaluate the concept of health information exchange, especially in terms of Meaningful Use. Pages 218–221	• Health information exchange is required to "get the right information to the right place at the right time." Meaningful Use will not be successful without it.
	• Health information exchange is used as both a verb, to exchange information, and a noun, the organization (HIE) providing exchange services.
	• Federal policy is to support the verb, the action of exchange, as opposed to identifying the organization that should be providing the exchange.
	• HIEs continue to have a difficult time being financially sustainable.
	  1. Providers are reluctant to exchange data with their competitors.
	  2. Services and standards are still evolving, creating both risk and an absence of value propositions.
	  3. Adoption of new reimbursement models, such as accountable care, shared-savings, and similar fee-for-value approaches, will make health information exchange very valuable for all stakeholders.
	• There are six primary types of HIEs.
	• There are numerous ways for health information exchange to reduce costs and improve outcomes under Meaningful Use.

8.5 Analyze the technologies required to support Meaningful Use. Pages 221–223	• The foundation for Meaningful Use is certified EHRs collecting and exchanging health information using ONC-supported standards. • A variety of private and public HIEs can provide connectivity to sources and users of a patient's health data. Direct Messaging—sharing health information in an encrypted, secure, and reliable way among healthcare professionals, similar to sharing a secure email. • Healtheway is the successor to the NHIN and NWHIN and is developing standards and a national health exchange. • Patient portals are a critical part of the infrastructure for achieving the goals of consumer-directed exchange and patient engagement.

chapter review

MATCHING QUESTIONS

Match each term with its definition.

_____ 1. **[LO 8.4]** accountable care organization

_____ 2. **[LO 8.5]** CPOE

_____ 3. **[LO 8.3]** Clinical Document Architecture

_____ 4. **[LO 8.1]** HHS

_____ 5. **[LO 8.4]** integrated delivery network

_____ 6. **[LO 8.1]** Meaningful Use

_____ 7. **[LO 8.3]** Continuity of Care Document

_____ 8. **[LO 8.3]** RxNorm

_____ 9. **[LO 8.3]** LOINC

_____ 10. **[LO 8.3]** standards

_____ 11. **[LO 8.4]** health information organization

a. Process by which a provider inputs requests into an electronic, automated system

b. XML-formatted document that is acceptable as a health record under Meaningful Use

c. Three-part legislation that aims to improve healthcare and security via data

d. Meaningful Use standard that identifies and codes laboratory observations, such as test results

e. Prescribed rules, approved by accrediting bodies, that govern how technologies interact

f. Federal agency helping implement HITECH and the Affordable Care Act

g. Database of drug names maintained by the Library of Medicine

h. Organizations which provide health data exchange within a particular region

i. Group of healthcare facilities that have networked together to provide better care through use of data

j. Hospitals that operate a group of facilities, such as clinics and long-term care settings

k. HL-7 standard that outlines how certain documents are formatted and structured

MULTIPLE CHOICE QUESTIONS

Choose the letter that best completes the statement or answers the question.

12. **[LO 8.1]** Which of the following is *not* part of Meaningful Use requirements?
    a. How vendors implement an EHR
    b. How providers use an EHR
    c. Technical certification of an EHR
    d. Certification of technicians installing an EHR

13. **[LO 8.1]** The stage of Meaningful Use with the objective that most focuses on care coordination is
    a. Stage 1.
    b. Stage 2.
    c. Stage 3.
    d. Care coordination is not a Meaningful Use objective.

14. **[LO 8.2]** What is encoder software?
    a. A technology used for making sure eSignatures are secure
    b. Software that assists with code assignment
    c. A tool for encrypting health records sent as attachments
    d. Software used for validating healthcare data

15. **[LO 8.2]** Which does a computerized MPI help reduce?
    a. Data collection
    b. Delinquent records
    c. Duplication
    d. Efficiency

16. **[LO 8.3]** The standard used for the coding and use of laboratory results is
    a. LOINC.
    b. SNOMED.
    c. ICD-10.
    d. CVX.

17. **[LO 8.3]** Beginning with Meaningful Use Stage 2, the standard that must be used for the capture and input of patient data into an EHR from a clinical encounter is
    a. LOINC.
    b. SNOMED.
    c. ICD-10.
    d. CVX.

18. **[LO 8.4]** In terms of health information exchange, the ONC policy is to
    a. develop statewide systems across the nation.
    b. directly support HIEs that are part of accountable care organizations.
    c. encourage health information exchange, "the verb."
    d. support Direct Messaging, because it is a national system.

19. **[LO 8.4]** Which is a benefit of health information exchange?
    a. Patient-generated data
    b. Electronic disease surveillance
    c. Reduction in redundant tests
    d. All of the above

20. **[LO 8.5]** Which is *not* typically part of a patient portal?
    a. Labs and test results
    b. Appointment scheduling
    c. Data from outside the health network
    d. Educational material and links

21. **[LO 8.5]** Which service exchanges patient data as part of an attachment?
    a. Healtheway
    b. Direct Messaging
    c. Availity
    d. HealthVault

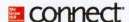 Enhance your learning by completing these exercises and more at http://connect.mheducation.com!

SHORT ANSWER QUESTIONS

22. **[LO 8.1]** What is the relationship between the stages of Meaningful Use for care coordination? Give examples of how care coordination will change as each stage of Meaningful Use takes effect.

23. **[LO 8.1]** Describe at least two specific ways the Meaningful Use of EHRs can lower healthcare costs.

24. **[LO 8.2]** Physicians' offices are smaller than hospitals; is chart tracking software necessary there? Why or why not?

25. **[LO 8.2]** Why do some hospitals fine or suspend physicians who have delinquent records?

26. **[LO 8.3]** What are the purposes of SNOMED and ICD-10? How is each being used under Meaningful Use?

27. **[LO 8.3]** Explain the relationship between health IT standards and interoperability.

28. **[LO 8.4]** ONC's policy is to encourage health information exchange, "the verb," not specific types of organizations. What are the results of this policy?

29. **[LO 8.4]** Describe why HIE organizations are having difficulty being financially sustainable.

30. **[LO 8.5]** Is Direct Messaging a suitable alternative to a national HIE network? Why or why not?

APPLYING YOUR KNOWLEDGE

31. **[LO 8.1]** Some providers may decide not to adopt EHRs but will stay with a paper-based records system. Would you be willing to go to a provider who was the last one in your community to go digital? Why or why not?

32. **[LO 8.2]** Jane Clooney arrives at your office and explains that a friend of hers called to tell her that she found a copy of Jane's laboratory test in the trash can at Dr. Seaford's office. Jane has never seen Dr. Seaford. She asks whether it is possible to know to whom her records have been released to outside of the hospital. How will you answer Jane, and what will you do to fulfill her request?

33. **[LO 8.3]** Two providers have two different EHR systems: one of them is certified under Meaningful Use standards, while the second is not certified. What are the implications for each of the providers? Whom can they share data with, and what is the effective functionality of each system?

34. **[LO 8.4]** What is the difference between *health information exchange* used as a verb and as a noun? Government policies focus on encouraging the verb. Is this the correct strategy?

35. **[LO 8.5]** There is no national health information exchange network. Why is the case? What are the benefits for having health information exchange at the local or regional level?

INTERNET RESEARCH

The ONC has a detailed dashboard tracking the progress made under Meaningful Use, available at http://dashboard.healthit.gov/. The dashboard is organized by the various programs under HITECH, as shown in Figure 8.8.

36. Using the HIT Dashboard, identify the latest percentage of office-based providers that have adopted EHRs across the nation and in your state. Identify the percentages for the same locations for hospitals adopting EHRs and for pharmacies actively e-prescribing.

37. Examine the results for the first exercise over time. How have your state's providers and hospitals done in terms of growth over the past three years? What about pharmacies actively e-prescribing?

38. Lab observations and results exchanged using the LOINC standard is another requirement of Meaningful Use. Using the HIT Dashboard, identify (a) the percentage of labs capable of sharing results outside their systems and (b) office-based providers with the capability of viewing lab results electronically. Do this for your state and the nation.

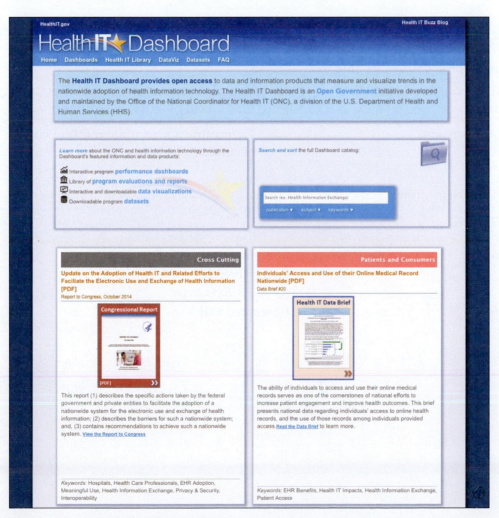

Figure 8.8   The Health IT Dashboard

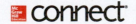 Enhance your learning by completing these exercises and more at http://connect.mheducation.com!

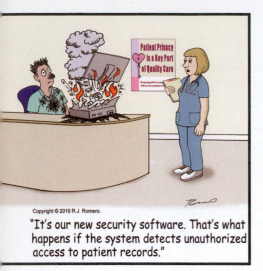

Copyright © 2010 R.J. Romero.

"It's our new security software. That's what happens if the system detects unauthorized access to patient records."

9

Privacy and Security of Digital Records

Learning **Outcomes**

When you finish this chapter, you will be able to:

9.1 Apply ethical standards of practice to patient scenarios.

9.2 Classify HIPAA privacy requirements.

9.3 Explain mechanisms used to secure data based on HIPAA regulations.

9.4 Determine appropriate methods of security compliance.

Key **Terms**

Accounting of disclosures
Audit trail
Court order
Directory information
Emancipated minor

Minimum necessary
Privacy breach
Subpoena duces tecum
Unsecured PHI

In a paper environment, keeping health information private, secure, and confidential internally was a challenge, since health information was typically shared internally by sending the paper record to the care unit, and it was difficult or impossible to know exactly who had read a patient's health record. A physical authorization was used to share the health information externally or was released as required by law. The patient's records remained in a tangible form, which, if needed by an outside entity, was copied and either faxed or mailed when requested.

The recent advances in the use of patient portals, electronic sharing among disparate healthcare providers, and the ability to share information through formal health information exchanges (HIEs) has blurred the lines and has increased HIM's responsibility in ensuring the release of complete and timely health information when there is a need for it. Advances have also escalated HIM's role in information security. Adequate safeguards must be in place to protect the security of electronic health information. The health information professional has a pivotal role in data security, including implementing measures to guard against unauthorized access, developing standardized processes, monitoring access, and investigating complaints.

9.1 Ethical Obligations

Ethical Duty to Patients

Healthcare professionals have an obligation to respect the privacy of patients as well as to respect their right to make decisions regarding their own physical, emotional, and psychological well-being. This being said, a physician or other healthcare professional cannot make informed decisions regarding diagnoses or care plans without accessing information from the patient or the patient's health record. Though health information is shared and accessed frequently, accessing only that which is necessary to diagnose and treat, while maintaining the patient's privacy and confidentiality, is the ethical duty of healthcare professionals, including health information professionals.

Anyone who works in a healthcare setting is required to sign a confidentiality agreement stating that any and all protected health information will be kept confidential regardless of whether it is oral, written, or maintained in electronic format. See Figure 9.1 for an example of a confidentiality agreement for healthcare workers. This applies not only to staff and physicians but also to volunteers, students, outside observers, and contractors. In addition, there is an ethical obligation to keep confidential all information one sees, hears, or documents. Physicians and other healthcare professionals take the Hippocratic Oath, which in effect states that nothing that is seen or heard will be repeated. As health information professionals, we are bound by the American Health Information Management Association (AHIMA) Code of Ethics, which states

> *A health information management professional shall: Preserve, protect, and secure personal health information in any form or medium and hold in the highest regards health information and other information of a confidential nature obtained in an official capacity, taking into account the applicable statutes and regulations.*

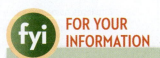

FOR YOUR INFORMATION

The complete AHIMA Code of Ethics is found at http://library.ahima.org/xpedio/groups/public/documents/ahima/bok1_024277.hcsp?dDocName=bok1_024277 and the HIMSS Business Practice Code of Ethics is found at http://www.himss.org/News/NewsDetail.aspx?ItemNumber=5017.

With the electronic exchange of health information among distinct healthcare providers and facilities, this ethical duty applies not only to the individual healthcare providers who care directly for the patient but also to the entities that enable the electronic exchange. HIEs must follow the same laws and regulations that cover healthcare providers and facilities.

Healthcare providers protect the patient's privacy not just because they are bound to do so through HIPAA or because it is an ethical duty, but because it is also a patient's right to expect that his or her privacy will be respected as well as the confidentiality of his or her health information.

The Patient's Right to Privacy

When one thinks of privacy in the healthcare field, HIPAA generally comes to mind. HIPAA resulted in standardization and clarification

---

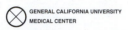 **GENERAL CALIFORNIA UNIVERSITY MEDICAL CENTER**   **CONFIDENTIALITY AGREEMENT**

> *Applies to all GCU Healthcare "workforce members" including employees, medical staff, and other healthcare professionals; volunteers; agency, temporary, and registry personnel; and house staff, students, and interns (regardless of whether they are GCU trainees or rotating through GCU Healthcare facilities from another institution).*

It is the responsibility of all GCU Healthcare workforce members, as defined above, to preserve and protect confidential patient, employee, and business information.

The federal Health Insurance Portability and Accountability Act (HIPAA) Privacy Law, the Confidentiality of Medical Information Act (California Civil Code § 56 et seq.), and the Lanterman-Petris-Short Act (California Welfare & Institutions Code § 5000 et seq.) govern the release of patient identifiable information by hospitals and other heathcare providers. The State Information Practices Act (California Civil Code sections 1798 et seq.) governs the acquisition and use of data that pertain to individuals. All of these laws establish protections to preserve the confidentiality of various medical and personal information and specify that such information may not be disclosed except as authorized by law or the patient or individual.

Confidential Patient Care Information includes: Any individually identifiable information in possession or derived from a provider of healthcare regarding a patient's medical history, mental, or physical condition or treatment, as well as the patient's and/or family members' records, test results, conversations, research records, and financial information. Examples include, but are not limited to:

- Physical medical and psychiatric records including paper, photo, video, diagnostic, and therapeutic reports;
- Patient insurance and billing records;
- Mainframe and department-based computerized patient data;
- Visual observation of patients receiving medical care or accessing services; and
- Verbal information provided by or about a patient.

Confidential Employee and Business Information includes, but is not limited to, the following:

- Employee home telephone number and address;
- Spouse or other relative names;
- Social Security number or income tax withholding records;
- Information related to evaluation of performance;
- Other such information obtained from the University's records which, if disclosed, would constitute an unwarranted invasion of privacy; or
- Disclosure of confidential business information that would cause harm to GCU Healthcare.

Peer review and risk management activities and information are protected under California Evidence Code section 1157 and the attorney–client privilege.

(continued)

Figure 9.1 **A Confidentiality Agreement for Healthcare Workers**

I understand and acknowledge that:

1. I shall respect and maintain the confidentiality of all discussions, deliberations, patient care records, and any other information generated in connection with individual patient care, risk management, and/or peer review activities.

2. It is my legal and ethical responsibility to protect the privacy, confidentiality, and security of all medical records, proprietary information, and other confidential information relating to GCU Healthcare and its affiliates, including business, employment, and medical information relating to our patients, members, employees, and healthcare providers.

3. I shall access or disseminate patient care information only in the performance of my assigned duties and where required by or permitted by law, and in a manner which is consistent with officially adopted policies of GCU Healthcare, or where no officially adopted policy exists, only with the express approval of my supervisor or designee. I shall make no voluntary disclosure of any discussion, deliberations, patient care records, or any other patient care, peer review, or risk management information, except to persons authorized to receive it in the conduct of GCU Healthcare affairs.

4. GCU Healthcare performs audits and reviews patient records in order to identify inappropriate access.

5. My user ID is recorded when I access electronic records and I am the only one authorized to use my user ID. Use of my user ID is my responsibility whether by me or anyone else. I will access only the minimum necessary information to satisfy my job role or the need of the request.

6. I agree to discuss confidential information only in the workplace and only for job-related purposes and to not discuss such information outside of the workplace or within hearing of other people who do not have a need to know about the information.

7. I understand that any and all references to HIV testing, such as any clinical test or laboratory test used to identify HIV, a component of HIV, or antibodies or antigens to HIV, are specifically protected under law and unauthorized release of confidential information may make me subject to legal and/or disciplinary action.

8. I understand that the law specially protects psychiatric and drug abuse records, and that unauthorized release of such information may make me subject to legal and/or disciplinary action.

9. My obligation to safeguard patient confidentiality continues after my termination of employment with the General California University.

I hereby acknowledge that I have read and understand the foregoing information and that my signature below signifies my agreement to comply with the above terms. In the event of a breach or threatened breach of the Confidentiality Agreement, I acknowledge that the General California University may, as applicable and as it deems appropriate, pursue disciplinary action up to and including my termination from General California University.

Print Name:	Signature:
Department:	Dated:

Routing: Please complete the form and return it to your hiring department.

of the information that is covered by patient right to privacy as well as the circumstances under which an authorization is and is not needed. Other regulations that govern a patient's right to privacy include the Medicare Conditions of Participation, The Privacy Act of 1974, and laws governing the confidentiality of alcohol and drug abuse records, both state and federal. There are instances when these rules and regulations conflict. As a general rule, the more stringent law must be followed; however, it is best practice to seek the opinion of the facility or practice legal counsel when this does occur, and the facility's written release of information policies must then reflect the advice given by the attorney. The HIPAA privacy rule, however, did resolve some inconsistencies and resulted in more standardized privacy regulations.

With the passage of HIPAA, patients gained the right to

- Receive notification of how their health information is used and to whom it is released for treatment, payment, and business operations, as well as circumstances that are required by law (for instance, reporting of communicable diseases)
- Authorize the use and release of their health records
- Expect hospitals, third-party payers, healthcare providers, and healthcare clearinghouses to safeguard their health information
- Request an accounting of all disclosures of their health information
- Expect that only information that is reasonably necessary to satisfy the reason for the disclosure is released
- Examine as well as obtain a copy of their health records and request corrections to documentation

In addition, because of HIPAA, those who violate a patient's right to privacy are held accountable in the form of civil and criminal penalties, should the patient's privacy be unlawfully breached.

Though HIPAA does protect the privacy of health information, it also allows for disclosure of some healthcare data for the public good—for instance, to public health agencies.

With the passage of HIPAA, healthcare providers must

- Notify individuals regarding their privacy rights and how their protected health information (PHI) is used or disclosed
- Adopt and implement internal privacy policies and procedures
- Train health facility staff (including physicians) to understand these privacy policies and procedures as appropriate for their functions within the covered entity
- Designate individuals who are responsible for implementing privacy policies and procedures and those who will receive privacy-related complaints (commonly known as privacy officers)
- Establish privacy requirements in contracts with *business associates* that perform covered functions
- Put or have in place appropriate administrative, technical, and physical safeguards to protect the privacy of health information
- Meet obligations with respect to health consumers exercising their rights under the privacy rule

Examples of business associates include

- A medical transcription company with which the hospital contracts for backlog transcription
- A company hired to perform an audit of diagnostic and procedural coding
- A certified public accounting firm performing an audit and having access to PHI
- The hospital's attorney, who has access to PHI

1. Why would it be nearly impossible to determine who has accessed a paper health record internally?
2. For what reason(s) might a patient request an accounting of disclosures of the PHI?

9.2 HIPAA Privacy Regulations

HIPAA affords people who leave their employer, for whatever reason, the ability to continue health insurance coverage. The patient is responsible for the payment of monthly premiums, however. The act also sets standards for storing, maintaining, and sharing electronic health information while ensuring the privacy and security of the information.

The HIPAA Privacy Rule

Individually identifiable patient information is protected under the HIPAA privacy rule. Individually identifiable data include the patient's name, address, phone number, email address, date of birth, Social Security number, and medical record number; account numbers tied to the patient; the patient's insurance identification numbers; the patient's fingerprints; photographs of the patient; and the name of the patient's employer. In the act, this is referred to as protected health information (PHI), which we discussed earlier in the chapter on external forces affecting health information.

Public persons who are easily identified—for instance, "the mayor Pittsburgh, PA"—are considered covered as well. Though the healthcare facility or provider owns the health record (in physical or electronic form), the patient owns the information in it and therefore has a right to authorize release or protect from release any information in which he or she is identified. PHI is protected, and the patient's authorization is necessary to release health information. However, information necessary to care for patients, collect payment for services, and operate a business is permitted to be used without authorization. This exception is known as treatment, payment, and operations, or TPO. The privacy rule applies to all covered entities, including healthcare providers (physicians, dentists, hospitals, nursing homes, chiropractors, pharmacies, psychologists, etc.), health plans (insurance companies, managed care plans, Medicare, Medicaid, veterans' health plans, etc.), and healthcare clearinghouses. There are also a number of other circumstances when release of information is required:

- Release as required by a **subpoena duces tecum**, **court order**, or other legal order (for instance, a search warrant)
- Public health surveillance, investigations, and interventions, such as reporting communicable diseases
- As otherwise required by federal, state, tribal, or local laws
- Health research, though certain conditions apply

Subpoena duces tecum A command issued by a clerk of the court or an attorney for someone to appear in person in court or a deposition, to bring any documents or papers noted in the *subpoena duces tecum*, and to give testimony.

Court order A written directive by a court judge that requires one to do something (for instance, appear in court or produce documents) or to *not* do something (for example, a restraining order).

- In the case of abuse, neglect, or domestic violence under certain circumstances
- For use in judicial and administrative proceedings, under certain circumstances
- Organ-procurement agencies for the purposes of facilitating transplant
- Health oversight agencies, such as state departments of health, for oversight activities authorized by law
- Disclosure of work-related health information as authorized by, and to the extent necessary to comply with, workers' compensation investigations

The initial compliance date with the privacy rule was April 14, 2003, with an extension to April 14, 2004, for smaller health plans.

Regardless of the presence of an authorization or as required in the previously listed circumstances, only the **minimum necessary** information to fulfill the reason for the request is released. Prior to HIPAA, authorizations stating the release of "any and all" records were honored; after HIPAA, the reason for the request must be documented in the authorization.

Minimum necessary The part of the HIPAA privacy rule that requires covered entities to make reasonable efforts to limit the patient-identifiable information released to only that which satisfies the intended purpose of the request for disclosure.

9.1 A DAY IN THE LIFE

Julie, the release of information coordinator at Memorial Medical Center, received an authorization from an attorney for the records of James Alexander. The authorization requested that "all records" of James Alexander were to be released to the attorney and that the purpose of the request was "investigation of an auto accident occurring on January 15, 2013." Upon review of the records, Julie noted that though Mr. Alexander had visited the hospital many times since 2010, only an emergency department visit on January 15, 2013, pertained to an auto accident. After matching the patient's signature on the authorization with one found in his records, Julie printed the documentation pertaining to the January 15, 2013, emergency department visit. She included a cover letter stating that the records pertaining to the auto accident that occurred January 15, 2013, were enclosed.

1. Julie received a letter from the attorney the following week, stating that the patient authorized the release of "any and all records." Construct a letter to the attorney, explaining why only certain records were released.

Accessing the minimum necessary information also applies internally. A physical therapist treating an inpatient may need to read the progress notes and orders of the orthopedic surgeon caring for the patient, but the consultation by a psychiatrist regarding the patient's mental status would generally not be considered necessary. The therapist has no need to read through the entire record unless information such as a psychiatric consult has bearing on the therapy prescribed for the patient.

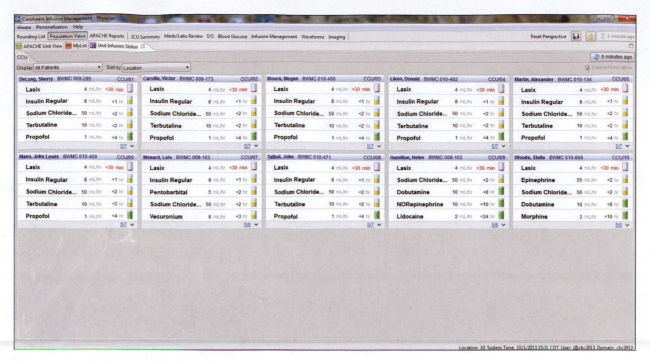

Figure 9.2 An Inpatient Bed Board or Census

Directory information may be released without written authorization unless the patient specifies otherwise. Directory information includes the fact that the patient is a patient (or an outpatient) in the hospital as well as his or her room number. Directory information also includes the condition of the patient, expressed in general terms, and the patient's religious affiliation. See Figure 9.2 for a screenshot of an inpatient bed board or census.

Notice of Privacy Practices

Patients must be notified of their rights under HIPAA, and that is accomplished through the patient's reading of, and signature of approval on, the Notice of Privacy Practices (NPP). The NPP must be in writing, must be signed by the patient, and must inform the patient how his or her health information will be used, the circumstances under which it may be released, that he or she may view or have copies of his or her health records, and that amendments may be requested (in writing), as well as the procedure for filing complaints with the Department of Health and Human Services. Patients need only sign an NPP one time for each facility or office in which they receive care, unless the facility or practice changes its NPP or if the patient wishes to make changes to what he or she has consented to—for instance, the individuals to whom his or her health information can be released.

HITECH Amendments

The passage of HITECH and the Omnibus Final Rule, with which compliance has been required since September 2013, necessitated increasing the scope of the privacy and security rules. Legal liability for noncompliance is enhanced under the HITECH amendments and provides for greater enforcement by the Office of Civil Rights.

Directory information
Covered entities, including hospitals, may maintain in a directory certain information about patients, such as the patient's name, the patient's location in the facility, the health condition of the patient (in general terms) that does not communicate specific medical information about the individual, and the patient's religious affiliation. The patient must be informed about the information to be included in the directory, and to whom the information may be released, in the notice of privacy practices and must have the opportunity to restrict the information or to whom directory information is disclosed, or opt-out of being included in the directory. The facility may provide the appropriate directory information, except for religious affiliation, to anyone who asks for the patient by name.

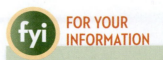

FOR YOUR INFORMATION

An example of a 2013 NPP document is found at http://www.hhs.gov/ocr/privacy/hipaa/npp_booklet_hc_provider.pdf.

HITECH requires mandatory penalties for "willful neglect." The act does not contain verbiage that defines willful neglect, however, and thus it may be decided on a case by case basis. The risk of being accused of willful neglect increases for healthcare providers that do not have strict privacy and security policies and/or do not have strong compliance plans in place.

The act increases monetary (civil) penalties for willful neglect. The fine is $250,000 but increases to $1.5 million in cases of repeat or uncorrected violations. A key enhancement of HITECH is that under certain conditions HIPAA's civil and criminal penalties now extend to business associates as well as covered entities.

As with HIPAA regulations, an individual cannot bring an action against a healthcare provider, but HITECH does allow a state attorney general to bring an action against a healthcare provider on behalf of his or her constituents.

Under HIPAA, oversight was also lax, but the Department of Health and Human Services (HHS) is now required to audit covered entities and business associates on a periodic basis.

Under the Omnibus Final Rule, patients' rights were expanded. For instance, as facilities and practices adopt a compliant EHR, covered entities will be required to provide the patient's health record in electronic form, when requested. Also, patients who are paying for their services in cash may instruct the provider not to bill their insurance and not to divulge any information about their services to the patient's health insurance carrier.

Authorizing the Release of PHI

The HIPAA privacy rule requires the authorization of the patient or his or her legal representative except as noted earlier in this chapter. A typical HIPAA-compliant authorization to release PHI is seen in Figure 9.3. Required elements of the authorization are

- The health information authorized for disclosure
- The name of the entity releasing the information (the hospital or the physician's practice, for example)
- The name of the receiving entity
- The purpose of the disclosure
- A statement informing the patient of
  - His or her right to revoke the authorization in writing
  - How to revoke the authorization
  - Any exceptions to the right to revoke
- A statement that the hospital cannot require the patient to sign the authorization in order to receive treatment or payment or to enroll or be eligible for benefits
- A statement that the information disclosed pursuant to the authorization may be redisclosed by the recipient of the information, and the information is no longer protected by federal privacy regulations

AUTHORIZATION TO DISCLOSE PROTECTED HEALTH INFORMATION

	For internal use only:
Memorial Medical Center **41515 Brownsville Road** **Anywhere, USA 77777** **(484-555-1156)**	**Date received** _____ **Date released** _____ **By**
Patient Name _____ **DOB** _____	**Medical Record Number** _____

I, _____, hereby authorize Memorial Medical Center to disclose information from my health record(s) as described below to:

Name of person/entity receiving information

_____

Address

_____

Purpose of disclosure

_____

Copies to be released:

Date(s) of encounter(s) from _____ to _____
Date(s) of encounter(s) from _____ to _____
Date(s) of encounter(s) from _____ to _____

The checked reports or documentation below may be released:

☐ Face sheet   ☐ Progress notes   ☐ Physicians' orders   ☐ Nurses' notes   ☐ Other

_____

☐ Summary   ☐ X-ray reports   ☐ EKG/echo   ☐ Lab results

_____

☐ Consultation   ☐ Op note   ☐ Mental health records

_____

☐ Discharge summary   ☐ History & physical   ☐ Substance abuse records

_____

I understand that I have the right to revoke this authorization at any time, except what has already been disclosed pursuant to this authorization. I understand that if I revoke this authorization I must do so in writing to the Health Information Department of Memorial Medical Center.

This authorization will expire on the following date _____ or in the following circumstance _____; otherwise it will expire 6 months following the date of signature below.

I understand the medical center cannot require me to sign the authorization in order to receive treatment or payment or to enroll or be eligible for benefits.

I am signing this authorization voluntarily. I understand that I may inspect or copy the information to be disclosed as provided by federal regulations. I understand that information disclosed may be re-disclosed without my authorization and may not be protected by federal privacy regulations.

Printed name of patient/legal representative

_____

Signature of patient/legal representative

_____

Legal representative's relationship to patient

_____

Date of signature

_____

Figure 9.3
A HIPAA-Compliant Authorization to Release Protected Health Information (PHI)

- A statement that the authorization will expire
  - On a specific date
  - After a specific amount of time
  - Upon a circumstance or an event related to the patient
- The signature of the patient and the date signed (see the discussion of emancipated minors, which follows); if the patient's representative signs the authorization, the authorization must include a description of that person's authority to act for the patient

In most states, the legal age of majority is 18 years old. If an individual is considered an **emancipated minor**, the patient may sign for himself or herself. *Emancipation* generally refers to patients under the age of 18 who live on their own (and are financially responsible for themselves) or individuals who are married and under the age of 18. In addition, minors may consent for their own treatment and to the release of health information relating to contraceptive management, testing and treatment for sexually transmitted diseases (including HIV), prenatal care and delivery services, and treatment for substance abuse or mental health care. Individual state laws vary, however, and the policies for release of information must clearly define the term *emancipated*, under what circumstances the minor's authorization will be accepted without parental authorization, and whether proof of emancipation is required (and in what form).

Emancipated minor A person, typically under the age of 18, who is no longer under a parent's control, financial or otherwise, and assumes responsibility for himself or herself.

9.2 A DAY IN THE LIFE

The following are typical requests for health information that Becky, the release of information coordinator at Memorial Hospital, handles each week. Discuss each of these scenarios, and state whether Becky did the right thing; explain why or why not.

1. The records of Cecelia Pike have been requested by a local attorney; an authorization was received and is signed by the patient's mother. The patient is 20 years old. Becky released the records using this authorization.
2. Neil Gustafson, the director of nursing at Memorial Hospital, called Becky to request the records of June Philips for her stay of February 3 to February 5, to investigate a matter that was brought to his attention about care June Philips received. Becky told Mr. Gustafson that she would first need an authorization signed by the patient.
3. A biller from the business office sent an email to Becky that Blue Cross has requested the progress notes for April 5 and 6 related to a patient, Howard Rawlings, before it will consider payment of the bill for that stay. Becky prints the progress notes for those dates and sends them to the biller.
4. Mike Redland is the human resources director; he has requested all the health records of Michelle Gesford, an employee in the human resources department.

(continued)

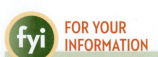

FOR YOUR INFORMATION

The terms *consent* and *authorize* are both used in the HIPAA privacy rule. Consent to use or release PHI is given by virtue of signing the facility's Notice of Privacy Practices. Authorization, on the other hand, is a specific document that gives permission to use or disclose PHI for a particular purpose other than for treatment, payment, or operations (TPO) or for disclosing PHI to an individual or entity (for example, an employer) specified by the patient.

5. Becky opened a request from an attorney, and the authorization was for "any and all" records of the healthcare of Lesli Simpson from June 8, 2010, through and including December 31, 2013. The purpose for the disclosure has a line through it.

9.2 THINKING IT THROUGH

1. Renee is 17 years old, has moved out of her parents' house, and supports herself. Can her mother sign for Renee's medical care or to receive copies of Renee's health records?

2. A copy of John's operative report was sent to Blue Cross because the claim is being reviewed for medical necessity for performing the procedure. John was not asked to sign an authorization to release the operative report to Blue Cross. Should John have signed an authorization to release his PHI? Explain your answer.

9.3 HIPAA Security Rule

Protecting the Integrity of Data

The HIPAA security rule instructs covered entities and business associates to provide appropriate administrative, physical, and technical safeguards to ensure the confidentiality, integrity, and security of electronic protected health information. Covered entities were required to comply with the security rules effective April 21, 2005; smaller covered entities were required to comply by April 21, 2006. The definitions of each from the HIPAA law are as follows.

Administrative safeguards include *"administrative actions, and policies and procedures, to manage the selection, development, implementation, and maintenance of security measures to protect electronic protected health information and to manage the conduct of the covered entity's workforce in relation to the protection of that information".* This type of safeguard includes ongoing education of all facility staff on HIPAA requirements and written acknowledgment of the facility's privacy and confidentiality policies by all staff. HIPAA also requires the designation of a privacy officer to develop the policies and procedures that ensure HIPAA compliance.

Physical safeguards include *"physical measures, policies, and procedures to protect a covered entity's electronic information systems and related buildings and equipment, from natural and environmental hazards, and unauthorized intrusion."* Examples include positioning computer screens so that they are only seen by staff, having a physical barrier between the public and the office areas that house computers, and locking down computers that are on movable carts.

Technical safeguards include *"the technology and the policy and procedures for its use that protect electronic protected health information and control access to it."* This includes a unique identifier and password for each user and automatic log-off from the computer after a specific period of time of inactivity.

Ensuring Data Security and Integrity

Covered entities should employ the HHS suggestions listed in this section for both administrative and technical safeguards. Although this is not an exhaustive list, the following should be included in a facility or practice security plan:

- Develop, document, and implement policies and procedures for assessing and managing risk to its electronic protected health information (ePHI).
- Periodically review risk analysis policies and procedures and update as necessary.
- Categorize information systems based on the potential impact to the facility or practice, should the system(s) become unavailable.
- Complete an accurate and thorough risk analysis, taking into account, for example, the occurrence of a significant event or a change in the business organization or environment of the facility or practice.
- Construct a documented program to mitigate the threats and vulnerabilities to ePHI identified through the risk analysis.
- Institute a risk management program that guards against the impermissible use and disclosure of ePHI.
- Document the results of risk analysis and distribute the results to those individuals who are responsible for mitigating the threats and vulnerabilities to ePHI identified through the risk analysis.
- Develop a formal security plan.
- Include a human resources policy requiring the discipline of staff members who have access to the facility's or practice's ePHI for violation of policies to prevent system misuse, its abuse, and any harmful activities that involve ePHI.
- Draft sanction policies and procedures as part of security awareness training programs for staff.
- Document policies and procedures for the review of information system activity.
- Regularly review information system activity.
- Appoint a senior-level staff member whose job it is to develop and implement security policies and procedures or act as a security point of contact.
- Share policies and procedures requiring safeguards to limit access to ePHI with those individuals and software programs appropriate for their role.
- Clarify policies and procedures for granting access to ePHI based on the software programs appropriate for given roles.
- Institute policies and procedures for the assignment of a unique identifier for each authorized user.
- Draft policies and procedures to enable access to ePHI in the event of an emergency.
- Document policies and procedures for creating an exact copy of ePHI as a backup.

- Require automatic log-off after a predetermined period of inactivity.
- Install mechanisms that can encrypt and decrypt ePHI.
- Audit control mechanisms that can monitor, record, and/or examine information system activity.

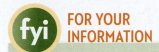

FOR YOUR INFORMATION

The full HHS Security Risk Assessment Tool for administrative and technical safeguards can be found at http://www.healthit.gov/providers-professionals/security-risk-assessment-tool.

9.3   THINKING IT THROUGH

1. What is meant by *data integrity?* Give an example.
2. Explain the difference between privacy and security.

9.4   Proving Compliance with Regulations and Reporting Noncompliance

What Is a Privacy Breach?

A **privacy breach** occurs when **unsecured PHI** is disclosed without the authorization of the patient/legal representative or as covered by law or regulation. HITECH requires notification for any unauthorized uses and disclosures of unsecured PHI.

Individual patients must be notified of any unsecured breach in writing by first-class mail or by email if the affected individual has agreed to receive such notices electronically. In addition, the secretary of the HHS must be notified of the breach through the HHS breach notification website. Breaches involving 500 or more patients require notification to HHS, which then results in the healthcare organization's or practice's name on the HHS website. Local media outlets must also be notified within a reasonable time following the breach, but in no case later than 60 days following the discovery of a breach when 500 or more individuals are affected.

There are exceptions to this stringent definition of a breach, including (1) unintentional acquisition, access, or use of PHI by a staff member or someone acting under the authority of a covered entity or business associate, if the access was made in good faith; (2) inadvertent disclosure by a covered entity or business associate of PHI by a person authorized to access PHI; and (3) the covered entity or business entity has a good faith belief that the person or entity receiving the unauthorized disclosure would not have been able to retain the information.

Breaches may be in the form of actual health records or in the form of reports that include data that identify the patient by name, medical record number, Social Security number, or other data element that could be tracked back to a specific patient or patients; thus, the terminology *privacy breach* or *data breach* may be used.

Audit Trails: Tracking Access and Disclosures

Another requirement of HIPAA is an **accounting of disclosures** made to external users as well as access to an individual's PHI by internal users upon request from the patient or legal representative.

Unsecured PHI Protected health information that has not been rendered unusable, unreadable, or indecipherable.

Privacy breach The acquisition, access, use, or disclosure of protected health information without appropriate authorization of the patient/legal representative or as required by law or allowed in HIPAA.

Accounting of disclosures A listing of all disclosures of protected health information about a patient that were not made as a result of treatment, payment, or operations or upon written authorization of the patient.

Healthcare facilities must keep a record of all releases of PHI made to external requestors, such as attorneys, other hospitals or healthcare providers, Social Security, and life insurance companies. This is often referred to as a correspondence log. Release of information software typically includes a means of reporting all releases.

As an internal safeguard, monitoring of internal access is required. **Audit trails** record each user who views health information internally and any changes that are made, as well as when they are made. Audit trails are important in compliance monitoring efforts as well as in investigating claims of unauthorized access. Figure 9.4 shows a correspondence log in an EHR that is used to track internal access to patient records.

Memorial Hospital Electronic Health Record **ACCESS LOG**					

Run date/time 11/30/2014 10:04:40
Run by: rs0175

RECORD: MRN: 019561   Account number: 10165868

User	Entry	Date Accessed	Time Accessed	Action
Mn1057	HPhys11/09/2014 09:32:14	11/09/2014	09:32:14	Created
Rk0619	NurNote11/09/2014 09:29:20	11/09/2014	09:32:18	Modified
Ng8926	NurNote11/09/2014 10:15:18	11/09/2014	10:15:18	Created
Ng8926	NurNote11/07/2014 08:14:32	11/09/2014	10:20:01	Accessed
Ng8926	VitSigns11/09/2014 10:20:12	11/09/2014	10:22:15	Deleted

Figure 9.4   **A Correspondence Log**

Avoiding Unauthorized Disclosures

Adequate education of staff (including physicians) is the best defense against unauthorized disclosures. Anyone with access to the health information of patients should understand HIPAA and HITECH, and they should be required to complete internal staff development on privacy and security. This is often accomplished through a video accompanied by a short quiz, and the staff member earns a certificate for having completed and passed the educational session.

In addition to staff education, clearly written policies regarding staff responsibility in ensuring that PHI remain private, confidential, and secure are necessary. Included in the policies should be consequences for accessing health information when it is not needed as part of one's job. Notification procedures should be in place when an internal breach does occur.

9.3   A DAY IN THE LIFE

A hospital administrator has received a letter from a former patient, Lyle Crafton, who is very upset and is threatening to bring legal action against the hospital, because his records were sent to a local attorney without his authorization. Upon review of the release of information log, it was determined that the records were indeed sent to a local

(continued)

attorney based upon a written request from the attorney that was accompanied by an authorization signed by Mr. Crafton. The release of information coordinator who released Mr. Crafton's records, the director of health information services (also the facility's privacy officer), the risk manager, and the hospital attorney met to review the circumstances surrounding the release. The attorney's letter clearly specified that the records requested were that of Lyle Crafton. The authorization was completed in its entirety and appeared to be legitimate. Upon review of the patient's signature against other signatures made by Lyle Crafton in his health record, the risk manager noticed, and the others agreed, that though very similar, there was some difference in the appearance of the signatures. By the end of the meeting, the validity of the signature on authorization had been questioned. The hospital attorney's recommendation was that a letter be written to Mr. Crafton that, based on review, the hospital staff acted properly in the release of his health information, since a valid request and authorization were received.

1. The release of information coordinator was not reprimanded. Why would he not be held accountable for releasing Mr. Crafton's records to the attorney?
2. Could this situation have been avoided? If so, how?

Medical Identity Theft

In February 2014, Kaiser Health News reported that during 2013 medical-related identity theft accounted for 43% of all identity thefts reported in the United States. Medical identity theft occurs when a name, a health insurance identification (policy) number, and/or a Social Security number are fraudulently used to obtain medical services. Identity theft may be committed by individuals who steal another's identity to be able to seek healthcare, by care providers to submit bogus claims to insurance plans seeking reimbursement for services that were not rendered, or by an individual to obtain narcotics or other drugs.

Healthcare facilities can help guard against medical identity theft by requiring picture identification and the patient's actual insurance card at each visit. Many EHRs include the ability to take and include the patient's picture in the health record itself (see Figure 9.5). None of these steps guarantee that medical identity fraud will not happen, but they can reduce the likelihood of its occurring. Biometrics, such as retina scans or fingerprints, may also be employed by some facilities, and these are "foolproof," since biometric data are impossible to fabricate. Once someone's medical identity is stolen, the thief's health history then becomes that of the victim, which is incredibly difficult to resolve.

Consumers should keep a close eye on all Explanations of Benefits (EOBs) received from insurance carriers once a claim has been filed to be sure the claim is legitimate. Also, consumers should ask questions of their providers regarding any charges that are not understood or

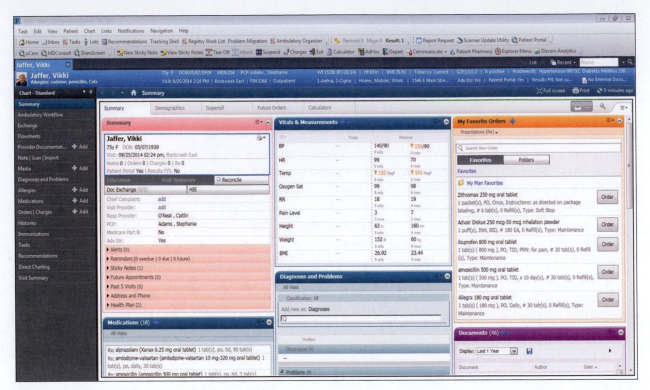

Figure 9.5 An EHR Record with a Patient Photo

that may not be legitimate. Patients have a right to request a copy of their health information and any associated itemized bills for services. As you will see in the next section, the use of patient portals by the patient or legal representative make monitoring one's own healthcare and charges much easier, although this provides a new challenge for health information staff.

Monitoring Patient Portals

Meaningful Use regulations require patients to have access to their health information electronically. The use of patient portals, whereby patients have access to their medical records at any time, has caused new concerns for health information professionals. In the past, the hospital's or practice's staff controlled what patients saw and when. For instance, if a record of a recent hospital stay was requested by the patient, but the record had not yet been completed, the patient was informed of that fact and that as soon as it became complete it would be released. With electronic record completion, and an electronic record, new procedures and policies need to be put in place, so that hospitals and/or practices still have the ability to control when the health record is set for release and what information will be included to the portal.

Also, the use of patient portals may increase the chance of unauthorized disclosure. Take, for instance, the record of William S. Smith III. He was recently a patient at Memorial Hospital due to congestive heart failure, and he has requested access to his health record through the portal. While reading through his records, he reads a consultation note, dictated by Dr. Brooks, about his recent bouts of depression. He has neither been seen by a Dr. Brooks nor been suffering from depression. He looks to the top of the page and reads that the name on the consultation report is William S. Smith Jr. The consultation report was dictated in Dr. Brooks's office and scanned into the wrong record.

In a paper record, this kind of error may have been caught during the process of final review, which is done before permanently filing the record. In an electronic record, some errors may not be so obvious, and therefore this type of error may not be caught, which in this case resulted in a privacy breach, though this type of breach is also possible in a paper environment.

Patient portals do bring new and different challenges to the health information staff, but as you will see in the chapter on the patient's role in healthcare, they have many advantages to the patient—access to his or her health history, billing information, and diagnostic test results and the ability to request prescription refills, to communicate with the staff and provider, and to make payments.

Privacy and security were—and in some cases are still—concerns in paper records just as they are now in electronic records. With paper records, however, these issues may have been taken for granted. Privacy and security are on healthcare's radar again as a result of HIPAA and more recently HITECH. Health information departments will encounter new challenges as the number of facilities, practices, and other healthcare settings moving to electronic records continue to rise and as the electronic exchange of health information increases. It is imperative to put in place formal policies and procedures to ensure the privacy and security of health information.

9.4 THINKING IT THROUGH

1. Give an example of a disclosure of secured data as opposed to unsecured data.
2. Assess ways a healthcare consumer can guard against medical identity theft. Have you taken or do you take steps to guard yourself against medical identity theft? Write a brief plan of how you do or will take these steps for you and your family.

chapter 9 **summary**

LEARNING OUTCOMES	CONCEPTS FOR REVIEW
9.1 Apply ethical standards of practice to patient scenarios. Pages 231–235	• Explain the use of a confidentiality agreement. • Name various codes of ethics. • Describe patients' rights regarding privacy. • Give examples of business associates under HIPAA.
9.2 Classify HIPAA privacy requirements. Pages 235–241	• List information that is considered private. • Differentiate between a *subpoena duces tecum* and a court order. • Name circumstances when health records are released without authorization and not pursuant to HIPAA. • What is meant by minimum necessary as it relates to HIPAA? Give examples of when it would apply. • Explain directory information. • What is a Notice of Privacy Practice? • How did the HITECH amendments change HIPAA requirements? • How did the Omnibus Final Rule expand patients' rights? • Name and explain the required elements of a HIPAA-compliant authorization for release of health information. • What is an emancipated minor?
9.3 Explain mechanisms used to secure data based on HIPAA regulations. Pages 241–243	• Name and describe the safeguards required by HIPAA. • Describe methods suggested by the HHS to safeguard health information.
9.4 Determine appropriate methods of security compliance. Pages 243–247	• Define a privacy breach and give examples. • Explain the responsibility of a covered entity when a breach does occur. • What is an accounting of disclosures? How does it differ from an audit trail? • How can unauthorized disclosures be avoided? • Explain medical identity theft. • What is HIM's role in monitoring patient portals?

chapter review

MATCHING QUESTIONS

Match each term with its definition.

_____ 1. **[LO 9.4]** privacy breach

_____ 2. **[LO 9.3]** HIPAA security rule

_____ 3. **[LO 9.2]** *subpoena duces tecum*

_____ 4. **[LO 9.4]** audit trail

_____ 5. **[LO 9.2]** minimum necessary

_____ 6. **[LO 9.2]** court order

_____ 7. **[LO 9.2]** emancipated minor

_____ 8. **[LO 9.1]** confidentiality statement

_____ 9. **[LO 9.4]** accounting of disclosures

_____ 10. **[LO 9.2]** directory information

_____ 11. **[LO 9.2]** Notice of Privacy Practices

a. Portion of HIPAA that requires appropriate administrative, physical, and technical safeguards

b. Document that healthcare employees must sign stating that all protected health information must be kept confidential

c. General facts that may release about a patient without written authorization

d. Patient, usually under 18, who assumes responsibility for himself or herself

e. Document, signed by the patient, stating he or she acknowledges how his or her health information will be used

f. Written document requiring the receiver to furnish relevant records

g. Acquisition, use, or disclosure of protected health information without appropriate authorization

h. Report of all electronic transactions performed by a user

i. Official direction issued by a court judge

j. Part of HIPAA that requires the limitation of the patient-identifiable information released for disclosure

k. List of all disclosures of PHI that were not made as a result of treatment, payment, operations, or written consent

MULTIPLE CHOICE QUESTIONS

Choose the letter that best completes the statement or answers the question.

12. **[LO 9.1]** An HIM professional is bound by the
    a. Hippocratic Oath.
    b. Notice of Privacy Practices.
    c. AHIMA Code of Ethics.
    d. Joint Commission Regulations.

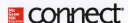 Enhance your learning by completing these exercises and more at http://connect.mheducation.com!

13. **[LO 9.1]** Healthcare workers must sign what type of document stating they will keep all patient identification confidential?
    a. HIPAA form
    b. Confidentiality statement
    c. Notice of Privacy Practices
    d. Consent

14. **[LO 9.1]** Which of the following is *not* true about patients' rights with regard to the passage of HIPAA?
    a. Patients may request an accounting of all disclosures.
    b. Patients may expect that only information that is reasonably necessary will be released.
    c. Patients may alter their medical record at any time.
    d. Patients will be notified of how their health information is used.

15. **[LO 9.1]** Which of the following is an example of a business associate?
    a. Facility cleaning personnel
    b. Facility receptionist
    c. Staff physical therapist
    d. Hospital attorney

16. **[LO 9.2]** Which circumstance requires an authorization to release protected health information?
    a. Payment for a Medicare claim
    b. Treatment by an occupational therapist
    c. Public health surveillance activities
    d. Performance improvement studies within the facility

17. **[LO 9.2]** A restraining order is an example of which of the following?
    a. *Subpoena duces tecum*
    b. A court order
    c. Notice of Privacy Practices
    d. An Office of Civil Rights declaration

18. **[LO 9.2]** Under the HITECH Act, civil penalties for willful neglect can range from
    a. $225,000 to $1.0 million.
    b. $250,000 to $1.0 million.
    c. $250,000 to $1.5 million.
    d. $250,000 to $2.0 million.

19. **[LO 9.3]** The HIPAA security rule instructs covered entities to provide all of the following safeguards *except*
    a. technical.
    b. administrative.
    c. electronic.
    d. operational.

20. **[LO 9.3]** Which type of safeguard would be demonstrated by using a unique identifier and password for each user and an automatic log-off from the computer after a time of inactivity?
    a. Security safeguard
    b. Administrative safeguard
    c. Technical safeguard
    d. Physical safeguard

21. **[LO 9.4]** The Jones Hospital wants to run a security review on the nursing staff. What could be used to identify all electronic transactions performed by the nurses?
    a. Accounting of disclosures
    b. An audit trail
    c. Notice of Privacy Practices
    d. A technical safeguard report

SHORT ANSWER QUESTIONS

22. **[LO 9.1]** Name and describe three examples of business associates.

23. **[LO 9.1]** List four rights patients gained with the passage of HIPAA.

24. **[LO 9.1]** Summarize the patient's right to privacy.

25. **[LO 9.2]** Discuss the enhanced legal liability for noncompliance under the HITECH Amendments.

26. **[LO 9.3]** List and describe the three safeguard categories covered under the HIPAA security rule.

27. **[LO 9.3]** Name and describe two types of administrative safeguards.

28. **[LO 9.3]** Name and describe two types of physical safeguards.

29. **[LO 9.4]** Summarize the process of HITECH notification for unauthorized uses and disclosures of unsecured PHI.

30. **[LO 9.4]** Compare and contrast an accounting of disclosure and an audit trail.

31. **[LO 9.4]** Discuss the benefits of using a patient portal.

APPLYING YOUR KNOWLEDGE

32. **[LO 9.1]** Using the Internet, go to the AHIMA website to locate and read the AHIMA Code of Ethics. Why do you think the AHIMA Code of Ethics is important for all HIM professionals to follow?

33. **[LO 9.1]** You have been recently hired to work in an HIM department of a local hospital. The hospital asks you to sign a confidentiality agreement. Discuss the importance of signing this document.

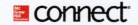 Enhance your learning by completing these exercises and more at http://connect.mheducation.com!

34. **[LO 9.1]** Discuss several differences in patients' rights after HIPAA was established.

35. **[LO 9.2]** Search the Internet for a sample Notice of Privacy Practices. Summarize how this document protects the patient and the facility.

36. **[LO 9.2]** Research the law in the state where you reside and define *emancipated minor*.

37. **[LO 9.3]** Select one of the HHS suggestions for administrative/technical safeguards. Discuss the importance of this safeguard and how it can be implemented in a facility.

38. **[LO 9.4]** Visit the OCR website and search for a recent health information breach. Summarize the details of the breach.

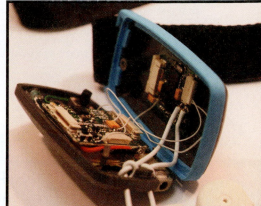

chapter **ten**

The Patient's Role in Healthcare

Learning Outcomes

When you finish this chapter, you will be able to:

10.1 Explain patient-centric healthcare.

10.2 Differentiate between a Personal Health Record and a patient portal.

10.3 Outline the uses of mHealth technologies in patient engagement

and adherence as well as the challenges these new technologies pose.

10.4 Illustrate the relationship between level of patient involvement in their care and patient outcomes.

Key Terms

Interactive personal (preventive) health record (IPHR)

Patient activation

Patient-centric healthcare

Patient engagement

Remote patient monitoring (RPM)

Telehealth

Wearables

Introduction

For the most part, it has been only in the past 20 or so years that patients have been comfortable questioning their physicians about their prescribed plan of care. Patients were not conditioned to think critically about their illness, prognosis, or treatment. With the advent of the Internet and a more open philosophy in the medical community that patient education and involvement have a positive effect on their overall healthcare, there has been a noticeable paradigm shift in this area. This chapter explores the concept of patient-centric care and its benefits as well as the technologies that have evolved to make this philosophy a reality.

10.1 | Patient-centric Healthcare

Patient-centric Defined

With Meaningful Use incentives as well as widely accepted and used electronic healthcare documentation systems comes more emphasis on patients as active participants in their own healthcare, also known as **patient engagement** or **patient-centric healthcare**.

> ### 10.1 A DAY IN THE LIFE
>
> Carlos Vasquez is a patient of Dr. Lewis's. He has hypertension, for which he takes Lisinopril. While visiting his daughter, who lives in another state, he realizes he has forgotten his medication. He visits an urgent care clinic near her home, and the physician there needs to know the dosage of his Lisinopril. It is the weekend, and Dr. Lewis is not available. The patient asks to use an office computer, logs into his patient portal, and retrieves the information needed by the urgent care physician.
>
> 1. What might have happened, had Mr. Vasquez not been able to access his medication history through the patient portal?

Patient engagement As defined by the National Institutes of Health, care that establishes a partnership among practitioners, patients, and their families (when appropriate) to ensure that decisions respect patients' wants, needs, and preferences and solicit patients' input on the education and support they need to make decisions and participate in their own care.

Patient-centric healthcare Increased interaction and communication between a team of healthcare providers and the patient to improve quality of care and outcomes.

Following the Patient—Data Flow

Gone are the days of data flowing by mail, fax machine, or telephone. In an electronic environment, through the use of health information exchanges as well as the patient's access to his or her own health information through a portal, information needed now, rather than an hour or a week from now, is often available quickly. Patients who are knowledgeable about the information available to them are likely to welcome more efficient, timely healthcare and are more likely to be willing participants in their own healthcare.

It is rare now that patients leave an outpatient radiology appointment without a CD containing the images taken during that appointment. Radiologists do not need to be in the same location where the films were taken; rather, they are often viewed remotely through a technology known as a picture archiving and communications system (PACS).

Transitions in Care

Continuity of care and coordination of care are both integral to improved healthcare. Traditionally, *continuity of care* referred to keeping the momentum going in improving a patient's health status through a continuous relationship with an identified provider. Today, care is rarely given by a single provider, and continuity of care has become the integration, coordination, and sharing of health information among different providers and their respective care teams. *Coordination* refers to using that health information in proactive, effective, and cost-efficient ways across the care management resources for all the stakeholders in the care continuity process.

Coordination is generally attributable to a central contact—increasingly, a team-based model typically led by a primary care physician (PCP). This is the basis of the patient-centered medical home (PCMH) model, which was discussed in the introductory chapter. The PCP is referred to as a gatekeeper, because he or she is the first point of contact for the patient and is often a generalist—an internist, a family practitioner, a pediatrician, or even a gynecologist. This is the healthcare provider who should be most familiar with the patient, including working knowledge of his or her complete medical, surgical, social, and family histories. What may go unnoticed by a physician who has never seen a patient before may be picked up in a matter of minutes by the patient's PCP.

As the patient transitions from that first line of care up through specialists, perhaps hospital visits, rehabilitation units, skilled nursing facilities, and even end-of-life care, the pieces of that patient's health can be gathered together seamlessly through the use of an EHR and health information exchanges.

10.1 THINKING IT THROUGH

1. How does the concept of "data following the patient" support changing the delivery of healthcare to a more patient-centric model?

2. How does the increased use of patient data across the transition of care change health information management?

10.2 The Patient Portal versus the Personal Health Record (PHR)

The terms *patient portal* and *Personal Health Record* are often used interchangeably, but there are distinct differences between the two. According to the Office of the National Coordinator for Health Information Technology (ONC), a Personal Health Record

(PHR) is designed to be set up and managed by the patient. A patient portal is web-based and is offered by the provider. A portal contains information from the EHR and other data selected by the provider. Typically, a portal has additional functionality, such as scheduling and prescription refills. The provider controls the portal.

The use of an EHR that supports a patient portal allows patients to more easily communicate with their physicians to ask about their care or to place health maintenance requests, such as prescription refills. Patients may also have access to their health information through the patient portal, which allows the patient or legal representative to monitor lab results, dates of last appointments, diagnoses, and the like. As explained earlier, patient portals, however, are not the same as Personal Health Records. Both have their place in healthcare, though there is much debate about the necessity and validity of a Personal Health Record now that the patient portal is supported by most EHR software and is part of Meaningful Use requirements.

Personal Health Records

Personal Health Records (PHRs) are kept by patients. They are not legal documents, and the accuracy and completeness are the responsibility of the patient or legal representative. The use of a PHR can help improve one's healthcare by providing physicians with information about the patient's medical history from multiple providers. When kept current, complete, and accurate, a PHR may also reduce duplication of testing and help the physician more efficiently map out the plan of care for that patient. Figure 10.1 shows the interface for the most popular PHR, HealthVault. Note that the information on this web page requires patient input.

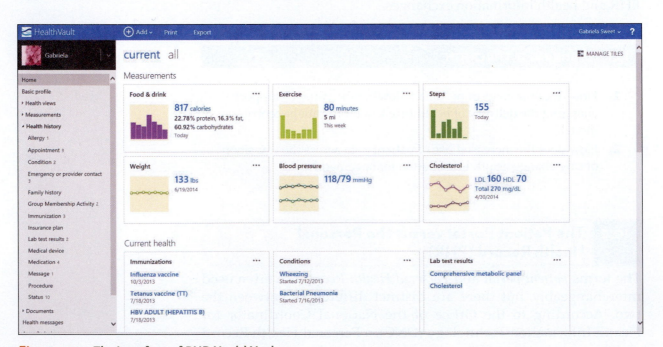

Figure 10.1 The Interface of PHR HealthVault

TABLE 10.1   Common PHR Contents

Identifying information	Insurance information	Medication allergies
Food and environmental allergies	Current list of medications, including dosages	Immunization record
Past surgeries	Past medical conditions	Conditions for which the patient is being treated, including chronic conditions (problem list)
Discharge summaries from hospital stays	Operative reports	Pathology reports
Laboratory test results	Radiology test results	EKG/echocardiogram and similar reports
Consultation reports	Advance directives	Physician office visit notes

Patients who travel often, or who see specialists as well as their PCP, may be more apt to compile a PHR and keep it with them at all times. PHRs may be basic, containing past medical and surgical histories and a list of current medications, or they may be very detailed, containing actual reports of surgeries and tests results. The top portion of Table 10.1 includes basic information, while the information below the bold line includes additional, more detailed content that can be in a PHR.

PHRs can be in paper format, web-based, or software-based and are available from third-party payers, through free or paid services.

Blue Button is another popular PHR, supported by the federal government. Initially, in 2010, Blue Button was established by the Veterans Administration (VA) to allow its patients to have access to portable health records. The name comes from a blue button logo that appears on a website and that is linked to a database with patient information. The initial success of the program resulted in its adoption by HHS in 2012, with ONC launching a Blue Button "pledge campaign" for businesses and consumers. Medicare also has established a Blue Button program.

Standards for transmission and sharing have been developed. Primarily, Blue Button is used for downloading and transmitting text records and basic information, such as allergies, medication lists, and diagnoses. As shown in Figure 10.2, iBlueButton, the mobile component of the Blue Button initiative, has the potential to integrate all parts of the healthcare system.

A more advanced form of the PHR is an **interactive personal (preventive) health record**, or **IPHR**. Unlike a traditional PHR compiled by the patient, an IPHR compiles information from the EHR and creates a summary for the patient that is in lay terms. A study conducted by a team at Virginia Commonwealth University in 2012 concluded that patients who used an IPHR were almost twice as likely to be up to date with clinical preventive services as those who did not (Krist).

Interactive personal (preventive) health record (IPHR) The summary of a patient's healthcare created by the EHR.

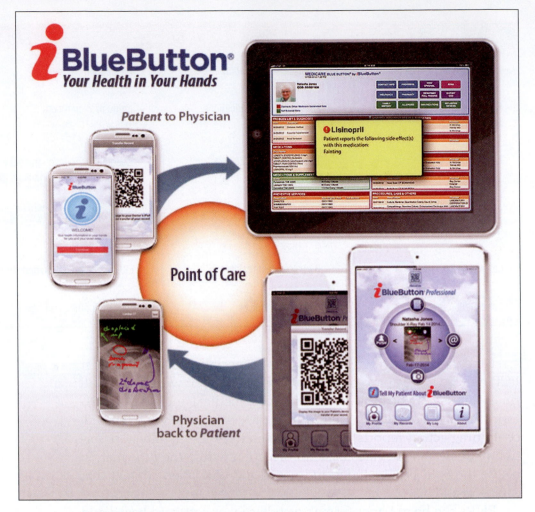

Figure 10.2 **Blue Button as an Integrator of Patient Records**

10.2 A DAY IN THE LIFE

Think of your own healthcare—do you have a PHR that documents your past medical and surgical histories? What are you allergic to? What immunizations have you had and when? Are there hereditary conditions in your family that you know about? Does your family know your medical history?

If you do not already have a PHR, locate a PHR through your insurance company, on the Internet, or through AHIMA. Complete what you can without any records from your physician's office records. Use the following questions to assess your personal health knowledge:

1. Are you fairly knowledgeable about your own health history, or are there large gaps in your knowledge?
2. Do you know your family's history, or do you have to ask a parent for more information?
3. Think back to a previous doctor's appointment when you were asked questions that you could not answer—would a PHR have helped in that situation?

Patient Portals

In contrast to PHRs, patient portals are more than simply a compilation of the patient's health history, immunizations, and allergies. Portals allow patients to make appointments, view laboratory or other diagnostic test results, request refills of prescriptions, and pay medical bills online. In the case of test results or other information that the patient may not fully understand, individual offices may place restrictions on what is and is not made available via the portal.

Portals have the added value of allowing patients to contact their physician's office to seek advice about current issues or to express complaints they are experiencing—for instance, cold symptoms—without making an office visit. The patient most often speaks with a nurse, who asks appropriate questions of the patient, speaks with the physician about the patient's complaint or question, and then relays the physician's recommendation to the patient, whether it is over-the-counter medications and home management, ordering a prescription, or the need to make an office appointment. Using the patient portal in this way is a form of triage that saves the insurance carrier, and often the patient, money; additionally, it allows the physicians and office staff to use their time more efficiently on patients being seen in the office. Frustration on the patient's part is also lessened, because he or she does not have to wait by the telephone for a return call from the office or to explain the complaint more than once.

Portals, however, are not without their challenges. "Tethered portals" are a major issue. There is limited sharing of data outside a health system, and most providers are offering their own portal "tethered" to their practice or health system. This means that if a patient sees multiple providers, he or she will have to log on to multiple provider portals to access a complete health record.

Meaningful Use, Patient Rights, Portals, and PHRs

Stage 2 of Meaningful Use requires providers to prove that at least 5% of their patients utilize a patient portal to view, download, or transmit their records. Stage 3, as proposed, goes even further, requiring patients to actively assist with assessing their own health information as found in their health record (as opposed to their PHR).

HIPAA gives patients the right to have private, secure health information as well as the right to

- Access, inspect, and copy health information
- Request corrections or amend health information
- Request accounting of disclosures of health information

The combined patient rights now afforded patients through HIPAA and Meaningful Use requirements mean increased patient involvement and encouragement of patient engagement as well as new and changing roles for health information professionals in ensuring privacy and security. These roles will be discussed in the chapter on expanding roles and functions of the health information management and health informatics professional.

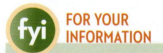

FOR YOUR INFORMATION

When a hospital system or other provider does not share patient information with other providers, a patient must use the portal provided by that provider to view or download his or her information. This is called a "tethered portal." It is linked only to that one provider. If a patient receives care from other providers, that patient will have to log on to multiple portals in order to get all of his or her health information.

Patient Acceptance and Adherence

Patients cannot or will not be involved in their own healthcare if they do not know that healthcare providers need and want their participation and compliance. A patient portal will not be used for its intended purpose if the patient is unaware of its existence. Medical practices and hospitals must educate their patients about the technology available to them through literature, signage, and the availability of computers in the office or facility, so that they can get started and seek assistance from staff, if necessary. Many healthcare facilities now have web pages on which basic information about the facility is available to the general public or to their patients. Providing information about the patient portal on the site is also an excellent tool to increase awareness.

Patients need to know not only that the technology is available but also how it can benefit them as well as their physician or healthcare community. If patients knew that they could check test results, send and receive messages to and from their physician, schedule appointments without playing phone tag, and receive reminders privately and securely, the issue of meeting the Meaningful Use requirement that 5% of patients actually use a patient portal would be a much easier goal to reach for healthcare providers. Figure 10.3 shows a sample of marketing information encouraging consumers to consider using a patient portal.

Perhaps most importantly, it is imperative that the physicians and the staff of the healthcare facility buy into the concept of a patient portal and the whole idea of patient engagement. Patients who sense that a physician is not on board are more likely to be bystanders rather than active participants.

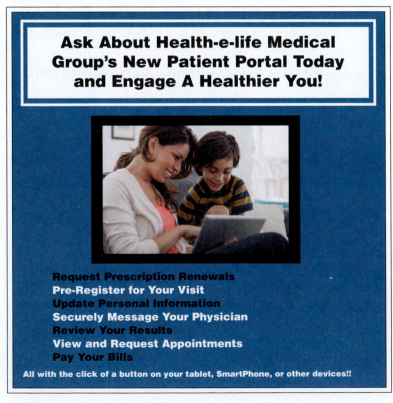

Ask About Health-e-life Medical Group's New Patient Portal Today and Engage A Healthier You!

Request Prescription Renewals
Pre-Register for Your Visit
Update Personal Information
Securely Message Your Physician
Review Your Results
View and Request Appointments
Pay Your Bills

All with the click of a button on your tablet, SmartPhone, or other devices!!

Figure 10.3   Encouraging Patients to Use a Portal

10.2 THINKING IT THROUGH

1. What are the major differences between a patient portal and a Personal Health Record (PHR)?
2. Is a patient portal or a PHR more useful? Why?
3. What strategies can be used to encourage patients to use PHRs or portals? Do you think that enough is being done?

10.3 Mobile Health (mHealth)

mHealth's Role in Healthcare

Innovation in technology is changing where and how healthcare can be delivered. At the forefront of this revolution are new devices and infrastructure that support the capture and transmission of health information outside the traditional care settings, such as a clinic or hospital. This area is being generally referred to as m(obile)Health. It ranges from visits using videoconferencing between caregivers and patients and home-based monitoring of an individual's vital statistics to wearable fitness bands or clinicians simply using tablets or other wireless devices during patient encounters.

Some of these applications are not new. **Telehealth** has been in use since the 1950s, but it was slow to take off. The high cost of networks and equipment combined with limits on diagnostic functionality were a barrier. Also, these types of patient encounters are seldom eligible for reimbursement by payers. There also were and still are licensing and credentialing issues if care is provided across state lines, liability and malpractice issues, privacy and security concerns, and a lack of training for physicians in telehealth. Successful applications of videoconferencing telehealth include providing services to patients in remote areas and less-developed countries, to individuals incarcerated in prisons, and even to astronauts (see Figure 10.4).

Telehealth The use of communication networks to provide services such as telemedicine, in which a clinician is in one location and the patient is in a second location.

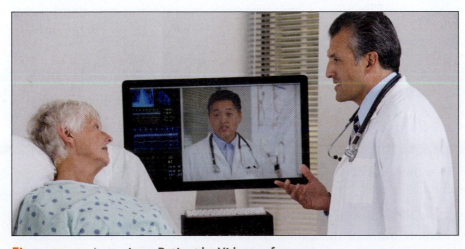

Figure 10.4 **Assessing a Patient by Videoconference**

Wearables Small health and fitness devices that can be worn on the body, similar to a bracelet, wristwatch, or pendant; they provide monitoring of physical activity, vital signs, or other information. Data from wearables are automatically captured and typically sent through a wireless network or Bluetooth connection to a smartphone.

Remote patient monitoring (RPM) The use of information technologies and communication networks to measure physiological data and perform tests from a location outside a clinic, such as at home, and send that information to healthcare professionals.

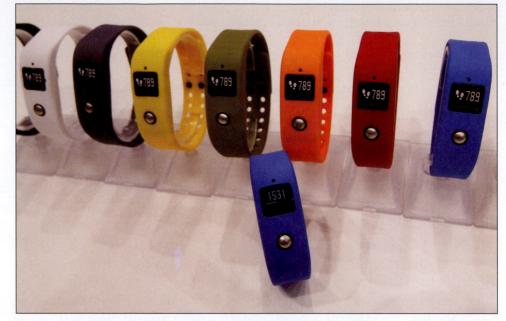

Figure 10.5   Runtastic® Combines Mobile Apps, Social Networking, Wearables, and an Element of Gamification

What has changed is the establishment of the Internet, wireless networks, low-cost portable devices, and the proliferation of applications. As a result, telehealth is being subsumed by a new and expansive category called mHealth—the use of wireless devices, such as smartphones and tablets, by patients and clinicians.

Current estimates indicate that more than 30,000 mHealth apps have been developed for smartphones and tablets. The most common type of app is for fitness, and popular ones, such as Runtastic, have recorded more than 85 million downloads. Runtastic has also expanded into the wearable business. Their Orbit 24-hour fitness tracker device was released in 2014 (see Figure 10.5). Also popular are nutrition and diet apps, such as Weight Watchers®, and apps for pregnancy.

A whole new category of devices has also been introduced: **wearables**. Wearable devices represent a new way to engage consumers and support wellness activities. Consumer-facing wearables are growing ever more popular, as tech startups and megacorporations alike are launching these products. Nike's FuelBand and FitBit® are two examples of wearables created by corporations that are sold directly to consumers (see Figure 10.6). These products do everything from tracking your physical activity to measuring the quality and quantity of your sleep, with the goal of promoting overall fitness by getting easy-to-use data in the hands of users. Expanding functionality, ease of use, a sleeker design, and decreasing prices for these devices should support their increased use.

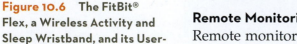

Figure 10.6   The FitBit® Flex, a Wireless Activity and Sleep Wristband, and its User-Friendly App

Remote Monitoring Devices

Remote monitoring of an individual with a chronic illness or someone who has recently been discharged from the hospital can result in better outcomes and lower costs. This is called **remote patient monitoring (RPM)**. Remote monitoring devices are similar to wearables but are larger, are more sophisticated, and need to be designed for higher reliability. Use of these devices also tends to be physician-directed as opposed to an independent initiative on the part of the patient; some insurance companies also reimburse patients for using these remote monitoring devices. Examples include a glucose meter and a cardiac monitor. BodyGuardian®, a remote cardiac monitoring platform using technologies pioneered by the Mayo Clinic, differs from a product like FitBit®, because it is designed to monitor a specific illness as opposed to indicators of general fitness (see Figure 10.7). Also, physicians and clinicians can access their

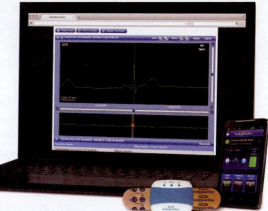

Figure 10.7 A Remote Cardiac Monitoring Platform Developed with Technologies Pioneered by the Mayo Clinic

patients' data and receive alerts if they show signs of distress. The US Food and Drug Administration distinguishes between mobile apps and wearables and more sophisticated medical mobile apps and remote monitoring devices. Medical mobile apps are defined as medical devices and are subject to regulatory approval and oversight before they are used.

Alerts and Monitoring

As mobile devices proliferate and their ability to capture health data in reliable and secure ways improves, there is the opportunity to do more with the data. One area of great promise is the emergency alert. Threshold levels or predictive measures can be used to identify a medical emergency and alert the patient, caregivers, clinicians, and emergency services. Or a potential medical emergency can be identified before an event occurs. Patients, caregivers, and medical staff can be alerted and can prevent or treat the situation in a timely fashion (see Figure 10.8).

Alerts can also be useful for monitoring patient adherence. For example, physicians could set up alerts for taking medicines properly, filling prescriptions, and attending follow-up appointments. These alerts are less urgent but likewise can be tracked by mobile devices and alerts generated and sent to caregivers, care coordinators, and social workers.

Remote Monitoring Devices, Wearables, and the Health System

It is still unclear as to how wearables, remote monitoring devices, and their various functionalities will be integrated into the health system. Currently, services are primarily provided through third-party monitoring services, similar to home security systems. There is no standard way to automatically integrate digital information from remote monitors into health information exchanges, EHRs, or PHRs. Integration varies by vendor and by the way in

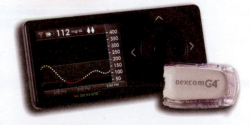

Figure 10.8 Dexcom®'s G4 Platinum Provides Continuous Glucose Monitoring and Alerts You to Potentially Dangerous Glucose Levels

which the remote monitoring device in question transmits patient health data. Essentially, interoperability between remote monitoring devices and EHRs, PHRs, and health information exchanges is a work in progress.

In the case of wearables, the situation is even less structured. Corporations have designed these technologies with the consumer in mind, but not the larger healthcare system. Three main challenges need to be overcome before wearables can be used as medical devices. First, wearables are not interoperable with EHRs or health information exchanges, but the data could be input into a PHR. Currently, the only way that wearable data are accessible to the physician is through the patient. Second, wearables are not currently accurate enough to be fully considered medical devices. Finally, both physician and patient must embrace engagement and a more patient-centric model of care. Future collaboration between health information professionals and the corporations developing these wearables may help overcome these limitations and represent new opportunities for health information professionals.

Like any technology, wearables and remote monitoring devices are subject to breaches in privacy and security as well as glitches that can compromise the quality of health data as well as patient privacy and security. With remote monitoring devices, companies are taking steps to prevent these issues. Since wearables are not regulated, however, they presently do not have to meet these requirements.

10.3 A DAY IN THE LIFE

John's elderly mother has been hospitalized several times from an arrhythmia, which is an irregular heartbeat. This condition is currently under control through medication, and she is living alone at her home. John is exploring ways to track his mother's status, so that she gets the medical assistance she needs in a timely fashion.

1. What are John's options in terms of mHealth solutions?
2. What are the advantages and disadvantages of each option?

10.3 THINKING IT THROUGH

1. Why did telehealth have trouble being widely used, and how is that changing?
2. What types of devices are used in mHealth? How do they differ? Do you think that eventually one device will be used for everything?
3. Explain how mHealth alerts can lead to lower costs and improved outcomes.

The goals of healthcare reform are to provide for better patient outcomes, lower costs, and a healthier population. These initiatives will be possible only by engaging and educating the patient. Patient-centric care is a developing area, and recent research is based on a framework that breaks this goal into two parts. The first is **patient activation**. This initial step involves getting the patient willing to participate in his or her own healthcare and wellness. This also involves ensuring that the patient or caretaker has the ability to understand what is involved and understand where educational and other supporting information is available. This is more about attitude than action.

The second goal is **patient engagement**. Patient engagement is about taking action such as dieting, exercising, using a PHR, or monitoring physical measures in order to be healthier.

Patient activation A patient's knowledge, skills, ability, and willingness to manage his or her own health and care.

Patient engagement A broad concept that combines patient activation with interventions designed to increase activation and promote positive patient behavior, such as obtaining preventive care or exercising regularly.

Chronic Disease Management

Research has shown that both patient activation and patient engagement lead to improved outcomes and lower costs. There are issues of cost and scale in identifying patients, customizing programs, individualizing programs, and changing behavior. Technology has the ability to make this economically feasible. For example, as shown in Figure 10.9, mHealth apps can be used to

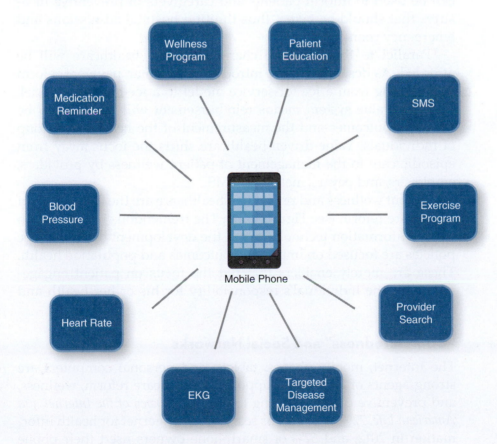

Figure 10.9 **Using Technology to Support Chronic Disease Management**

target patients, track data, communicate with patients and caregivers, and support treatment, behavior modification, and education.

As described in the introductory chapter, the treatment of chronic diseases, such as diabetes and hypertension, represent a great cost. This cost will increase with an aging population and other demographic shifts. Treatment, prevention, and wellness are critical to reduce healthcare expenses, which are spiraling out of control.

Wellness and the Role of Digital Health

A healthy population has many benefits to a society, including a higher quality of life, greater productivity, and lower healthcare costs. All these are critical to the United States. Healthcare costs are unsustainable at their current rate of growth and are changing the demographics of the country. Healthcare reform and technological innovation are providing the foundation for creating a massive change in society.

The development of a high-tech infrastructure based on digitized health data provides the ability to get health information to the right place at the right time. This capability supports a paradigm shift in favor of placing the patient at the center of the care process and providing access to the relevant data to all caregivers across the continuum of care. Patients will have access to their health information through patient portals and PHRs on a variety of devices at any time they choose. Predictive analytics and alerts can be used to inform patients and caregivers of preventive measures that should be taken, thus limiting hospital admissions and emergency room use.

Parallel to this shift are changes in how healthcare will be afforded. As described in the introductory chapter, payment reform is migrating from a fee-for-service model to a fee-for-value model. A fee-for-value system means reimbursement will increasingly be based on outcomes and the measurement of the health of a group of individuals. Value-driven healthcare shifts the focus away from episodic care to the management of patient wellness by providers, employers, and payers, including CMS.

Patient wellness and preventive healthcare are the foundation of healthcare reform (see Figure 10.10). The tremendous investment in health information technology and the development of new public policies are focused on improving outcomes and population health. These are merely enablers that put the focus on patient engagement and the individual's responsibility for his or her health and wellness.

"Connectedness" and Social Networks

The Internet, mobile phones, tablets, and personal computers are strong agents of change in supporting healthcare reform, wellness, and preventive care. According to the *Pew Survey of the Internet and American Life,* 72% of US adults searched the Internet for health information in 2012, and 52% of smartphone owners used their phone

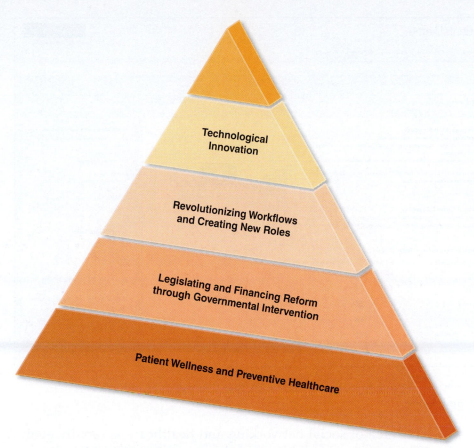

Figure 10.10 Patient Wellness and Preventive Healthcare Are the Foundation of Healthcare Reform

for looking up health information. Specific diseases, conditions, and treatments were the most commonly searched items, follow by information on providers and physicians. This information suggests a promising trend, with the caveat that there is always an issue of accuracy and veracity, depending on the source of the information on the Internet.

Combined with mobile apps, patient portals, and PHRs, the use of the Internet is a critical component of supporting healthcare delivery and patient wellness. This use of technology demonstrates the "connectedness" of individuals when considering their healthcare and provides direct patient empowerment. The Internet offers basic information for patient education, support groups, treatment options, physician and hospital reviews, and related details. The Internet, along with other aspects of mHealth, serve as a trigger for getting a patient active in his or her healthcare and taking proactive steps to maintain or improve his or her overall health.

Social networks play an important role in engagement. Whereas Facebook provides an opportunity to connect, healthcare websites, such as those of WebMD, Yahoo! Health, and Mayo Clinic, are specialized and have the advantage of content oversight and moderators. Other targeted websites, such as PatientsLikeMe, take a medical condition–specific approach, and provide specific information, support, and networking opportunities (see Figure 10.11).

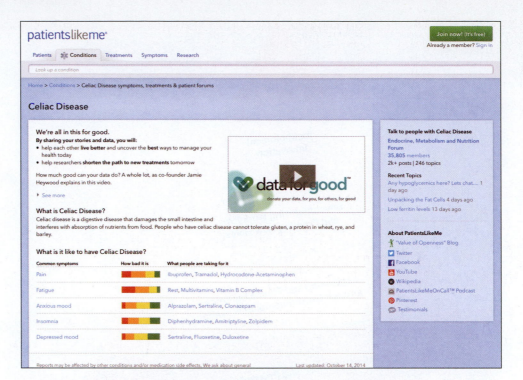

Figure 10.11 **Search for Other People with Your Disease or Symptoms on PatientsLikeMe**

This area of social networking and healthcare is rapidly evolving. The number of unique monthly visitors to WebMD alone is 80 million. There has been little research into the role of social networks and health websites on patient behavior or outcomes. It is clear, however, that social networks could provide direct support for patient engagement.

10.4 **A DAY IN THE LIFE**

A family member recently diagnosed with diabetes mellitus asked you for advice on what he should do.

1. Do you think patient engagement is important in managing one's healthcare? What would you say?
2. How could mHealth help him or her?
3. If this family member asked for advice on using social media, what would you suggest?

10.4 **THINKING IT THROUGH**

1. What is the difference between patient activation and patient engagement?
2. Why is patient engagement so important in chronic disease management?
3. How are social networks being used to improve health outcomes and achieve the goal of healthier populations?

chapter 10 **summary**

LEARNING OUTCOMES	CONCEPTS FOR REVIEW
10.1 Explain patient-centric healthcare. Pages 254–255	• Patient-centric healthcare is a change in the delivery of services that places an emphasis on the healthcare consumers as active participants engaged with the full range of their caregivers. 1. Patient-centric care is a goal of Meaningful Use. 2. HIT provides an infrastructure that enables patient-centric care. 3. Continuity and coordination of care are supported by patient-centric models.
10.2 Differentiate between a Personal Health Record and a patient portal. Pages 255–261	• A patient portal is a secure web-based site controlled by a provider where patients can access designated information from the provider's EHR and other functionality. 1. A portal contains diagnoses, lab results, discharge summaries, immunizations, and imaging study reports. 2. A portal typically contains other information and functionality, such as the ability to schedule appointments and make payments, refill prescriptions, email providers, and gain access to insurance claims data and online forms. • A Personal Health Record is managed by the patient and can contain information from a variety of sources typically input by the patient. 1. PHRs can be paper format, web-based, or software-based. • Both portals and PHRs are designed to increase patient engagement, adherence, and outcomes. 1. Meaningful Use Stage 2 requires that providers demonstrate that 5% of patients are viewing, downloading, or transmitting their health record.
10.3 Outline the uses of mHealth technologies in patient engagement and adherence as well as the challenges these new technologies pose. Pages 261–264	• The term *mHealth* refers to devices and infrastructure that support healthcare delivery outside a traditional setting, such as a clinic or hospital. • Telehealth is the original mHealth service, consisting of a traditional provider/patient encounter using audio and video connections over a distance. • The advent of the Internet and mobile devices has enabled an explosion in health applications consumers can conveniently use. • Remote monitoring devices can be used for real-time clinical measures for chronic disease management to create alerts. • Wearable devices can be used to encourage fitness and allow individuals to monitor their vital measures.

LEARNING OUTCOMES	CONCEPTS FOR REVIEW

10.4 Illustrate the relationship between level of patient involvement in their care and patient outcomes. Pages 265–268	• There are two parts to patient engagement.
	  1. Activation is the patient's knowledge, skills, ability, and willingness to manage his or her own health and care.
	  2. Patient engagement is a broader concept that combines patient activation with interventions designed to increase activation and promote positive patient behavior, such as obtaining preventive care or exercising regularly.
	• Patient engagement is a key part of healthcare reform, especially for chronic disease management.
	• Social networks, including websites, support groups, and other forms of messaging, are playing an important role in education, wellness initiatives, and self-management in patient engagement.

chapter review

MATCHING QUESTIONS

Match each term with its definition.

_____ 1. **[LO 10.3]** wearable

_____ 2. **[LO 10.3]** telehealth

_____ 3. **[LO 10.4]** patient activation

_____ 4. **[LO 10.4]** patient engagement

_____ 5. **[LO 10.3]** mHealth

_____ 6. **[LO 10.4]** Blue Button

_____ 7. **[LO 10.1]** PACS

_____ 8. **[LO 10.2]** patient portal

_____ 9. **[LO 10.3]** remote monitoring

_____ 10. **[LO 10.2]** PHR

a. Interventions designed to increase patient activation and promote positive patient behavior

b. Wireless devices used to track an individual's vital measurements and take action based on that information

c. Technology allowing films and images to be viewed from remote locations

d. Secure, web-based site where patients can access designated information from a provider's EHR

e. Small health and fitness devices that can be worn on the body, similar to a bracelet, wrist-watch, or pendant, and provides monitoring

f. New devices and infrastructure that support the capture and transmission of health information outside the traditional care settings

g. Patients' knowledge, skills, ability, and willingness to manage their own health and care

h. Personal Health Record, supported and marketed by the federal government

i. Information managed by the patient that contains information similar to an electronic health record (EHR)

j. Use of communication networks to provide services, such as in telemedicine, in which a clinician is in one location and the patient is in a second location

MULTIPLE CHOICE QUESTIONS

Choose the letter that best completes the statement or answers the question.

11. **[LO 10.1]** *Continuity of care* refers to
    a. sharing health information with the patient.
    b. sharing information within a single health system.
    c. sharing information with all providers involved with a patient.
    d. sharing information with all care teams involved with a patient.

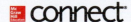 Enhance your learning by completing these exercises and more at http://connect.mheducation.com!

12. **[LO 10.1]** Care coordination is the basis for
    a. the patient-centered medical home model.
    b. the Meaningful Use model.
    c. mHealth.
    d. health information exchange models.

13. **[LO 10.1]** Radiologists who are viewing a CT scan from a remote location are using
    a. PACS.
    b. PCP.
    c. PHR.
    d. patient portals.

14. **[LO 10.2]** A patient portal is
    a. controlled by the patient.
    b. controlled by the provider.
    c. untethered.
    d. vendor neutral.

15. **[LO 10.2]** A Personal Health Record can be
    a. software.
    b. web-based.
    c. paper.
    d. all of these.

16. **[LO 10.2]** Common content in a Personal Health Record does not include
    a. insurance information.
    b. discharge summaries.
    c. pathology reports.
    d. physician profiles.

17. **[LO 10.3]** All of the following are reasons that telehealth has had limited success *except*
    a. insurance companies seldom pay for tele-visits.
    b. lack of physician training in using telehealth.
    c. medical licensing issues for services crossing state lines.
    d. telehealth cannot use the Internet because of HIPAA issues.

18. **[LO 10.3]** Sophisticated remote monitoring devices and applications
    a. are not regulated by the US Food and Drug Administration.
    b. are often designed for a single function, such as measuring blood sugar levels.
    c. cannot automatically send alerts to caregivers.
    d. do not work in rural areas.

19. **[LO 10.3]** The most popular mHealth application for smartphones is
    a. fitness.
    b. diet and nutrition.
    c. glucose monitoring.
    d. pregnancy.

20. **[LO 10.4]** mHealth supports healthcare reform by
    a. increasing the incidence of episodic care.
    b. making it easier to measure fees charged for services.
    c. replacing a PHR.
    d. helping get the right information to the right place at the right time.

21. **[LO 10.4]** Patients should use the Internet for all of the following *except*
    a. joining support groups.
    b. seeking information on providers and physicians.
    c. finding information on specific diseases and conditions.
    d. substituting medical advice in place of actually visiting a physician for treatment and professional advice.

SHORT ANSWER QUESTIONS

22. **[LO 10.1]** Explain the concept of the patient being part of the "healthcare team."

23. **[LO 10.1]** Describe how transitions in care have evolved from one location to multiple locations.

24. **[LO 10.1]** Identify the elements of continuity of care.

25. **[LO 10.2]** Contrast PHRs and patient portals.

26. **[LO 10.2]** Describe the content commonly found in a PHR.

27. **[LO 10.2]** Explain how "tethered" portals are complicating patient engagement.

28. **[LO 10.3]** Search the Internet for mHealth apps. Select one and summarize how it operates. What is an advantage of using this app?

29. **[LO 10.3]** Assess the uses for each category of mHealth device.

30. **[LO 10.4]** Discuss the relationship between healthcare costs and chronic diseases in the United States.

31. **[LO 10.4]** Describe the role social networks play in patient engagement.

APPLYING YOUR KNOWLEDGE

32. **[LO 10.1]** How does health information management support transitions in care? Give examples of how data following the patient can lead to improved outcomes and lower costs.

33. **[LO 10.2]** Why do you think Meaningful Use Stage 2 requires providers to prove that patients are downloading, viewing, or transmitting their records through a portal?

34. **[LO 10.3]** More than 30,000 healthcare mobile apps have been developed. Do you think they are being used after being downloaded? Will they have an impact on patient engagement?

35. **[LO 10.4]** Discuss the two-step process of patient activation and patient engagement. Which is the more difficult? Develop and detail strategies for both activation and engagement.

36. **[LO 10.4]** Describe how social networks can be used for healthcare purposes. What are some innovative ways for social networks to be used?

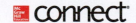 Enhance your learning by completing these exercises and more at http://connect.mheducation.com!

chapter **eleven**

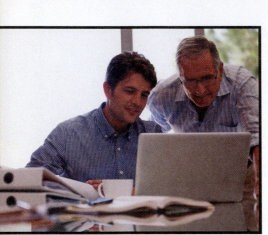

Expanding Roles and Functions of the Health Information Management and Health Informatics Professional

Learning Outcomes

When you finish this chapter, you will be able to:

11.1 Discuss how traditional health information management roles are expanding as a result of electronic health records and patient-centric healthcare.

11.2 Explain the new health information management roles that are emerging as

a result of electronic health records and patient-centric healthcare.

11.3 Assess the steps that health information professionals need to take to progress and evolve in their careers.

Key Terms

Certified Health Data Analyst (CHDA®)
Disease registry
General equivalence mapping (GEM)
ICD-10-CM/PCS implementation or conversion specialists

Structured data
Unstructured data

With an aging population, an increase in health information technology, and more individuals with access to healthcare insurance coverage, the need for professionals to organize and manage health information will grow. In addition, the profession itself is forecasting that large numbers of baby boomer professionals will retire in the next 10 to 15 years, leaving a shortage of health information and health informatics professionals. The US Department of Labor's 2014 *Occupational Outlook Handbook* projects an increase in the need for health information technicians of 22% from 2012 to 2022, which is a much faster rate of growth than the average for all occupations. As the complexity of electronic systems and the need for accurate, timely data increase, the educational level of health information professionals will also rise. This is a very exciting time for the healthcare profession as a whole, and for the health information management and informatics profession, in particular.

With so many changes occurring in the healthcare field—from the expanding role of data in ensuring quality healthcare to the changing models for reimbursement—the opportunities for health information and informatics professionals are also expanding. This chapter will explore traditional roles that are undergoing a metamorphosis and new roles in managing data and information. Finally, the steps that professionals must take to forward their careers in today's healthcare environment will also be addressed.

11.1 Expanding Roles in an Electronic, Patient-centric Environment

Database and Registry Management

Healthcare delivery is shifting from episodic care with paper-based records to proactive, preventive care with digital (electronic) records. One of the major advantages of digital records is that they make it easy to undertake sophisticated analysis, to track trends over time, and even to make predictions. Digital records require storing data in a standardized format in a database, which needs to be managed and used.

Health information professionals have traditionally been involved with ensuring the standardization and integrity of patient data as well as analyzing the data they collect. Think back to the chapter on functions, careers, and credentials of the health information professional. Abstracting and record processing, whether working with a registry, a Master Patient (Person) Index (MPI), or any other type of database, has long been an integral part of the health information professional's role. The recent changes in healthcare have simply resulted in a greater need and ability to record and analyze patient data.

Let's look at registries as an example. Until recent years, registries included mainly logs of births, deaths, trauma cases, and implantable devices. Now, **disease registries** are an increasingly important database used in healthcare. These new and expanding registries need individuals to develop and maintain them. Work on registries allows health information professionals to apply traditional functions in exciting new ways—to support public health and performance-based care—as the role of registries in healthcare shifts and expands.

Disease registry A large collection or registry belonging to a healthcare system or public health entity that contains information on different chronic health problems or diseases affecting patients in a system. This registry helps manage and log data on chronic illnesses and diseases. All data in the disease registry are logged by healthcare providers and can be used to perform benchmarking measures on healthcare systems.

Registries have developed in specific structures, such as diabetes registries, cancer registries, and childhood immunization registries. Figure 11.1 shows sample output from a diabetes registry.

Registries can be used to track a single patient or a patient population with a specific diagnosis. Thus, a patient can be benchmarked against, or compared to, other patients in terms of treatment and clinical measures, or the total disease-specific population can be benchmarked against standards or the performance of other providers. Benchmarking and registry data are important, because reimbursement will increasingly be based on performance measures. For example, CMS is no longer providing reimbursement or is lowering reimbursement for Medicare patients readmitted to the hospital within 30 days for some conditions based on the threshold of an excess readmission ratio. Therefore, if a hospital has a higher percentage of readmissions than measures established by CMS, the hospital will receive no or a lower reimbursement for that patient.

A registry can also be used to identify issues in care delivery and improve performance by clinicians and others across the continuum of care. A disease registry can predict potential problems

Patient: Carlton, Roberta   DOB: 07/15/1961   Age: 53

	Goal	2/15/2013	8/12/2013	2/11/2014	8/9/2014
Weight	Less than 185 lbs.	199	190	195	191
Blood Pressure	Less than 140/80	140/82	135/70	140/85	150/88
Lab Tests					
HbA1c (sugar for 3 months)	Less than 7%	7.1	7.4	7.1	8.0
LDL (bad cholesterol)	Less than 100	100	130	150	150
HDL (good cholesterol)	More than 40	41	42	40	38
Triglycerides	Less than 150	150	160	200	220
Medications					
Aspirin	81 mg daily	Yes	Yes	Yes	Yes
HCTZ	25 mg daily	Yes	Yes	Yes	Yes
Preventive Medicine		Status	Most Recent Exam	Due	
Eye Exam (prevents blindness)	Yearly	Current	08/9/2014	08/10/2015	
Foot Exam (prevents amputations)	Yearly	Current	08/9/2014	08/10/2015	
Urine Microalbumin (monitors for kidney failure)	Yearly	Current	08/9/2014	08/10/2015	
Flu Shot (preventive for influenza)	Yearly	Current	08/09/2014	08/2015	
Vaccines		Status			
Pneumovax (prevents pneumonia)	Given once unless first shot before age 65, then give second shot	Given 08/12/2013			
ZOSTAVAX®	Given once after the age of 50.	Declined			

Clinic Report

Patients Meeting Goals on Most Recent Tests

Clinic ID		HbA1c	LDL	B/P	All 3 Same Time
Clinic X	% patients met goal	59%	69%	55%	27%
All Clinics	% patients met goal	56%	62%	57%	23%
Goals		<7	<100	130/80	

	Goals	All Clinics Averages	Clinic X Averages
Number of Patients		22,262	311
Number of Visits		130,263	1285
Blood Pressure	130/80	131/76	128/75
Eye Check	One time a year	25%	47%
Foot Check	One time a year	34%	64%
A1c	<7	7.2	7.1
Total Cholesterol	<200	171	165
LDL	<100	93	86
HDL		46	43
Non-HDL	<130	125	122
Triglycerides	<150	167	176
Urine Microalbumin	One time a year	35%	59%
Flu Shot	One time a year	21%	58%

Figure 11.1   A Disease Registry Report for an Individual Patient and a Clinic

with a resulting intervention that may prevent a medical issue from becoming acute. The goal of the disease registry is to support better outcomes, lower costs, and promote a healthier population.

The mounting importance and versatility of registries in the age of digital health records have increased the demand for new workers as well as new skill sets for current employees. First, registries data need to be processed once they are gathered; otherwise, they cannot be used to create reports. Health information professionals must code and abstract the mounting quantities of data being collected by registries. The data must also meet all the privacy, security, and other HIM requirements discussed throughout this text. For example, the data must meet federal and state regulations to be viable for deeper analysis, such as benchmarking. The evolving nature of database work allows HI professionals to expand traditional skill sets while using them toward exciting new ends.

Health Data Analyst

Although data analysis has traditionally been a function of health information professionals, EHRs and a shift toward patient-centric care have only increased the importance of data analytics in healthcare. The sheer quantity of data now being collected and the variety of those data are staggering. Someone needs to ensure that all these data become actionable information. Data analysts are responsible for identifying trends or patterns of disease or utilization of services. They collect and validate data. They are typically responsible for writing summaries and presenting findings in a way that can be understood by others who are not knowledgeable in the subject area.

As data analysis becomes more critical, the data analytics function of health information management professionals will become more prominent, either within existing functions or as new jobs. AHIMA saw the need to encourage HIM professionals to expand their data analytics skills and, in 2008, created the **Certified Health Data Analyst (CHDA®)** certification. This certification is becoming increasingly prevalent, particularly among health information management professionals with bachelor's or master's degrees.

An HIM professional's knowledge of how and when data are collected in the healthcare cycle, as well as the definition of each piece of data, gives him or her insights into details that someone with only a theoretical knowledge of data analysis might miss. For example, if a hospital administrator asks for the facility's readmission rate, an HIM professional would know to ask the administrator what he or she is attempting to glean from the results. From the administrator's answer, the HIM professional would then ask, "Readmissions within what time period?" or "Readmissions for the same or different diagnoses?" or "Readmissions by nursing unit, by attending physician, or an aggregate total?"

With the impending conversion to ICD-10-CM/PCS, another role or skill in data analytics that has emerged is mapping, also known as a crosswalk, from one coding system to another. This mapping of

Certified Health Data Analyst (CHDA®) A professional certification sponsored by AHIMA to recognize professionals who have the training and experience to acquire, manage, analyze, interpret, and transform data into accurate, consistent, and timely information.

TABLE 11.1 An Example of ICD-9-CM to ICD-10-CM GEM

ICD-9-CM TO ICD-10-CM GEM ENTRY FOR COMPLEX ENDOMETRIAL HYPERPLASIA

2013 Entry	Updated 2014 Entry	Comment
621.32 Complex endometrial hyperplasia without atypia To/from **N85.02** Endometrial intraepithelial neoplasia [EIN]	**621.32** Complex endometrial hyperplasia without atypia To/from **N85.01** Benign endometrial hyperplasia	The updated entry is a closer match. The ICD-10-CM index entry *Hyperplasia, hyperplastic > endometrium, endometrial (adenomatous) (benign) (cystic) (glandular) (glandular-cystic) (polypoid) > complex (without atypia)* refers to N85.01. The entry has also been added to the ICD-10-CM to ICD-9-CM GEM.

Source: CMS. Gems2014 Update Summary.

General equivalence mapping (GEM) Forward (ICD-9-CM to ICD-10-CM) and backward (ICD-10-CM to ICD-9-CM) mappings of each code found in both coding systems. GEMs are also created for ICD-9-CM to/from ICD-10-PCS for procedural codes.

diagnosis and procedural coding is known as **general equivalence mapping (GEM)**, which was created by CMS. Table 11.1 illustrates ICD-9-CM to ICD-10-CM GEM for complex endometrial hyperplasia.

In order to compare "apples to apples," the data gathered with the legacy system, ICD-9, must be mapped to the newly instituted system, ICD-10 (and vice versa); otherwise, data collected using ICD-10 is not comparable to data collected using ICD-9, and vice versa. The ability to map in either direction is known as bi-directional mapping. One-to-one mapping is not always the case, however—some diagnosis or procedural codes map to more than one code in the opposite coding system, known as one-to-many mapping. Extensive experience and training in both ICD-9 and ICD-10 coding are necessary in order to understand that one-to-one or one-to-many relationship. Healthcare facilities must anticipate the volume of certain diagnoses or procedures based on historical figures—a mapping activity that will likely be performed by individuals with a coding background. Third-party payers are also anticipating the change to ICD-10, and they are likely to need the expertise of coders to perform this function as the transition evolves.

HIM professionals with data analytics skills will likely face challenges, such as the transition from ICD-9 to ICD-10, in the coming years. Data analysts with a strong HIM background, but who lack IT expertise, will often work with someone from health informatics to write reports or use database management programs. Data analytics skills will only make an HIM professional more marketable as we continue to shift toward an EHR-driven, patient-centered healthcare model. Data analytics also represents a key area of expansion of the health information management profession.

Coding/Clinical Documentation Improvement (CDI) Specialist

The role of coder was discussed several times in the early chapters of this text and has been an HIM role for years. Several factors have come together to evolve and expand the role of the coder. First, the implementation of EHRs has led to a massive expansion of data that can and need to be coded. Second, the move toward ICD-10-CM/

PCS has increased the complexity of coding, which allows it to create a truer picture of a patient's diagnosis and the procedures performed. Third, in a healthcare system evolving toward a patient-centric model, the increased detail and specificity of health record documentation have become of paramount importance.

Coders have traditionally performed, as described earlier, a document improvement function. The coder reads the documentation in a health record and then assigns diagnosis and procedural codes according to what has been documented. Documentation that is not thorough or precise is brought to the physician's attention, but in such a way that he or she is not led to document anything that cannot be substantiated. Documentation improvement will increasingly become part of a coder's role, especially as coding becomes more automated. Like the role of medical transcriptionists, the role of the coder will increasingly become to verify and check the quality of data.

The role of clinical documentation improvement specialist (CDI) originally expanded out of coding, but it is also becoming increasingly important as a distinct career. In this time of transition, CDI specialists will work with physicians and other practitioners to implement new clinical documentation improvement practices and to analyze new digital workflows. Although CDI specialists will rely on a knowledge of coding and communication skills as before, they will also have to develop new skills and a current knowledge of ever-changing regulations in today's changing healthcare environment. The roles of the coder and the clinical documentation improvement specialist are evolving in new and interesting ways in the face of change; clearly, they will continue to have an important—if altered—position on the healthcare team in the future.

Auditor

The quality and integrity of data—whether **structured data** or **unstructured data**—are imperative to the healthcare system. Auditors are the professionals who review the work of any type of healthcare provider or professional to ensure the accuracy, timeliness, and appropriateness of documentation, coding, or any other function that is documented and measurable.

In addition, government regulations and accrediting agency standards, as well as the requirements of third-party payers, must also be monitored, and auditors must ensure that data conform to these various standards, requirements, and regulations. Auditing may be performed internally by supervisory or compliance staff or as part of a peer review system. Auditing may also be performed by third-party payers or consulting agencies contracted by the facility to review compliance with acceptable practice. Some of the HIM-related reviews include inpatient and outpatient coding, Medicare Severity Diagnosis Related Group (MS-DRG) or Ambulatory Payment Classification (APC) assignment, and proper release of information. Auditors not only review and monitor but also educate, so that discrepancies, inconsistencies, and errors do not continue.

Structured data Data that fit a particular model or format and can be tracked as part of a database. Examples include diagnosis or procedural codes in ICD or CPT format, a patient's age, and a laboratory value.

Unstructured data Data in the form of words or audio files that cannot be tracked in a database. Examples include the text of an email, written narratives, and audio files from speech/voice recognition technology.

The auditor looks for trends, such as the same coder or coders making errors or the same doctor or doctors recording incomplete documentation that does not support MS-DRG assignment. Often, staff are intimidated by someone looking at their work, yet the results of an audit can very well result in positive outcomes for the staff, as in the case of positive findings that result in an excellent performance appraisal or, where improvement is needed, a recommendation that ongoing education of coding staff would result in higher coding accuracy. Though this may seem like more work initially, it should be seen as a benefit to coders, because the cost of continuing education is provided by the facility, the coders' knowledge is enhanced, and they instantly become more marketable by staying current in their field. External auditors not only report coders' issues but also review their findings regarding the quality of the documentation in the health records with the chief of medical staff and often with the physicians as a group, which in turn may make the coder's job a bit easier.

Professionals who choose to pursue auditing as a career undergo ongoing professional development, because continuing education is a necessity if one is to monitor and educate others about documentation shortcomings. Currency with government memorandums and transmittals is a requirement for the same reason. Auditing requires a strong grasp of Standard English, because written reports and oral presentations are part of an auditor's job description.

A certain number of years of coding experience, whether internal or external, are necessary to become an auditor. External auditors often travel—some in a particular region, some all over the United States.

The job of the auditor has changed as a result of electronic records and automated processes. For instance, the increase in available data allows the auditor to look for trends by coder or trends by diagnosis or procedure. The auditor can more easily look for problem areas even before opening a record. Also, auditors are more likely to work off-site now that the EHR is more the norm than the exception; for example, the education of providers or coders can be accomplished through live or recorded webinars, rather than on-site education.

Release of Information Coordinator

Patients are growing increasingly educated about their own healthcare and want to have a more active role in it, including accessing their health information. More and more, patients inquire about how to access their health records as well as how to use other patient portal functionality, such as setting up appointments, accessing their patient accounts, and communicating with their healthcare team. New job responsibilities for release of information coordinators include enlightening patients about the information and functions available to them through the portal, educating them on how to sign up to use the portal, walking through the steps in using the portal, and showing them how to keep their health information private and secure in whatever format their patient information is accessed.

Healthcare facilities that see the value in assisting patients with their portals will be providing customer service, which in the end may also increase the percentage of patients utilizing the patient portal functionality—a requirement of Meaningful Use Stage 2. Marketing of the patient portal, and the services offered through the release of information staff, is a first step in providing this valuable customer service. Providing marketing materials to particular populations of patients, such as those with cancer or chronic illnesses, is a good starting point to get the word out about the value of access to their own healthcare records.

11.1 A DAY IN THE LIFE

Jane is the release of information coordinator at a community hospital. She has been there for close to 30 years and has seen many changes through the years. Prior to the hospital's conversion to an electronic release of information tracking system and the EHR, every aspect of Jane's job was manual. In a typical day, she opened the mail and logged every request into a paper journal, which included the date received, the patient's name, the patient's medical record number (which she needed to locate in the hospital's MPI), the requestor's full name, and the type of request (physician, hospital, insurance, attorney, disability, law enforcement, patient, etc.). After opening all the mail, which could be as few as 10 or as many as 20 requests, she sorted the requests in order of priority, which by policy was physicians, hospitals, other healthcare facilities, insurance, disability, law enforcement, patients, attorneys, and then all others. Not only did she receive requests through the mail, but she also had walk-in requests from patients and *subpoena duces tecums* were delivered in person; the billing office forwarded any insurance requests it received through interoffice mail. Of course, she read each request to see if there was a date by which the records were needed. A *subpoena duces tecum*, for example, requiring the record to be presented at a court hearing in three days needed to be expedited, if all requirements of the *subpoena duces tecum* were met. Every request and corresponding authorization had to be reviewed to ensure that HIPAA, state, and federal regulations as well as facility policies were met. Any that did not meet the requirements needed to be returned to the requestor, along with a letter explaining the reason the request had not been filled.

After opening and logging the mail, Jane worked on manually pulling the records she needed to fill requests remaining from previous days' mail and any from the current day that needed to be filled immediately. She had to assess each request to determine what could be copied based on the authorization signed by the patient or legal representative, and she had to ensure that the correct patient's records were pulled. The bulk of her day was spent photocopying all the requested records. Some were just a few pages; others were for an entire record, which could be several inches thick, or for just certain

(continued)

parts of a record, which meant dismantling the record and locating the individual reports requested. Once the pages were photocopied, Jane had to put the record back together in the correct order. Then, she refiled the records, placed a cover letter and a copy of the original request in an envelope addressed to the recipient, and updated the correspondence log to show the date the records were mailed. All this had to be done with 100% accuracy and within the time frame stated in the facility policy: within two business days for requests from physicians, hospitals, or other healthcare providers; within four days for insurance and disability requests; and within seven days for all others. She then took all the mail to the mailroom, where all the outgoing mail was weighed and stamped. The next day, Jane started over again with the entire process. Keeping to the seven-day maximum turnaround time was often difficult, so when necessary, the file room staff retrieved and refiled records for Jane, and another HIM technician who had been trained in the entire process was pulled from his job as a record analyst.

Fast-forward to 2009, when Jane's job was made easier through automated correspondence tracking. The job of opening and logging the mail was cut nearly in half, because the correspondence software interfaced with the MPI, and she no longer had to look up each patient's medical record number. Using the software, Jane ran a daily report that sorted the requests by priority, so that she could more easily organize her day and she could see at a glance the requests that were coming up on the turnaround time limits.

Between 2010 and 2012, the facility converted to an EHR, further changing Jane's job by eliminating the need to pull records manually and copy paper in many cases. However, she still has to pull some records and manually copy them when the requested records are older than 2010.

Records that are electronic no longer need to be retrieved from file—Jane can access the patient's EHR and, with a few clicks of the mouse, print out the requested documents. Now that electronic faxing has been instituted, there is no longer a need to print anything, if the requested record is electronic and the requestor has the capability to receive faxes either electronically (from computer to computer) or on a fax machine. For patients who utilize the EHR's patient portal feature, Jane is able to send the requested documents to the portal, if they aren't already there, in which case she corresponds through email with the patient or mails the patient instructions on how to access his or her portal and the specific documents he or she has requested.

With the advent of automated processes, Jane now receives close to half of the requests electronically through an email address, available on the hospital's website, specifically set up for requests for health information. The number of requests Jane receives has increased by about 15% since 2009, and though the automated processes make her job much easier, she is still kept busy every day, and the analysis technician works with Jane 16 hours a week.

(continued)

1. Complete a flow chart of the processes Jane used prior to automation and after.
2. What factors can be attributed to the increase in requests Jane has seen since 2009?
3. Jane now has more contact with patients, in person and electronically. Why is that?

Population Management Researcher

Health informatics is the practice of information and knowledge management across clinical healthcare and public health domains. Put simply, it is using the digital data collected in a healthcare-related setting by turning the data into information and using that information in a meaningful way. This data-to-information (which in turn is knowledge) concept has always occurred in healthcare, which is fundamentally evidence-based. But the digitization of records and the use of computerized systems and analytics have changed the processes, information structure, and knowledge possessed. Thus, health informatics concerns the methods and output of the very leading edge of health information management.

Once information has been made usable, informatics is involved in analysis, assessment, and reporting. These functions include data extraction, analytics, and evaluation. The scope of the data used ranges from healthcare delivery to payment. Under Meaningful Use requirements and payment reform, informatics will play an increasingly important role in directly supporting patient care, measuring performance, and shaping processes.

Related to health informatics is health information technology. HIT develops and supports the infrastructure used in healthcare delivery, which is increasingly computerized and networked. Health informatics uses the data, information, and knowledge that can be extracted and otherwise synthesized in an interconnected delivery network. The function of the health informatics professional is to apply information systems and information management to support clinical information technology and medical research.

Healthcare has always been research-driven. Investigation has historically involved the areas of pharmaceuticals, treatment protocols, and other elements of direct patient care. Now, however, the healthcare system is being redesigned. There is a need to understand how best to engineer this redesign, making research more critical and broadening its scope. Many areas of business research, such as process re-engineering and change management, need to be understood within the healthcare context. Other new areas, including consumer engagement and consumer satisfaction, involve the patient. Virtually every chapter of this book has topics that require research into how they are affected and should evolve, given the changes in the healthcare system.

The amount of research in healthcare will increase as healthcare reform changes the delivery paradigm. There will continue to be positions for individuals trained with research design and methodology skills in undertaking both applied research and more academic research. Training in research is an important skill when coupled with knowledge of the industry.

11.2 A DAY IN THE LIFE

Mary Johnson works for the Department of Medicaid in her home state. Hers is one of the states that expanded Medicaid under the ACA to include previously uninsured individuals. The result is that the number of lives covered by Medicaid in the state has almost doubled, and costs to the taxpayers have risen. The state has initiated a new program whereby Medicaid patients with chronic diseases, such as diabetes, are assigned to a primary care doctor who is supposed to be proactive in partnering with the patient to manage the patient's health.

Mary's job is to measure the effectiveness of this program. She must design a research plan, collect data, and analyze the results.

1. How does this represent an expanding area of work for informatics and health information professionals?
2. What type of training do you think is necessary for Mary to undertake this work successfully?
3. The work includes data extraction and reporting. Are these health informatics or health information management skills? How does this work represent a blending of the fields?

Educator

Health information and informatics professionals have an educational background related to the methods used to gather, analyze, archive, and protect health information. In years past, records were kept in paper format through manual processes. Since the latter part of the 20th century, health records have been increasingly kept electronically. Health information practitioners have transitioned from paper to electronic records and from manual to electronic means of processing and keeping health records. The educational foundations of the health information field have also gone through an extensive transition; rather than only the management of health information, there are now health informatics programs as well. Though the trend is toward electronic methods, the basic concepts and procedures done manually are still necessary, because not all healthcare facilities are fully electronic—some choose to maintain dual manual and electronic systems. Also, computers do go down, and therefore at least temporary reversion to manual means is occasionally necessary.

Educators and educational programs have had to alter already full curriculums to cover electronic systems and the technology that comes with them while still covering manual systems, at least at a cursory level.

Health information management and health informatics programs, referred to as HIIM programs, are found at the associate, baccalaureate, and master's degree levels. There is a shortage of qualified teaching personnel. Those teaching in HIIM programs are not always trained as educators; thus, practitioners often think they are not qualified to teach. Teaching at the college level, or becoming a director of an educational program, requires learning an entirely new skill set, yet the underlying knowledge of health information and informatics and the experience as a practitioner are necessary to train the next generation of HIM and HI practitioners.

Many who choose to move from practitioner to educator do so by first becoming an adjunct instructor. Adjuncts teach one or two courses per term, either in a classroom (face-to-face) setting or online. This gives the individual a chance to test the waters and provides additional income.

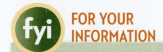

FOR YOUR INFORMATION

The term *HIIM program* is used to refer to educational programs that cover health information management or health information or health informatics (or a combination of all three).

11.3 A DAY IN THE LIFE

I'm Marcia, HIM practitioner turned HIM educator. Why did I make the move from practitioner to professor? After working in the HIM field for 13 years in many different roles ranging from supervisor and quality improvement analyst to director, I decided to make a career change. After deep reflection, I realized that I enjoyed learning and sharing knowledge; therefore, the field of education became appealing. To gain experience to see if this would be a good fit for me, I became a guest lecturer at the HIM program that educated me. Luckily, I enjoyed the experience.

There are several reasons I moved from practitioner to professor, but the one that sticks out the most is that it was a way for me to give back to a profession that provided many great career opportunities for me. I love talking with students and encouraging them to pursue an HIM career. The other reasons I made the career switch is the flexibility that teaching allows, the opportunity to continue learning and to get advanced degrees, and the satisfaction obtained from knowing that you have made a difference in someone's life. The education field has also pushed me to do things out of my comfort zone and realize and accept that it is fine to make mistakes. I have learned so much through my mistakes.

What is the skill set needed to become a professor? The best way for me to present an answer to this question is by listing those skills I think are important to succeed as an educator.

1. Lifelong learner (you must love learning; you may have to go back to school)
2. Patience (you must have patience; students will test your patience, even if you are teaching online)
3. Share knowledge (realizing that all learners are different and therefore you must be creative in finding ways to reach all learners)
4. Communication skills (written, presentation, and soft skills are essential)
5. Competent in HIM

(continued)

6. Flexible, adaptable (change is occurring everywhere in every industry; you must be flexible to survive)
7. Genuine (your concern and care toward the students goes a long way)
8. Competent in technology (education and HIM are both becoming high-tech)

As an educator, the majority of my day is spent preparing for class. Preparing for class may include researching a topic, finding current literature surrounding the topic, deciding which format to deliver the content, preparing the presentation, developing assignments, and grading assessments. In addition, a great deal of time is spent responding to student inquiries and advising and mentoring students.

1. Assess your own skills and career goals. Do you have the skills and desire to one day be an HIM educator?
2. As a student, think of educators who have made a significant impression on you. Do they have skills or traits not listed in this feature that have had a positive impact on you? What are they?

11.1   THINKING IT THROUGH

1. Explain why the role of the release of information specialist has changed as a result of electronic health records and Meaningful Use.
2. Why are data so important in research activities?
3. How do registry data impact reimbursement?

11.2   Health Information Professionals' New Roles and Responsibilities in an Electronic, Patient-centric Health System

ICD-10-CM/PCS Implementation or Conversion Specialist

ICD-10-CM/PCS implementation or conversion specialists
Individuals who are proficient at ICD-10-CM/PCS coding who plan and coordinate the conversion to ICD-10-CM/PCS in healthcare facilities, insurance companies, or clearinghouses. Responsibilities include choosing the content of and time frame for training facility staff and care providers and assessing the needs of the facility (including the need for additional training in documentation for providers or in human disease and anatomy and physiology for the coders).

The transition from ICD-9-CM to ICD-10-CM/PCS has been long and complicated, since the implementation date for ICD-10 changed more than once. At the time of this writing, the implementation date is October 1, 2015. Re-engineering of internal processes has been planned and to some extent implemented, then stopped in its tracks due to the continued delay in ICD-10 implementation. This delay in transition has resulted in the need for **ICD-10-CM/PCS implementation or conversion specialists**. Because ICD-9 will become the legacy system, the need for this position will continue even after the conversion has occurred. Individuals in this role must, of course, be proficient in both ICD-9 and ICD-10 coding, while having a sound knowledge of disease processes discussed earlier. In addition, he or she must have excellent communications skills, because upper management, physicians, other clinicians, and, of course, the coders must be apprised of timetables, documentation requirements, coding changes, and similar tasks that will be affected by this transition.

Service Provider (Vendor) Staff

Health information–related software service providers (vendors) are seeing an increase in EHR installations and conversions, and with that comes a need for staff possessing knowledge of health information as well as health informatics. Health information and informatics professionals understand record content requirements, data flow, record retention, and the reimbursement cycle; therefore, they are instrumental in ensuring a smooth, efficient EHR transition as well as post-implementation support. Previous experience in managing HIM departments or performing HIM functions in a healthcare setting is an asset to EHR and related service providers, because such experience provides firsthand knowledge of day-to-day routines, workflow, areas of bottlenecks, and other HIM functions. An informatics background is important in ensuring that the content is available when and where it is needed in a secure electronic framework. A person with an HIM background may work with a hospital or practice to determine its electronic needs and wants, to assess the current system, to configure a new system, to plan the new system implementation (project management), and/or to train staff. Often, graduates of health informatics programs hold these positions, because they possess IT and health information knowledge and skills.

Health information and informatics professionals are also sought by companies specializing in EHR software, voice recognition practice management, encoders, and release of information software.

A growing area of opportunity for employment is in health information exchanges (HIEs). These organizations provide the network and services that allow providers and other stakeholders to exchange data, as well as offering services such as disease registries, patient alerts, and patient portals. HIEs are vendors of services, and there are numerous new work roles for programmers, analysts, and data managers. HIEs were discussed in detail in the chapter on Meaningful Use.

11.4 A DAY IN THE LIFE

Hannah Wilson has worked as a health information manager at a hospital for more than a decade. When the hospital installed EHRs, Hannah was selected as a super-user, someone who learns the system and is part of a team that teaches others to use EHRs within the organization. The vendor of the EHR was so impressed with Hannah that it offered her a job traveling from hospital to hospital, installing the EHR systems and training others on how to use the system.

1. How does Hannah's background in HIM provide the skills needed for this position?

2. How does this position differ from a traditional HIM role? Is there training that would make a HIM professional suited for this type of job?

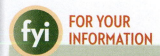

FOR YOUR INFORMATION

Super-users are employees who learn a new technology system, such as an EHR; they help others learn the system and take a leadership role in integrating the system within the organization. Super-users typically have high-level rights and permissions to make changes or adjust computer settings and access, for instance, network or system administrators.

Health Informaticist

A health informaticist has some things in common with a health information manager. However, the fundamental difference is that the health informaticist has special technical skills in computer interfaces, database management, business intelligence applications, report writing, and analytics (these areas were described in the registry section of this chapter). However, informatics goes beyond registries to include the manipulation, interpretation, and assessment of health information in many contexts, such as public policies, public health, financial management, and business process assessment.

Various databases, including registries, are becoming more important, because their effective use supports the healthcare reform goals of improved patient outcomes, lower costs, and improved public health. Among the roles of informaticists is the aggregation of data in a valid and usable structure and the undertaking of data analyses. The principal uses for databases, besides billing and financial reporting, are patient and population reports, performance assessment, benchmarking, and predictive analytics.

The process of analysis involves gathering the data into a database. This is a complicated process, because it involves exchanging information, usually from hardware and software developed by different vendors. All interfaces must be based on industry standards and are typically customized. Once centralized, the data must be standardized both in structure and through the use of a common vocabulary. Cleaning and maintaining the data in a registry are complex tasks.

Data extraction from a registry is also a specialized and complex practice. Queries bringing the required data together must be written and reports constructed. This requires expertise in business intelligence applications, such as SQL and Crystal Reports. Often, in the past, reports were based on paper records and required manual extraction. The data then had to be transformed into input for special software programs. Today, healthcare can use standard business applications that make the process quicker but require training.

Reports must be developed in conjunction with clinicians and other specialists—using highly refined healthcare terminology and an understanding of clinical processes. Thus, workers in this area need technical skills plus a good understanding of healthcare and medical terminology.

Once reports are created from a database, they can be used. This may be the case of a physician using a report in a patient encounter, or it may be a performance assessment of a physician or hospital against benchmark measures for chronic disease management or other outcomes. Reports also need to be created and sent to CMS, insurance companies, public health, and state Medicaid offices. Applications can also be developed that are predictive, either at the individual or the population level—for example, flagging a chronic condition for preventive care based on trends and measurements. Or at the population level, a registry can flag an infectious outbreak, such as the flu, by surveillance of diagnosis, or so-called syndromic surveillance.

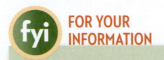

FOR YOUR INFORMATION

Cleansing data is identifying and correcting data that are corrupt, inaccurate, or incomplete within a database.

The knowledge and skills needed by workers in this area are specialized. Interface specialists, who allow various systems to communicate, must understand standards and HL-7 programming. Database maintenance and standardization are additional areas. Critical to the process are individuals who can extract data using SQL or a comparable business intelligence application and produce reports that are valid, reliable, and usable by various stakeholders. Finally, analysts are required to interpret the reports and turn them into actionable information and knowledge.

Evolving technologies and objectives in healthcare research have created the new role of the health informaticist as well as positions for those who support them in a technical capacity.

11.5 A DAY IN THE LIFE

A large primary care practice has implemented an EHR and needs to attest to its ability to meet CMS clinical quality reporting requirements under Meaningful Use Stage 2. Although its EHR should be able to generate these reports automatically, the practice wants to hire a local professional who can extract the required reports and provide custom reports to the doctors in the practice. It decides to hire a health informaticist staff to manage a patient database and to provide both the reports required by CMS and those requested by clinical staff (such as summary reports on the treatment of patients with diabetes).

1. What skills should a person have in order to succeed in this position?
2. How are traditional business intelligence skills, such as SQL programming, becoming mainstreamed in healthcare?
3. What analytical skills are required in this role (beyond database management and data extraction)?

Chief Knowledge Officer/Information Governance Officer

The integrity of health record documentation is a key responsibility of the health information professional. Someone in this profession is the most knowledgeable about what must be documented as required by government regulations, accrediting standards, and third-party payers and as required to protect the legal interests of patients, healthcare providers, and healthcare facilities. In an electronic environment, where data are collected in both structured and unstructured formats, it is the health information management and informatics staff that must attest to the validity, reliability, and integrity of electronic data. The HIM staff attests to the completeness of the record and the accuracy of the coded data, and the informatics staff attests that the electronic record has not been tampered with and that the data added or edited have been appropriately authenticated through signature and date stamp or electronic signature. The quality of healthcare cannot be assessed without data to prove it.

Information (data) governance involves overseeing, monitoring, and controlling data collection. Individual facilities and health enterprises are giving information governance responsibilities to health information/informatics directors; new titles, such as chief knowledge officer or information governance officer, are also becoming more common. This individual advocates for quality documentation and processes that lead to interdisciplinary and interdepartmental collaboration, which results in documentation that accurately reflects the diagnosis, treatment, and outcome of each patient encounter. He or she is responsible for developing policies that cover the appropriate use of copy-and-paste or template usage. Education of all hospital or office staff, including physicians, should be a priority, as should the ongoing monitoring of compliance with the policies.

11.2 THINKING IT THROUGH

1. Why is database and registry management both an expanding and an emerging role for health information professionals?
2. Why is there a need for information or data governance as a result of an electronic system?

11.3 Health Information Education and Beyond

The maintenance of health information, paper or digital, requires knowledgeable individuals who want a career in healthcare but prefer the "business" side of it, rather than patient care. The concepts covered in this text are not exclusive to hospitals and physicians' practices. Long-term care, hospice, home health agencies, urgent care centers, ambulatory surgical centers, outpatient diagnostic centers, and rehabilitation facilities are all bound by licensure, federal regulations, and in many cases accreditation standards. Health records must be kept on every patient for every encounter, and the records need to be tracked, maintained, coded, and analyzed, just as in the hospital environment. Also, digitization and automation are increasingly adopted in these settings. Thus, the expanding and emerging roles of health information and health informatics may be seen in these organizations as well.

Preparing for a Career in Health Information Management or Informatics

As mentioned earlier in this chapter and in the chapter on functions, careers, and credentials, three degree levels are available to the aspiring health information professional, as well as various certificates (which were discussed in the early chapters of this text). Here we will concentrate on the degrees, the key courses taken in those curriculums, and the current and future position responsibilities one may be able to attain at that degree level.

The first is a two-year degree culminating in an associate degree. If you graduate from a Commission on Accreditation for Health Informatics and Information Management Education (CAHIIM)– approved associate degree program, you can take the national exam to become a Registered Health Information Technician® (RHIT®). Along with general education courses (e.g., English, math, social sciences, humanities) the curriculum typically includes courses in

- Medical terminology
- Anatomy and physiology
- Human disease
- Pharmacology
- General office software (word processing, spreadsheets, presentation software)
- Fundamentals of health information principles
- Electronic record-keeping
- Legal aspects of health information, HIPAA and other disclosure regulations
- Quality assessment methodologies
- Basic and advanced ICD coding
- HCPCS coding (CPT and Level 2)
- Supervision of health information services
- Healthcare statistics
- Healthcare reimbursement
- Computer technology
- A combination of practicum and/or internship opportunities

The positions requiring an associate-level education include, but are not limited to, those listed in Table 11.2:

TABLE 11.2	Common Associate-Level Positions
Health information specialist	Retrieval and archival of documents, quality monitoring for record completion, electronic health record processes
Release of information coordinator	Processes written or electronic requests for health information, ensures information is released only with valid authorization or as required by law, assists patients with patient portal access
Patient access specialist	Makes appointments, registers patients, collects and enters demographic and administrative data, verifies insurance
Insurance/billing positions	Insurance verification, insurance authorizations, medical claim filing, follow-up of medical claims
Coder	Inpatient or outpatient: codes diagnoses and procedures using ICD and HCPCS coding systems and MS-DRG, APC, or other reimbursement methodology

(continued)

TABLE 11.2	Common Associate-Level Positions *(continued)*
Quality improvement specialist	Reviews health records against predetermined criteria for clinical indicators
Trainer	Instructs staff on the use of EHR or other health information–related software
Registrar	Cancer, trauma, birth defect, and so on: collects data on all patients appropriate for a specific type of registry, including identification of appropriate cases, data abstracting, reporting of cases to state registries, statistical report preparation, follow-up of cases, ensures regulatory requirements are met
Transcriptionist	Transcribes reports from physicians' dictation or edits output from speech recognition software
Medical office administrator	Day-to-day management of a physician's practice

Individuals wishing to perform the duties in the previous list, but at a management level or in larger institutions, should seek at least a baccalaureate degree and take the RHIA® exam. The curriculum includes the associate-level curriculum but at a higher academic level and with additional coursework in problem solving, team building, change management, project management, performance standards, data security methods, systems development, database architecture and design, electronic communications technology and design, research protocols, inferential statistics, and data quality assessment and integrity.

The positions for which a bachelor's degree is typically needed include those listed for the associate degree at a higher organizational level, as well as the following:

- Department director
- Information security manager
- Compliance officer
- Privacy officer
- Data quality manager
- Project manager
- Reimbursement cycle manager
- Coding manager
- Department operations manager
- Transcription manager

Though a bachelor's degree is considered the terminal degree in health information management, in recent years master's programs have been gaining momentum. Individuals seeking a master's degree in health information will gain knowledge as in the previously discussed educational levels but will specifically gain skills in data structure and design, policy development relating to information (particularly electronic), information management system planning, workflow (clinical and administrative), operations management, and efficient, cost-effective management of information processing. The positions for which a master's degree is typically required include those under the bachelor's degree at a higher organizational level or in a healthcare enterprise, as well as the following:

- Vice president or executive of information privacy and security
- Department chairperson or program director (at a college or university)
- Vice president or executive of informatics
- Chief compliance officer
- Chief knowledge officer

Health informatics programs are generally at the master's degree level, although associate and bachelor's programs are incorporating informatics into their curriculums. The main emphasis of these programs is information systems, including the analysis, design, implementation, and management of the entire system. In addition, the structures, function, and transfer of information internally and externally are under the purview of a health informatics professional's responsibility.

Another avenue to advancement in the health IT realm is the Certified Healthcare Technology (CHTS) exam, which when passed shows proficiency in health IT in order to assume roles in workflow assessment, selection of software and hardware, work with vendors, system testing and system installation, diagnosis of IT problems, and staff training. This proficiency exam is offered through AHIMA.

The Healthcare Information Management Systems Society (HIMSS) IT certifications include the Certified Associate in Healthcare Information and Management Systems (CAHIMS), with a target audience of professionals with five years' experience in the field of health IT, and the Certified Professional in Healthcare Information and Management Systems (CPHIMS), which would be of interest to professionals with more than five years of health IT experience.

Any healthcare facility or healthcare software provider may hire health informatics or information management (HIIM) professionals, though hospitals continue to be the main employers. In addition to healthcare facilities and software providers, health information professionals may also be employed by law firms specializing in medical malpractice, insurance companies, government agencies, or research firms specializing in healthcare.

All professionals have to pay their dues—they do not start at the top of the corporate (or in this case healthcare) ladder; they earn promotions or seek out positions in organizations at a higher organizational level. The key word is *earn*—a professional's education does not end when a college diploma is in hand or when a certification exam has been passed. Learning and professional growth continue by earning higher degrees and taking advantage of continuing education, by attending professional association meetings and networking with other professionals, and by being an *active* member of a professional association by holding office, serving on committees, presenting at conferences, or writing articles for professional journals or authoring a book, for example. In addition, it is important to keep up with healthcare news in the mainstream media as well as through professional journals, by mentoring others who are new to the field, and by making a commitment to lifelong learning.

11.6 A DAY IN THE LIFE

Joette received her associate degree in health information management in 1998. After graduation, she had a hard time finding a job, because her area of interest was coding in a hospital, but she was being passed up by others who had inpatient coding experience. After about four months, she landed a position as a coder in an internal medicine practice with four physicians and two physicians' assistants. She had thought long and hard about taking the position, because she really wanted the fast pace of a hospital, but she figured that in a small practice she would have room for advancement.

She has enjoyed her job at the practice and has found it fulfilling, for the most part. After a few years, she was promoted to the lead coder position. She thought again about trying to find an inpatient coding position, but she liked the close interaction with the physicians, office staff, and often patients. Joette decided to enroll in an online bachelor's program in HIM, which she completed in 2006. She received much encouragement from the physicians at the practice, which then totaled eight physicians, and the practice was continuing to grow. She was promoted to business office manager in 2008, supervising the work of five coders and three billers.

The physicians in the practice are very forward-thinking and rely heavily on data. Every month at the office staff meetings, which included the physicians, she presented a topic on documentation or coding. Joette had been instrumental in the practice's preparations for ICD-10-CM. She had studied to become a CCS-P® (coding credential specializing in physicians' practice coding) and then became an AHIMA-approved ICD-10-CM trainer. Two of the managing partner physicians approached Joette in 2013, asking whether she would be interested in attaining her master's degree in health administration or health informatics, because the current office manager was planning to retire in two years and the role of the officer manager was expanding, particularly since the office was just about to the point of being paperless, and its EHR was in need of updating, as were the office's procedures and policies.

(continued)

The practice offered to pay for her master's degree. She thought about it and is currently enrolled in a master's program in health informatics. Her career path is summarized in Figure 11.2. The practice has just hired another physician and a physician's assistant; Joette has been tasked with investigating new EHR and practice management software, and the physicians are contemplating opening another office in a neighboring town. Joette is quite happy that she took the coder position at the practice, despite her initial hesitation. She found that she did not have to be a coder in a hospital in order to be challenged and to expand her career goals.

1. What about Joette do you think caused the managing partners to take note of her potential growth within the practice?

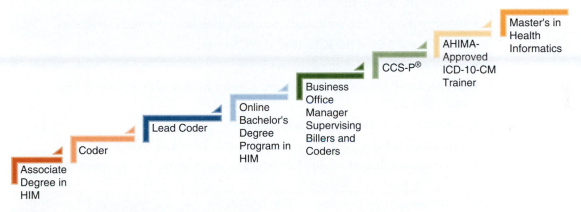

Figure 11.2   Joette's Career Trajectory

11.3   THINKING IT THROUGH

1. A relative is graduating from high school this year and is contemplating her educational future. She attended a college fair, and has decided she wants to pursue a career as a medical coder. She comes to you for advice since she knows you have been in the healthcare field for a long time. What level of education might you recommend for her? Why?

2. Joseph has a bachelor's degree in HIM and is an RHIA®, and has been working as a project manager in the IT department of Community Hospital as it converts from one EHR to another. He would like to be recognized for his health IT expertise as well as his HIM expertise, and at the moment cannot afford to begin a master's degree. What options does Joseph have to prove his expertise?

chapter 11 summary

LEARNING OUTCOMES	CONCEPTS FOR REVIEW
11.1 Discuss how traditional health information management roles are expanding as a result of electronic health records and patient-centric healthcare. Pages 275–286	• What is a disease registry? What role does the health information/informatics professional play in the development and maintenance of a disease registry? How can the data gathered from a disease registry affect reimbursement? • What is a service provider? Give examples. • Why would someone with a background in HIM or HIT be an asset to service providers? • Explain the role of the clinical data analyst. • Identify the role of the clinical documentation improvement specialist. • Identify the role of the ICD-10-CM/PCS implementation specialist. • Why is auditing of data necessary? • Define *health informatics*. How does it differ from health information management? • What role do data play in research? • Differentiate between applied research and theoretical research. • What impact does the role of an educator have on the health information and informatics profession? • What impact has Meaningful Use had on the role of a release of information specialist?
11.2 Explain the new health information management roles that are emerging as a result of electronic health records and patient-centric healthcare. Pages 286–290	• Discuss new roles and functions in database management that are emerging due to an electronic environment and Meaningful Use. • Explain the training necessary for and the role of a health informaticist. • What is the role of information (data) governance?
11.3 Assess the steps that health information professionals need to take to progress and evolve in their careers. Pages 290–295	• List the typical positions or duties held by persons holding an associate, bachelor's, or master's degree in health information or informatics management. • Differentiate between the RHIT® and the RHIA® credentials. • What are the positions often held or that are emerging for each credential? • What courses are taken in each? • What are the credentials that are available to individuals who are in the health IT realm rather than the more traditional HIM realm? • How can a health information/informatics professional ensure career growth?

chapter review

MATCHING QUESTIONS

Match each term with its definition.

_____ 1. **[LO 11.2]** health informaticist

_____ 2. **[LO 11.1]** certified health data analyst

_____ 3. **[LO 11.1]** structured data

_____ 4. **[LO 11.3]** registrar

_____ 5. **[LO 11.1]** disease registry

_____ 6. **[LO 11.3]** release of information coordinator

_____ 7. **[LO 11.1]** CDI specialist

8. **[LO 11.2]** ICD-10 consultant

_____ 9. **[LO 11.3]** Registered Health Information Technician

_____ 10. **[LO 11.1]** unstructured data

a. Collection of information on different chronic health problems

b. Data in the form of words or audio files that cannot be tracked in a database

c. Professional who is proficient at coding and who plans and coordinates the conversion to the new coding system

d. Professional who has graduated from an approved CAHIIM program and passed the AHIMA national exam

e. Professional who has technical skills in computer interfaces, database management, report writing, and analytics

f. Professional who transforms data into information

g. Professional who collects data on all patients appropriate for a specific type of registry

h. Professional who implements new clinical documentation improvement practices

i. Data in a format that can be tracked in a database

j. Professional who processes requests for health information

MULTIPLE CHOICE QUESTIONS

Choose the letter that best completes the statement or answers the question.

12. **[LO 11.1]** Jane works at her local hospital. Her job is to log and manage data on chronic illnesses and diseases. What is Jane working with on a daily basis?

a. Unstructured data

b. A disease registry

c. CMS regulations

d. Joint Commission regulations

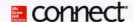 Enhance your learning by completing these exercises and more at http://connect.mheducation.com!

13. **[LO 11.1]** Data analysts are responsible for
    a. itemizing patient bills.
    b. identifying trends or patterns of diseases.
    c. programming EHR templates.
    d. obtaining clinical information from patients.

14. **[LO 11.1]** Professional certification sponsored by AHIMA to recognize professionals who have the training and experience in data is
    a. Registered Health Information Technician.
    b. Registered Health Information Administrator.
    c. Certified Health Data Analyst.
    d. Clinical Documentation Improvement Specialist.

15. **[LO 11.1]** Data that fit a particular model and can be tracked as part of a database are called
    a. unstructured data.
    b. vital statistics.
    c. voice recognition technology.
    d. structured data.

16. **[LO 11.2]** The principal uses for databases besides billing and financial reporting are all of the following *except*
    a. patient reports.
    b. performance assessment.
    c. joint Commission requirements.
    d. predictive analytics.

17. **[LO 11.2]** Professionals who interpret reports and turn them into actionable information are called
    a. programmers.
    b. coders.
    c. analysts.
    d. auditors.

18. **[LO 11.3]** What is the acronym of the HIMSS IT certification targeted to IT professionals with five years' experience?
    a. CPHIMS
    b. CHTS
    c. CAHIMS
    d. RHIT®

19. **[LO 11.3]** The Registered Health Information Administrator (RHIA®) exam requires which level of education?
    a. Associate degree
    b. Bachelor's degree
    c. Master's degree
    d. Doctorate

20. **[LO11.3]** Which position usually requires a bachelor's degree?
    a. Transcriptionist
    b. Privacy officer
    c. Coder
    d. Release of information specialist

SHORT ANSWER QUESTIONS

21. **[LO 11.1]** List three goals of a disease registry.

22. **[LO 11.1]** Describe the role of the health informatics professional.

23. **[LO 11.1]** Discuss why it is important for auditors to undergo continuing education.

24. **[LO 11.1]** List three factors that have expanded the role of the coder.

25. **[LO 11.2]** Describe the required skills of an ICD-10 conversion specialist.

26. **[LO 11.2]** Discuss why health information and informatics professionals are recruited by EHR software vendors.

27. **[LO 11.2]** What has caused the need for ICD-10-CM/PCS conversion specialists?

28. **[LO 11.2]** What is the fundamental difference between a health information specialist and a health informaticist?

29. **[LO 11.3]** Compare and contrast the AHIMA curriculums of the associate degree level and the bachelor's degree level.

30. **[LO 11.3]** What actions can a health information management/informatics professional take to further his or her career?

APPLYING YOUR KNOWLEDGE

31. **[LO 11.1]** Discuss the increased demand for new workers within registries.

32. **[LO 11.1]** Summarize the job of an auditor as a result of electronic health records and automated processes.

33. **[LO.11.1]** Compare and contrast structured data and unstructured data. Give an example of each.

34. **[LO 11.2]** Discuss what type of healthcare-related entities use reports generated by provider databases.

35. **[LO 11.2]** Search the Internet for EHR service vendors that might employ health information management professionals, and list several.

36. **[LO 11.3]** Choose one HIM position, requiring an associate degree, that interests you the most. Describe what appeals to you about this position.

37. **[LO 11.3]** What factors do you think have contributed to the master's-degree-level programs gaining momentum?

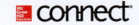 Enhance your learning by completing these exercises and more at http://connect.mheducation.com!

abbreviations and acronyms

a

AAAASF American Association for Accreditation of Ambulatory Surgery Facilities

AAAHC Accreditation Association for Ambulatory Health Care

ACA Affordable Care Act

ACHC Accreditation Commission for Health Care, Inc.

ACOs Accountable care organizations

ACS American College of Surgeons

ADT Admissions, discharges, and transfers

AHA American Hospital Association

AHDI Association for Healthcare Documentation Integrity

AHIMA American Health Information Management Association

ALA American Library Association

ALS Amyotrophic lateral sclerosis

AMA Against medical advice

AMA American Medical Association

AMIA American Medical Informatics Association

AMRA American Medical Record Association

AOA American Osteopathic Association

AOA/HFAP American Osteopathic Association/ Healthcare Facilities Accreditation Program

APCs Ambulatory Payment Classifications

ARLNA Association of Record Librarians of North America

ARMA American Record Management Association

ARRA American Recovery and Reinvestment Act

ART Accredited Record Technician

ASC Ambulatory surgery centers

ASTM American Society for Testing Materials

b

BCBSA Blue Cross and Blue Shield Association

BI Business intelligence

BMI Body mass index

c

CAC Computer-assisted coding

CAH Critical Access Hospital

CAHIIM Commission on Accreditation for Health Informatics and Information Management Education

CARF Commission on Accreditation of Rehabilitation Facilities

CCA Certified Coding Associate

CCD Continuity of Care Document

CCR Continuity of Care Record

CCS Certified Coding Specialist

CCS-P Certified Coding Specialist—Physician-based

CCU Cardiac care unit

CDA Clinical Document Architecture

CDC Centers for Disease Control and Prevention

CDI Clinical documentation improvement

CDIP Certified Documentation Improvement Practitioner

CDS Clinical Decision Support

CDs Compact Discs

CEUs Continuing Education Units

CHAMPUS Civilian Health and Medical Program of the Uniformed Services

CHAP Community Health Accreditation Program

CHDA Certified Health Data Analyst

CHINS Clinical Health Information Networks

CHIP Children's Health Insurance Program

CHPS Certified in Healthcare Privacy and Security

CHTS Certified Healthcare Technology Specialist

CIHQ Center for Improvement in Healthcare Quality

CIOs Chief information officers

CMI Case mix index

CMS Centers for Medicare and Medicaid Services

CNPs Certified nurse practitioners

COPD Chronic obstructive pulmonary disease

CoPs Conditions of Participation

CPOE Computerized physician order entry

CPT Current Procedural Terminology

CRNAs Certified Registered Nurse Anesthetists

CT Computerized axial tomography

CTR Certified Tumor Registrar

CVX Vaccine Administered

d

DIRECT Directed Exchange or Direct Secure Messaging

DMADV Define, measure, analyze, design, and verify

DMAIC Define, measure, analyze, improve, and control

DME Durable medical equipment

DNV Healthcare Det Norske Veritas Healthcare

DO Doctor of Osteopathy

DOB Date of birth

DRG Diagnosis related group

DRS Designated record set

e

EBM Evidence-based medicine

ED Emergency department

EIN Employer identification number

EKG Electrocardiogram

eMAR Electronic medication administration record

EMPI Enterprise Master Persons Indices

EMR Electronic medical record

EOBs Explanations of Benefits

ePHI Electronic Protected Health Information

EPOs Exclusive provider organizations

eSignature Electronic signature

ESRD End-stage renal disease

f

FFS Fee-for-service

FFV Fee-for-value

g

GEM General equivalence mapping

GNP Gross national product

h

H&P History & physical exam

HAC Hospital Acquired Conditions

HCFA Health Care Financing Administration

EHR Electronic health record

HEW Department of Health, Education, and Welfare

HFAP Healthcare Facilities Accreditation Program

HHA Home health agencies

HHS Department of Health and Human Services

HI Health information

HIE Health information exchange

HIM Health information management

HIMSS Healthcare Information Management Systems Society

HIO Health Information Organization

HIPAA Health Insurance Portability and Accountability Act

HIT Health Information Technology

HITECH Health Information Technology for Economic and Clinical Health Act

HL-7 Health Level Seven

HMOs Health maintenance organizations

HPI History of present illness

HPID Health Plan Identifier

HRRP Hospital Readmission Reduction Program

i

I&O Input and output

ICD International Classification of Diseases

ICD-10-CM International Classification of Diseases, 10th revision, Clinical Modification

ICD-10-PCS International Classification of Diseases, 10th revision, Procedure Coding System

ICD-9-CM International Classification of Diseases, 9th revision, Clinical Modification

ICU Intensive care unit

IDN Integrated delivery network

IFHIMA International Federation of Health Information Management Associations

IM Information Management

IPA Independent Practice Association

IPHR Interactive personal (preventive) health record

IPPS Inpatient Prospective Payment System

IRS Internal Revenue Service

IT Information technology

l

L&D Labor and delivery

LOINC Logical Observation Identifiers Names and Codes

LPNs Licensed practical nurses

m

MA Medical assistant

MAR Medication Administration Record

MD Medical doctor

mHealth Mobile Health

MI Myocardial infarction

MPI Master Patient (Person) Index

MRI Magnetic resonance imaging

MS-DRG Medicare Severity Diagnosis Related Group

MSSP Medicare Shared Savings Program

n

NCRA National Cancer Registrars Association

NDC National Dental Codes

NHIN/NWHIN Nationwide Health Information Network

NICU Neonatal intensive care unit

NISO National Information Standards Organization

NLP Natural language processing

NPI National Provider Identifier

NPP Notice of Privacy Practices

o

ONC Office of the National Coordinator for Health Information Technology

OPPS Outpatient Prospective Payment System

OPT Outpatient treatment

OR Operating room

p

P4P Pay-for-performance

PACS Picture archiving and communication systems

PACU Post-anesthesia care unit

PAs Physicians' assistants

PCMH Patient-centered medical home

PCP Primary care physician

PDCA Plan, Do, Check, Act

PDSA Plan, Do, Study, Act

PET Positron emission tomography

PHI Protected health information

PHM Population health management

PHR Personal Health Record

PMP Project Management Professional

POA Present on Admission

POS Point of service

PPE Professional Practice Experience

PPOs Preferred provider organizations

PPS Prospective payment system

PQRI Physician Quality Reporting Initiative

PROs Peer Review Organizations

PSROs Professional Standards Review Organizations

q

QI Quality Improvement

QIOs Quality Improvement Organizations

r

RAC Recovery audit contractor

RADT Registrations, admissions, discharges, and transfers

RBRVS Resource-based relative value scale

RC Record of Care, Treatment and Services

REC Regional extension center

RHC Rural health clinics

RHIA Registered Health Information Administrator

RHIT Registered Health Information Technician

RNs Registered nurses

ROI Release of Information

ROS Review of systems

RPM Remote patient monitoring

RRA Registered Record Administrator

RRL Registered Record Librarian

s

SNOMED-CT Systematized Nomenclature of Medicine—Clinical Terms

SOW Scope of work

SSDI Social Security Disability Insurance

t

TEFRA Tax Equity and Fiscal Responsibility Act of 1982

TJC The Joint Commission

TPO Treatment, payment, and operations

u

UHDDS Uniform Hospital Discharge Data Set

v

VA Veterans Administration

VBP Hospital Value-Based Purchasing

w

WHO World Health Organization

WORM Write once, read many

x

x-rays Plain films (radiographic images)

a

Accountable care organizations (ACOs) Groups of doctors, hospitals, and other healthcare providers that come together voluntarily to give high-quality care using a fixed payment model; they work collaboratively and accept collective accountability for costs and the quality of care.

Accountability measures A Joint Commission system that measures quality and accountability for treatment of certain diagnoses—for instance, myocardial infarction (MI).

Accounting of disclosures A listing of all disclosures of protected health information about a patient that were not made as a result of treatment, payment, or operations or upon written authorization of the patient.

Accreditation Voluntary assessment by an accrediting agency that proves a healthcare facility exceeds the minimum requirements set by licensing agencies.

Administrative data Nonmedical data, such as patient identifiers, insurance-related data, authorizations, and business correspondence.

Admission, discharge, and transfer (ADT) system Electronic tracking of the registrations, admissions, discharges, and transfers occurring in a hospital at any given time. It is sometimes referred to as RADT (*R* for "registration").

Advance directive A document listing a patient's wishes, should he or she be unable to make decisions for himself or herself, or the naming of an individual who is authorized to do so.

Affordable Care Act (ACA) Healthcare reform with the goal of improving quality of care and affordable healthcare coverage through health insurance exchange, new payment models, initiatives to improve-care and the expansion of Medicaid to millions of low income citizens; provides healthcare consumers with stability and flexibility of healthcare coverage.

Allowed charges The maximum amount Medicare (or other third-party payer) will reimburse for services.

Ambulatory Payment Classifications (APCs) The classification system used by Medicare and Medicaid to calculate payment for hospital ambulatory (outpatient) encounters.

American College of Surgeons (ACS) A professional association of physicians specializing in surgery, founded in 1913, with the purpose of improving quality of care by setting patient care and surgical education standards.

American Hospital Association (AHA) A professional association of hospitals with the purpose of improving medical care through advocacy, education of healthcare leaders, and tracking of trending healthcare-related issues.

American Medical Association (AMA) A professional association of physicians founded in 1847 with the purpose of developing standards for medical education, improving public health, establishing medical ethics, and advancing the study of science.

Apgar score A newborn assessment done at one minute and five minutes after birth to assess the newborn's respiratory function, heart rate, muscle tone, reflexes, and skin color.

Attending physician The physician responsible for the care of the patient while hospitalized.

Audit trail A reporting of all electronic transactions performed by a user (through use of the user's log-in ID), including individual patient records accessed, the date and time of access, the length of time the user was in the record, and whether the data were viewed, entered, edited, or deleted.

Authentication In a paper record, the signature of the person who wrote an entry in a health record, showing authorship; in a digital environment, the security process of verifying an individual's right to access a system or portion of it.

Autopsy An examination performed after death to examine organs and tissue in order to determine cause of death.

b

Bar code A machine-readable code consisting of vertical parallel bars and white space, which is converted to identification. Every scanned document contains a bar code identifying the patient and encounter to which the document belongs and matches that document to the correct patient and encounter within the EHR.

Benchmarking Comparing the performance or outcomes of a provider or facility to that of a similar provider or facility. Examples include infection rate, death rate, and occupancy percentage.

Business associate An individual or organization with which a covered entity contracts to perform functions or duties that involve the use or disclosure of individually identifiable health information.

c

Cancer registry A database of all patients diagnosed or treated for cancer in a hospital; the hospital registry data are submitted to a state cancer registry, then reported to the Centers for Disease Control and Prevention (CDC).

Care provider A physician, physician's assistant, dentist, psychologist, nurse practitioner, or midwife; these individuals can diagnose and give orders for diagnostic or therapeutic services.

Case mix index (CMI) The average relative weights of all the MS-DRGs representative of the severity of all patients admitted to a facility.

Centers for Medicare and Medicaid Services (CMS) Formerly known as the Health Care Financing Administration (HCFA), CMS manages Medicare and Medicaid claims and regulates Medicare and Medicaid programs.

Centralized registration   Type of hospital registration in which all patients presenting for any type of care are registered through one central area, regardless of the type of care being sought.

Certified Health Data Analyst (CHDA®)   A professional certification sponsored by AHIMA to recognize professionals who have the training and experience to acquire, manage, analyze, interpret, and transform data into accurate, consistent, and timely information.

Change management   A structured approach for ensuring that changes in an organization are thoroughly and smoothly implemented and that the benefits of change are achieved.

Charting by exception   Documentation based on occurrences that are out of the norm or documentation of complaints voiced by the patient. Examples include a patient stating that his pain is worse than it had been, the fact that a patient was combative, and the fact that a patient walked to the bathroom without calling for assistance, even though he was to be non-ambulatory.

Claims data   Billing codes that physicians, pharmacies, hospitals, and other healthcare providers submit to payers. These data have the benefit of following a relatively consistent format and of using a standard set of ICD-9/10 codes.

Clearinghouse   An organization or entity (public or private) that processes data into a standardized billing format and checks for inconsistencies or other errors in the claims data.

Client/server   The use of computers in a network where functions are split between server tasks and client tasks; the client computer makes requests of the more powerful server computer in order to undertake local processes.

Clinical data   Data found in a health record that are of a medical nature—past medical or surgical history, vital signs, test results, physician progress notes, nurses' notes, and so on.

Clinical decision support (CDS)   Case-specific computerized alerts, clinical guidelines, and current resources regarding diagnosis and treatment options, based on the data found in individual patient records.

Clinical Document Architecture (CDA)   CDA is a standard from HL-7 to support interoperability and exchange. CDA defines the characteristics of a clinical document, including semantics, encoding, and structure.

Clinical documentation improvement (CDI)   The review of health records, usually concurrently, to ensure that the documentation in the health record is at the level of specificity that allows for code assignment that accurately depicts the patient's diagnoses and procedures performed.

Cloud-based solution   Service in which software and data are stored on remote computers and accessed by a local computer through the Internet, typically using a browser.

Commission on Accreditation for Health Informatics and Information Management Education (CAHIIM)   An independent accrediting organization whose mission is to serve the public interest by establishing and enforcing quality Accreditation Standards for Health Informatics and Health Information Management (HIM, 2014) educational programs (CAHIIM, 2014).

Compliance   Adherence to rules—for instance, regulations and standards; also refers to the culture of an organization to provide high-quality, cost-effective, efficient healthcare that operates within the requirements of regulatory, accreditation, and other requirements.

Compliance officer   A position responsible for monitoring activities that are susceptible to fraud, misuse, or overutilization.

Computer-assisted coding (CAC)   Computer software that improves the efficiency and quality of coding by assessing documentation and suggesting possible code choices, which are then verified by the coder.

Computerized physician order entry (CPOE)   Electronic means of ordering tests and medications that also provides clinical advice about the drug, the dosage, and any contraindications.

Conditions of Participation (CoP)   Regulations that healthcare facilities and providers must meet in order to receive reimbursement from Medicare and Medicaid.

Continuity of Care Document (CCD)   Based on the CDA standard, the CCD is the standard for the actual health record. It is an XML-based document and has been selected as one of two formats (the other being CCR) accepted under Meaningful Use. The CCD is more commonly used than the CCR standard and has greater traction with vendors and providers because it supports more applications.

Continuity of Care Record (CCR)   Developed by medical practitioners through the American Society for Testing Materials (ASTM), the CCR consists of a patient care summary with defined elements. CCR is XML-based and designed to be exchanged and easily usable by providers and patients. It is one of two health record standards (the other being the CCD) that is acceptable under Meaningful Use.

Copy (cut) and paste   The copying of data from a previous encounter that may or may not be accurate for the current encounter.

Core measurement system   A Joint Commission initiative used to measure the quality and safety of healthcare.

Court order   A written directive by a court judge that requires one to do something (for instance, appear in court or produce documents) or to not do something (for example, a restraining order).

Covered entity   Any healthcare provider or contractor that transmits in electronic form any individually identifiable health information.

Critical Access Hospital (CAH)   A hospital that has no more than 25 inpatient beds; maintains an annual average length of stay of 96 hours or less for acute inpatient care; offers 24-hour, 7-day-a-week emergency care; and is located in a rural area at least 35 miles' drive away from any other hospital or other Critical Access Hospital; the CoP regulations for CAHs differ from those for hospitals that are not CAHs.

Current Procedural Terminology (CPT)   The coding system used to convert narrative procedures and services performed in an outpatient setting to numeric form.

d

Data analysis   The process of systematically applying statistical and/or other techniques to describe and illustrate, condense and recap, and evaluate data. (Source: HHS definition.)

Database management   The maintenance of digital data stored in computer systems to ensure accuracy, access, availability, usability, and security.

Data mining   The search for and extraction of large amounts of data for the purpose of turning it into useful information through data analysis.

Decentralized registration   Type of hospital registration in which there are multiple points of patient access, depending on the type of care being sought—inpatient admission, emergency department, outpatient diagnostics, ambulatory surgery, and so on.

Deemed status   By virtue of achieving accreditation status, a facility is also in compliance with the CoP.

Deficit Reduction Act   Legislation passed with the intent to reduce growth in Medicare and Medicaid spending and decrease the number of fraudulent Medicare and Medicaid claims.

Delinquent records   Records that remain incomplete after 15 or 30 days post-discharge or encounter.

Demographic data   Administrative data that identify the patient—name, date of birth, address, and gender.

Department of Health and Human Services (HHS) The federal agency responsible for ensuring the provision of vital human services and health protection to Americans.

Designated record set (DRS)   As defined by HIPAA, any records maintained by a covered entity that are used for patient care or to make payment decisions, such as health records, billing records, insurance enrollment records, insurance claims, and coverage decisions.

Diagnosis related group (DRG)   A system that classifies patients into groups based on a patient's principal and secondary diagnoses, procedures performed, and other factors and determines the amount reimbursed to the hospital by Medicare, Medicaid, and other third-party payers.

Digitized health records   Health records kept in an electronic binary format.

Direct Messaging   Also known as DIRECT, Directed Exchange, or Direct Secure Messaging, a health information network initiative used by providers to easily and securely send patient information—such as laboratory results, patient referrals, or discharge summaries—directly to another healthcare professional. This information is sent over the Internet in an encrypted, secure, and reliable way among healthcare professionals who already know and trust each other, and is commonly compared to sending a secured email.

Directory information   Covered entities, including hospitals, may maintain in a directory certain information about patients, such as the patient's name, the patient's location in the facility, the health condition of the patient (in general terms) that does not communicate specific medical information about the individual, and the patient's religious affiliation. The patient must be informed about the information to be included in the directory, and to whom the information may be released, in the notice of privacy practices and must have the opportunity to restrict the information or to whom directory information is disclosed, or opt-out of being included in the directory. The facility may provide the appropriate directory information, except for religious affiliation, to anyone who asks for the patient by name.

Disaster recovery planning   Consists of having a backup infrastructure to support business continuity after a disruptive event. In healthcare, minimal recovery service levels are defined, such as access to patient records within a targeted time frame.

Disease registry   A large collection or registry belonging to a healthcare system or public health entity that contains information on different chronic health problems or diseases affecting patients in a system. This registry helps manage and log data on chronic illnesses and diseases. All data in the disease registry are logged by healthcare providers and can be used to perform benchmarking measures on healthcare systems.

Document imaging/scanning   The process of digitizing images of documents into computer-readable format.

Durable medical equipment (DME)   Medical equipment meant to be used for long periods, such as hospital beds, hearing aids, orthotics, and prostheses.

e

eHealth management   The processes and policies that govern the digital collection, maintenance, and archiving of data.

Electronic health record (EHR)   An EHR captures more information than an EMR and is designed to be exchanged and used at any point of care, following the patient. EHRs need to meet Meaningful Use standards.

Electronic medical record (EMR)   An EMR provides a digital record of the traditional chart used within one location. It does not meet the certification requirements of Meaningful Use because of its limited functionality.

Electronic signature (eSignature)   A digitized signature placed on a chart entry through the use of a personal identification number (PIN).

Emancipated minor   A person, typically under the age of 18, who is no longer under a parent's control, financial or otherwise, and assumes responsibility for himself or herself.

Encoder software   Technology used to assign ICD or CPT codes based on the coder's input of terms.

Enterprise system   A health system, made up of a hospital or hospitals, physicians' practices, long-term care facilities, outpatient (ambulatory) diagnostic and therapeutic facilities, and the like.

e-Record A patient's medical history, diagnostic test results, images, and clinical notes stored digitally in a database.

Evidence-based medicine (EBM) Diagnostic and treatment protocols based on proven research and documented best practice.

f

Fee-for-service Billing for healthcare services after the services have been provided (retrospectively) according to the facility's or office's actual fees for each service.

g

General equivalence mapping (GEM) Forward (ICD-9-CM to ICD-10-CM) and backward (ICD-10-CM to ICD-9-CM) mappings of each code found in both coding systems. GEMs are also created for ICD-9-CM to/from ICD-10-PCS for procedural codes.

Grouper software Technology used to categorize an inpatient admission or an outpatient encounter into a payment classification.

h

Healthcare Facilities Accreditation Program (HFAP) A voluntary accreditation program used by the American Osteopathic Association, which, like The Joint Commission, holds deemed status for Medicare.

Healthcare professional Generally refers to a nurse, medical assistant, or other technician who directly cares for the patient.

Healtheway The successor to the Nationwide Health Information Network, a nonprofit organization chartered to operationally support the eHealth Exchange, a rapidly growing community of exchange partners who share information under a common trust framework and a common set of rules. Healtheway leads in the development and implementation of strategies that enable secure, interoperable nationwide exchange of health information.

Health informatics The practice of information and knowledge management across clinical healthcare and public health domains.

Health information exchanges (HIEs) The organizations that provide the infrastructure and services allowing for the movement of health-related data between nonaffiliated stakeholders based on nationally established standards.

Health Information Organization (HIO) A health information exchange organization that provides services only in a smaller region, usually a metropolitan area.

Health Information Technology for Economic and Clinical Health Act (HITECH) Legislation resulting from the ARRA that provides incentives to providers and hospitals that adopt or upgrade existing electronic health record (EHR) systems and associated technologies and use them in specified ways.

Health information technology (HIT) The framework on which health information is collected, stored, exchanged, and reported.

Health Insurance Portability and Accountability Act (HIPAA) A law consisting of five rules—privacy, security, data sets and electronic transaction standards, administrative simplification, and enforcement and compliance; it impacted healthcare in general and the health information profession in particular more so than any piece of legislation since Medicare and Medicaid.

Health Level Seven (HL-7) HL-7 international is a standards body focused on the exchange, integration, sharing, and retrieval of electronic health information that supports clinical practice and management. HL-7 programming is critical to interfaces between systems to allow interoperability. HL-7 is an exchange format.

Health plan A health insurance company that reimburses for medical care in all or in part.

Health Plan Identifier (HPID) A unique identifier assigned to every health plan that controls its own business activities, actions, or policies or that is controlled by entities that are not health plans; the effective dates for use of the HPID are November 5, 2014, for large plans and November 5, 2015, for small plans.

Hill-Burton Act Legislation that supplied funding for the modernization of existing hospitals and the building of new ones, in exchange for which hospitals provided care at a reduced rate or for free to patients who did not have the ability to pay.

History of present illness (HPI) The symptoms or circumstances leading the patient to seek medical intervention.

Hospitalist A physician, employed by a hospital and is typically a board-certified internist or family practitioner, responsible for admitting patients, following and assessing patients as needed, and writing orders as necessary.

Hospital Acquired Conditions (HAC) Diagnoses that appeared after a patient was admitted but which perhaps should not have occurred—for instance, a urinary tract infection in a patient who was catheterized while hospitalized or a fall that resulted in a fracture.

Hospital Quality Initiative A program developed by the Department of Health and Human Services to "ensure quality health care for all Americans through accountability and public disclosure."

Hospital Readmission Reduction Program (HRP) Part of the Affordable Care Act (ACA), a program that requires CMS to reduce payments to hospitals with excessive readmission rates.

Hospital Value-Based Purchasing (VBP) A pay-for-performance method in which hospitals are rewarded for providing high-quality, cost-effective care and meeting performance measures for quality and efficiency.

Hybrid record Health record maintained in paper format, electronic format, and/or in the form of recordings or tracings derived from diagnostic tests.

i

ICD-10-CM/PCS implementation or conversion specialists Individuals who are proficient at ICD-10-CM/PCS coding who plan and coordinate the conversion to ICD-10-CM/PCS in healthcare facilities, insurance companies, or clearinghouses. Responsibilities include choosing the content of and time frame for training facility staff and care providers and assessing the needs of the facility (including the need for additional training in documentation for providers or in human disease and anatomy and physiology for the coders).

Incident (occurrence) report Data collected about any abnormal occurrence involving a patient, a visitor, or an employee that detail the circumstances surrounding the incident and are used in the facility's internal investigation.

Independent Practice Association (IPA) A group of physicians that contracts with a managed care organization to provide care at a pre-determined, pre-negotiated (often reduced) rate.

Individually identifiable health information Data that identify a patient, such as name, address, date of birth, and gender.

Information (data) governance The specification of decision rights and an accountability framework to ensure appropriate behavior in the valuation, creation, storage, use, archiving, and deletion of information; it includes the processes, roles and policies, standards, and metrics that ensure the effective and efficient use of information in enabling an organization to achieve its goals (*Gartner*, 2013).

Information security The administrative, technical, and physical safeguards put in place to ensure the validity and safety of digital data.

Informed consent Patient consent required for invasive surgical procedures and any treatment or procedure that carries a risk to the patient; informed consent provides explanation of the procedure/treatment to be performed and the reason for it; in other words, the risks and benefits of the procedure/treatment, alternatives to the procedure/treatment and their risks and benefits, and the name(s) of the healthcare provider(s) performing the procedure/treatment.

Integrated delivery network (IDN) A network of hospitals and physicians organized under a single parent company for the purpose of providing care across the full continuum of a patient population's needs.

Interactive personal (preventive) health record (IPHR) The summary of a patient's healthcare created by the EHR.

Interface A program that allows two or more similar or different devices to communicate and be interoperable.

International Classification of Diseases, 9th revision, Clinical Modification (ICD-9-CM) A classification system used to convert narrative diagnoses and procedures to numeric form for statistical and reimbursement purposes.

International Classification of Diseases, 10th revision, Clinical Modification (ICD-10-CM) A more specific and scalable classification system for coding of diagnoses that, though approved for use in the United States, has not yet been implemented at the time of this writing.

International Classification of Diseases, 10th revision, Procedural Coding System (ICD-10-PCS) A more specific and scalable classification system for coding of inpatient procedures that, though approved for use in the United States, has not yet been implemented at the time of this writing.

Interoperability The ability of two or more systems to exchange data and to use the information once it has been received.

j

Jukebox A means of storing multiple optical disks using a robotic arm that loads and unloads optical disks for delivery of requested health records.

l

Legacy systems Prior computer or business systems used to accomplish the tasks now accomplished by a new system; often, legacy systems continue to be partially used during system upgrade cycles.

Legal health record The health record, identified by facility policy, that is considered the official business record and that would be presented if subpoenaed.

Licensure Regulations regarding the minimum requirements to practice medicine or provide medical services; they vary from state to state.

Lifetime reserve days A one-time bank of a maximum of 60 days of inpatient service days after the use of the first 90 benefit days per spell of illness. Lifetime reserve days can be split among more than one inpatient hospitalization.

Logical Observation Identifiers Names and Codes (LOINC) LOINC is a standard required under all stages of Meaningful Use. LOINC is used to identify and code laboratory observations (e.g., test results) to be exchanged between labs, providers, and other stakeholders.

m

Managed care insurance plans Insurance plans that promote quality, cost-effective healthcare through the monitoring of patients, preventive care, and performance measures.

Master Patient (Person) Index (MPI) A permanent listing of all patients who have been admitted to or received care in a healthcare facility; it is the key to locating patient records in a facility and is maintained permanently.

Meaningful Use The section of HITECH meant to increase the effective use of electronic health records through monetary incentives to adopt and use certified technology.

Medicaid Title XIX of the Social Security Act of 1935; Medicaid provides financial assistance for healthcare coverage to poor and indigent populations.

Medical record number   A unique numeric identifier for each patient seen in a health facility; sometimes referred to as a health record number.

Medical staff bylaws   A set of policies that define the code of conduct, categories of medical staff membership, rules and regulations related to individual departments with which they may be affiliated, and health information–related policies.

Medical transcriptionist   A healthcare professional who converts the recorded dictation of care providers into typed report form using word processing software.

Medicare   Title XVIII of the Social Security Act of 1935; Medicare provides financial assistance for healthcare coverage to persons 65 years of age and over, to persons who are disabled, and to those with end-stage renal disease.

Medicare Prescription Drug Improvement and Modernization Act of 2003 (MMA)   This act provides Medicare beneficiaries with financial assistance in paying for prescription medications.

Medicare Severity Diagnosis Related Group (MS-DRG)   A revision to the Medicare reimbursement system, which takes into account severity of illness and resource utilization.

Medicare Shared Savings Program (MSSP)   A CMS program that facilitates coordination and cooperation among providers to improve the quality of care provided to Medicare fee-for-service beneficiaries and to reduce unnecessary cost through participation in an ACO.

Medication Administration Record (MAR)   Documentation of each medication administered, the dosage, the route of administration, the time and date administered, and the name of the person administering the medication.

mHealth   The sending and receiving of health information using a mobile phone, mobile device, or other wireless device.

Minimum necessary   The part of the HIPAA privacy rule that requires covered entities to make reasonable efforts to limit the patient-identifiable information released to only that which satisfies the intended purpose of the request for disclosure.

n

National Provider Identifier (NPI) number   A unique 10-digit number that identifies each care provider on all administrative or financial transactions—for instance, claim forms.

Natural language processing (NLP)   The ability of a computer to understand what is written in an EHR or to understand human speech.

Notice of Privacy Practices (NPP)   Written notification, which must be signed by the patient/legal representative, that communicates how PHI is used, disclosures made without the need for authorization, the patient's rights regarding PHI, the persons to whom PHI may

be released, and the covered entity's legal duties with respect to that information.

Nursing assessment   The documentation of a nursing interview and exam performed immediately or shortly after admission that details information such as means of admission (by wheelchair, ambulatory, etc.), reason for admission, events leading to admission, presence of chronic conditions, current medications, drug allergies, person to contact in case of emergency, and whether the patient can perform typical activities of daily living.

o

Observation   A patient status used when the patient's condition does not warrant an inpatient level of care but does require observation by medical personnel. Observation typically lasts from 24 hours to no more than 48 hours.

Office of the National Coordinator for Health Information Technology (ONC)   Located within the office of the secretary of Health and Human Services, the ONC is the federal agency promoting a national health information technology infrastructure and overseeing its development.

Omnibus Budget Reconciliation Act of 1986   The act that focused on substandard care and resulted in the requirement that PROs report substandard care to licensing agencies.

Omnibus Final Rule to the HITECH Act   Legislation that updates and clarifies the requirements in the HITECH Act.

Outguides   In a manual record-keeping system, these are cardboard or plastic folders that take the place of health records that have been removed from file. They include the date the files were removed and the locations to which the files were taken.

Outlier   Within the prospective payment system, an inpatient encounter that has an abnormally long length of stay or abnormally high costs associated with it.

Outpatient Prospective Payment System (OPPS)   A system used by Medicare and Medicaid for payment of hospital ambulatory (outpatient) encounters based on an ambulatory (as opposed to inpatient) payment system.

p

Pathologist   A physician whose specialty is dealing with the analysis of a tissue sample to establish a diagnosis.

Patient activation   A patient's knowledge, skills, ability, and willingness to manage his or her own health and care.

Patient census   The number of inpatients occupying beds at any given time.

Patient-centered medical home (PCMH)   A healthcare model that involves the patient and family in the care of the patient; care is rendered in a team approach.

Patient-centric   Communications, information sharing, and decision making that includes the patient and is managed by both the patient and the provider.

Patient-centric healthcare   Increased interaction and communication between a team of healthcare providers and the patient to improve quality of care and outcomes.

Patient engagement   As defined by the National Institutes of Health, care that establishes a partnership among practitioners, patients, and their families (when appropriate) to ensure that decisions respect patients' wants, needs, and preferences and solicit patients' input on the education and support they need to make decisions and participate in their own care.

Patient portal   A secure website where a patient can access information from a provider's EHR, such as diagnoses, lab results, discharge summaries, immunizations, and imaging study reports. A portal typically contains other information and functionality, such as the ability to schedule appointments, refill prescriptions, email clinicians, check insurance claims data, make payments, and gain access to online forms.

Patient rights acknowledgement   A listing of guarantees that a patient should expect, including the right to privacy, the right to make one's own medical decisions, the right to refuse treatment, and the right to be treated fairly.

Patients' rights   Patients have the right to know who their healthcare team consists of, the right to privacy and confidentiality, the right to be informed about their diagnosis and treatment, the right to refuse treatment, the right to actively participate in their care plan, and the right to be cared for in a safe environment, free from abuse. Patients also have the right to read or have a copy (paper or electronic) of their health record, the right to know who has accessed their health record, and the right to request an amendment to their health record.

Payer   An entity other than the patient who pays for or finances healthcare services. These include insurance companies, the Centers for Medicare and Medicaid Services, and self-insured employers.

Peer review   The review of a professional's work by another in the same profession or specialty. For example, an RN specializing in orthopedic nursing is not a peer of an RN specializing in obstetrics and does not qualify to perform a peer review of the orthopedic nurse's work.

Peer Review Organizations (PROs)   Organizations that replaced PSROs to perform medical necessity and quality of care monitoring.

Personal Health Record (PHR)   A paper record, a website, or software that contains information similar to that in an electronic health record (EHR), such as diagnoses, medications, and medical history. The patients can also add information themselves, such as notes from other clinicians (e.g., specialists), their personal notes and observations, and data from home monitoring devices or other sources. The patient or the patient's caregiver determines who has access to a PHR.

Physician extenders   Providers of healthcare who have advanced education and can diagnose as well as give orders; includes physicians' assistants, certified nurse practitioners, certified registered nurse anesthetists, and nurse midwives.

Physician Quality Reporting Initiative (PQRI)   A voluntary pay-for-performance incentive program.

Pioneer ACO Program   An ACO model for hospitals and care providers who have experience with coordinating care for patients across the continuum of care (across different care settings).

Plan, Do, Check, Act (PDCA)   The steps of a data-driven quality improvement process to identify reasons for variation, to make plans for improvement, to check results, and to implement the improvements, coined by W. Edwards Deming.

Plan, Do, Study, Act (PDSA)   The statistical model introduced by Walter Shewhart.

Point of care   The physical location where a healthcare professional delivers services to a patient.

Population health management (PHM)   Clinical and financial activities undertaken to improve health outcomes and to lower costs for a defined group of individuals.

Post-anesthesia care unit (PACU)   The unit to which a patient is transferred following surgery for monitoring of vital signs and condition post-surgery.

Pre-authorization   The requirement of some managed care plans that patients seek authorization (approval) for testing or admission in order for the insurance to pay for the services (providing that other requirements, such as medical necessity, are met).

Premium   The amount paid (typically monthly or quarterly) to an insurer for health insurance, either directly to the insurance carrier for solo coverage or through payroll deductions as part of a group health insurance plan.

Present on Admission (POA)   Chronic or comorbid conditions, such as the presence of diabetes mellitus or hypertension, which the patient contracted prior to admission.

Primary care physician (PCP)   A family practitioner, an internist, or a pediatrician who manages a patient's basic healthcare needs and coordinates care with specialists under a managed care insurance plan.

Privacy   The right to be left alone and to expect that one's health information is available only to those who have a need to access it.

Privacy breach   The acquisition, access, use, or disclosure of protected health information without appropriate authorization of the patient/legal representative or as required by law or allowed in HIPAA.

Privacy officer   A higher-level position dealing with compliance with privacy laws, investigation of potential breaches in confidentiality, and monitoring of the facility's release of information practices.

Professional Standards Review Organizations (PSROs)   Organizations charged with monitoring the medical necessity of hospital admissions and the quality of care rendered to Medicare and Medicaid patients.

Project management   The application of knowledge, skills, and techniques to execute projects efficiently and effectively.

Property and valuables inventory   A listing of all the personal property (clothing, jewelry, prosthetic devices, wallet, money, etc.) the patient had on his or her person when arriving in the hospital room.

Prospective payment system (PPS)   A fixed reimbursement system based on the diagnosis related group (DRG) assigned to each inpatient stay; used by Medicare and Medicaid reimbursement and some third-party payers.

Protected health information (PHI)   Any piece of data that identifies a patient as well as the clinical data tied to the patient.

Provider network   A network of hospitals, physicians, ambulatory clinics, and so forth with which a managed care insurance plan contracts to provide services to enrollees at an agreed-upon reduced rate, saving the enrollee out-of-pocket expenses for medical care; often referred to as "in network."

q

Qualitative analysis   A review of documentation to ensure that it is complete, thorough, and accurate.

Quality Improvement Organizations (QIOs)   Entities with which CMS contracts to review medical care, based on health record documentation, and to assist Medicare and Medicaid beneficiaries with complaints about quality of care issues and to implement improvements in the quality of care available throughout healthcare facilities.

Quantitative analysis   The review of a health record to ensure that required documentation is complete and a part of the record—for instance, a history and physical report or an operative report—but it does not include a review of the quality of the documentation.

r

Record retention plan   A written policy that documents the length of time a healthcare facility retains its health records, the form (medium) in which the records will be kept, and the location(s) of the records.

Recovery audit contractor (RAC)   A position resulting from the Medicare Modernization Act of 2003, with the purpose of recovering improper Medicare payments.

Regional extension center (REC)   An organization funded by the HITECH Act to assist providers by extending EHR adoption training and support services, offering guidance in EHR implementation, troubleshooting related technical issues, and meeting Meaningful Use.

Reimbursement cycle   The processes that take place from the time a patient is registered for care to the time the services are paid, whether paid by the patient or through insurance.

Remote patient monitoring (RPM)   The use of information technologies and communication networks to measure physiological data and perform tests from a location outside a clinic, such as at home, and send that information to healthcare professionals.

Resource-based relative value scale (RBRVS)   The reimbursement method used by Medicare and Medicaid to reimburse physicians according to a fee schedule that is based on weights assigned to resources used to provide the services, including the cost of work performed, the expenses incurred to operate a medical practice, and the cost of malpractice insurance, and that is adjusted based on the geographic region where the practice is located.

Revenue cycle managers   Those responsible for the functions that lead to an efficient, effective revenue cycle from the time a patient is registered for care until the bill is paid in full.

Review of systems (ROS)   A body system–by–body system set of questions asked of a patient regarding symptoms he or she may be experiencing.

Risk management   Internal activities performed with the goal of minimizing risk exposure through the identification, evaluation, control of, and response to errors or injuries that could occur or have occurred in order to lessen the facility's liability and to finance incidents for which the facility is found liable.

RxNorm   RxNorm provides for the normalization of names for clinical drugs used in pharmacy management and drug interaction software. RxNorm is required for pharmacy databases and messaging under Meaningful Use. RxNorm was developed and maintained by the US National Library of Medicine.

s

Scope of work (SOW)   The work plan for QIOs, which changes every three years, intended to improve the efficiency, effectiveness, economy, and quality of services provided to Medicare and Medicaid patients.

Security rule   The HIPAA rule that protects PHI through standard procedures and methods of storage, access, and transmission, as well as through auditing for security breaches.

Six Sigma   Developed by Motorola in 1986, a data-driven method for improving processes that involves the five-step process define, measure, analyze, improve, and control.

Spell of illness   A period of consecutive days beginning with the first day on which a Medicare beneficiary begins inpatient hospitalization or extended care (long-term care) services and ending with the close of the first period (up to 90 days) through 60 consecutive days in which the patient is neither a hospital inpatient nor a patient in a skilled nursing facility.

Standards   A prescribed set of rules or formats for how technologies operate and interact. Standards are approved by recognized industry bodies or can evolve *de facto*. In healthcare, standards exist for programming languages, operating systems, data formats, communication protocols, and electrical interfaces.

Straight numeric (sequential) filing   Records are filed in sequential numeric order.

Structured data   Data that fit a particular model or format and can be tracked as part of a database. Examples include diagnosis or procedural codes in ICD or CPT format, a patient's age, and a laboratory value.

Subpoena duces tecum   A command issued by a clerk of the court or an attorney for someone to appear in person in court or a deposition, to bring any documents or papers noted in the *subpoena duces tecum*, and to give testimony.

Systemized Nomenclature of Medicine-Clinical Terms (SNOMED-CT)   SNOMED is an established international standard for clinical medical terms to allow for common definitions in electronic data. This standard is part of EHR requirements under Meaningful Use Stage 2. SNOMED must be used for coding the data input from the medical encounter. It is a terminology that contains more than 300,000 medical term concepts to accurately record an encounter or care episode.

Systems management   The administration and maintenance of a distributed computer system across an organization, such as a hospital system.

t

Tax Equity and Fiscal Responsibility Act of 1982 (TEFRA)   Legislation that resulted in a shift from fee-for-service reimbursement to a prospective payment system.

Telehealth   The use of communication networks to provide services such as telemedicine, in which a clinician is in one location and the patient is in a second location.

Template   A preformatted document, found in software, that prompts structured responses in the EHR.

Terminal digit filing   Breaking a medical record number into segments of single or multiple digits, with filing based on the last segment as the primary file placement, followed by the middle segment, and then the first segment.

The Joint Commission (TJC)   Formerly known as The Joint Commission on Accreditation of Hospitals, a voluntary accrediting agency holding deemed status by Medicare.

Third-party payer   Often referred to as an insurance carrier or company; includes Medicare, Medicaid, Blue Cross/Shield, TRICARE, CHAMPVA, and any of the private health insurers.

TRICARE   Formerly known as the Civilian Health and Medical Program of the Uniformed Services (CHAMPUS), healthcare coverage for active armed services personnel, dependents, and retirees who receive care outside military treatment facilities; the federal government pays a portion of the healthcare costs.

u

Uniform Hospital Discharge Data Set (UHDDS)   Defined data elements that are required to be collected on all hospital discharges.

Unit record   System in which all records for one person are filed together under one medical record number in one location.

Unsecured PHI   Protected health information that has not been rendered unusable, unreadable, or indecipherable.

Unstructured data   Data in the form of words or audio files that cannot be tracked in a database. Examples include the text of an email, written narratives, and audio files from speech/voice recognition technology.

Utilization management   The review and management of the appropriateness of admissions and facility services.

v

Vaccine Administered (CVX)   CVX is the standard used for immunization messages. The Centers for Disease Control and Prevention (CDC) develops and maintains CVX codes under HL-7. The use of CVX standards is required for the immunization objectives encompassed under Meaningful Use.

Verbal order   An order given to a nurse either in person or over the phone, then later authenticated by the physician or physician extender.

Voice recognition   Software that recognizes the dictation of a care provider or other professional and converts the speech to text.

w

Wearables   Small health and fitness devices that can be worn on the body, similar to a bracelet, wristwatch, or pendant; they provide monitoring of physical activity, vital signs, or other information. Data from wearables are automatically captured and typically sent through a wireless network or Bluetooth connection to a smartphone.

Workflow   A well-defined sequence of activities undertaken in order to achieve a work outcome.

WORM technology   WORM is an acronym for "Write once, read many," meaning that records may be read numerous times, but nothing on the disk can be altered in any way.

chapter 1

Beeuwkes, M., Buntin, S., and Blumenthal, M. (2010). Health Information Technology: Laying the Infrastructure for National Health Reform. *Health Affairs, 29*(6): 1214–1219.

Centers for Medicaid and Medicare Services. *National Health Expenditure Projections 2012–2022.* Retrieved from http://www.cms.gov/Research-Statistics-Data-and-Systems/Statistics-Trends-and-Reports/NationalHealthExpendData/downloads/proj2012.pdf.

Obamacare: Enrollment Numbers and Medicaid Expansion. Retrieved from http://www.cnn.com/interactive/2013/09/health/map-obamacare/.

Patient-Centered Medical Home Cyberinfrastructure: Current and Future Landscape. (May 2011). *American Journal of Preventive Medicine, 40*(5, Suppl. 2): S225–S233. Retrieved December 20, 2013, from http://www.ajpmonline.org/article/S0749-3797%2811%2900067-5/fulltext.

Patient-Centered Primary Care Collaborative. (February 2007). *Joint Principles of the Patient-Centered Medical Home.* Retrieved December 20, 2013, from http://www.pcpcc.net.

Riley, G., and Lubitz, J. (2010). Long Term Trends in Medicare Payments in the Last Year of Life. *Health Services Research Journal,* April: 565–576.

Shi, L., and Singh, D. (2008). *Delivering Health Care in America: A Systems Approach,* 4e. Jones and Bartlett Publishers. Sudbury, MA.

Squires, D. (May 2012). *Explaining High Health Care Spending in the United States: An International Comparison of Supply, Utilization, Prices and Quality.* The Commonwealth Fund. Retrieved from http://www.commonwealthfund.org/~/media/Files/Publications/Issue%20Brief/2012/May/1595_Squires_explaining_high_hlt_care_spending_intl_brief.pdf.

Understanding Publicly Available Healthcare Data. (2013). *Journal of AHIMA, 84*(9): expanded web version. Retrieved December 19, 2013, from http://library.ahima.org/xpedio/idcplg?IdcService=GET_HIGHLIGHT_INFO&QueryText=%28Understanding+Publicly+Available+Healthcare+Data%29%3Cand%3E%28xPublishSite%3Csubstring%3E%60BoK%60%29&SortField=xPubDate&SortOrder=Desc&dDocName=bok1_050345&HighlightType=HtmlHighlight&dWebExtension=hcsp.

What Is an Accountable Care Organization? Retrieved from http://www.accountablecarefacts.org/topten/what-is-an-accountable-care-organization-aco-1.

World Health Organization. (April 2011). *Global Status Report on Noncommunicable Diseases 2010.* Retrieved from http://www.who.int/nmh/publications/ncd_report2010/en/.

chapter 2

AHIMA. (August 2013). Celebrating 85 Years of AHIMA. *Journal of AHIMA,* 84(8): 28–31.

AHIMA. (2013). *Who We Are: Mission, Vision, and Values.* Retrieved December 26, 2013, from http://www.ahima.org/about/aboutahima?tabid=mission.

AHIMA. *Information Governance.* Retrieved December 28, 2013, from http://www.ahima.org/topics/infogovernance?tabid=overview.

AMIA. (2013). *About AMIA.* Retrieved December 28, 2013, from http://www.amia.org/about-amia.

CAHIIM. (2014). Home page. Retrieved June 17, 2014, from http://cahiim.org/index.html.

EHR Incentives & Certification: How to Attain Meaningful Use. HealthIT.gov. Retrieved December 26, 2013, from http://www.healthit.gov/providers-professionals/how-attain-meaningful-use.

Garets, D., and Davis, M. (October 2005). *Electronic Patient Records: EMRs and EHRs.* Healthcare Informatics Online. Retrieved December 28, 2013, from http://www.providersedge.com/ehdocs/ehr_articles/Electronic_Patient_Records-EMRs_and_EHRs.pdf.

Gartner IT Glossary. (2013). Retrieved June 17, 2014, from http://www.gartner.com/it-glossary/information-governance/.

HIM. (2014). Home page. Retrieved from http://cahiim.org.

HIMSS. (2013). *Healthcare Information Management Systems Society (HIMSS): About HIMSS.* Retrieved December 28, 2013, from http://www.himss.org/AboutHIMSS/index.aspx?navItemNumber=17402.

Recovery Audit Contractors and Medicare. *The Who, What, When, Where, How and Why?* Retrieved June 17, 2014, from http://www.cms.gov/.../Recovery-Audit-Program/Downloads/RACSlides.pdf.

United States Department of Labor, Bureau of Labor Statistics. (2013). *Occupational Outlook Handbook.* Retrieved December 28, 2013, from http://www.bls.gov/ooh/healthcare/medical-records-and-health-information-technicians.htm.

chapter 3

AMIA. (2012). Definition of Biomedical Informatics and Specification of Core Competencies for Graduate Education in the Discipline. *Journal of the American Medical Informatics Association, 19:* 931–938.

HHS. (2012) *Responsible Conduct in Data Management: Data Analysis.* Retrieved from http://ori.hhs.gov/education/products/n_illinois_u/datamanagement/datopic.html.

Hsiao, Chun-Ju, and Esther Ming. (2014). Use and Characteristics of Electronic Health Record Systems Among Office-Based Physician Practices: United States, 2011-2013. NCHS Data Brief. January 2014. Retrieved from http://www.cdc.gov/nchs/data/databriefs/db143.pdf.

Mind Tools. *Change Management: Making Change Happen Effectively.* Retrieved August 6, 2014, from http://www.mindtools.com/pages/article/newPPM_87.htm.

Office of the National Coordinator for Health Information Technology. *Meaningful Use Stage 1 Requirements.* Retrieved August 6, 2014, from http://www.healthit.gov/policy-researchers-implementers/meaningful-use-stage-2.

Office of the National Coordinator for Health Information Technology. *Regional Extension Centers.* Retrieved August 6, 2014, from http://www.healthit.gov/providers-professionals/regional-extension-centers-recs.

chapter 4

AHIMA. (September 2010). Fundamentals for Building a Master Patient Index/Enterprise Master Patient Index (Updated). *Journal of AHIMA.* Retrieved from http://library.ahima.org/xpedio/idcplg?IdcService=GET_HIGHLIGHT_INFO&QueryText=%28Fundamentals+for+Building+a+Master+Patient+Index%2fEnterprise+Master+Patient+Index%29%3Can

d%3e%28xPublishSite%3csubstring%3e%60BoK%60%29
&SortField=xPubDate&SortOrder=Desc&dDocName=
bok1_048389&HighlightType=HtmlHighlight&dWebExtens
ion=hcsp.

AHIMA. (November 2010). *Managing the Transition from Paper to EHRs.* Practice Brief.

AHIMA. *Planning for the Unthinkable: AHIMA Introduces Disaster Recovery Toolkit.* Retrieved from http://journal.ahima.org/2013/08/28/planning-for-the-unthinkable-ahima-introduces-disaster-planning-and-recovery-toolkit/.

Gartee, R. (2011). *Health Information Technology and Management.* Upper Saddle River, NJ: Pearson.

LaTour, K. M., and Echenwald Maki, S. (2010). *Health Information Management: Concepts, Principles, and Practice.* Chicago: AHIMA.

Williams, B. K., and Sawyer, C. S. (2010). *Using Information Technology: A Practical Introduction to Computers & Communications.* New York: McGraw-Hill.

chapter 5

American Medical Association. *HIPAA Violations and Enforcement.* Retrieved January 31, 2014, from http://www.ama-assn.org/ama/pub/physician-resources/solutions-managing-your-practice/coding-billing-insurance/hipaahealth-insurance-portability-accountability-act/hipaa-violations-enforcement.page?

Clark, J. S., and Eisenberg, J. L. (2013). *The Joint Commission Survey Coordinator's Handbook.* Danvers, MA: HCPro.

CMS. *Conditions of Participation State Operations Manual: Appendix A.* Retrieved January 31, 2014, from https://www.cms.gov/Regulations-and-Guidance/Guidance/Manuals/downloads/som107ap_a_hospitals.pdf.

The Joint Commission. *Accreditation Publicity Kit.* Retrieved February 2, 2014, from http://www.jointcommission.org/accreditation/accreditation_publicity_kit.aspx.

The Joint Commission. (2014). *What Is Accreditation?* Retrieved February 4, 2014, from http://www.jointcommission.org/accreditation/accreditation_main.aspx.

Miaoulis, William M. (March 2010). Access, Use, and Disclosure: HITECH's Impact on the HIPAA Touchstones. *Journal of AHIMA,* 81(3): 38–39, 64.

Patient Advocate Foundation. *Managed Care Answer Guide.* Retrieved January 31, 2014, from http://www.patientadvocate.org/requests/publications/Managed-Care.pdf.

State Board of Health. *Rules and Regulations for the Licensure of Hospitals in Virginia.* Retrieved February 2, 2014, from http://www.vdh.virginia.gov/OLC/Laws/documents/2011/pdfs/2011%20complete%2012vac5-410%20hospital.pdf.

State of Rhode Island and Providence Plantations Department of Health. *Rules and Regulations for Licensing of Hospitals.* Retrieved February 2, 2014, from http://sos.ri.gov/documents/archives/regdocs/released/pdf/DOH/7022.pdf.

chapter 6

Centers for Medicare and Medicaid Services. (2014). *State Operations Manual. Appendix A—Survey Protocol, Regulations and Interpretive Guidelines for Hospitals.* Retrieved February 14, 2014, from http://www.cms.gov/Regulations-and-Guidance/Guidance/Manuals/Downloads/som107ap_a_hospitals.pdf.

The Leapfrog Group. (2014). *Computerized Physician Order Entry.* Retrieved February 13, 2014, from http://www.leapfroggroup.org/56440/SurveyInfo/leapfrog_safety_practices/cpoe.

Peden, A. (2012). *Comparative Health Information Management,* 3rd ed. Clifton Park, NY: Delmar Cengage Learning.

Wiedemann, L. (2010). CPOE Lessons Learned. *Journal of AHIMA,* 81(10): 54–55.

chapter 7

AHIMA. (2011). Fundamentals of the Legal Health Record and Designated Record Set. *Journal of AHIMA,* 82(2): expanded online version.

AHIMA. (2013). Patient Access and Amendment to Health Records (Updated). *Journal of AHIMA,* 84(10): expanded online version.

AHIMA. (2013). Understanding Publicly Available Healthcare Data. *Journal of AHIMA,* 84(9): expanded online version.

Centers for Medicare and Medicaid Services. (2014). *Medicare 2014 Costs at a Glance.* Retrieved March 17, 2014, from http://www.medicare.gov/your-medicare-costs/costs-at-a-glance/costs-at-a-glance.html#collapse-4810.

Dooling, Julie A., and Warner, Diana. (2014). Determining If Continuity of Care Documents Are Part of the Health Record. *Journal of AHIMA,* 88(2): 50–51.

Healthgrades, Inc. (2013). *The Right Hospital. The Right Doctor. The Right Care.* Retrieved February 26, 2014, from http://articles.healthgrades.com/about/.

Hospital Compare. (2014). Medicare.gov. Retrieved February 26, 2014, from http://www.medicare.gov/hospitalcompare/search.html.

iSixSigma. (2014). *What Is Six Sigma?* Retrieved February 21, 2014, from http://www.isixsigma.com/new-to-six-sigma/getting-started/what-six-sigma/.

The Joint Commission. (October 2013). *Accountability Measures List.* Retrieved February 22, 2014, from http://www.jointcommission.org/assets/1/18/2013_Accountability_Measures.pdf.

The Joint Commission. (2014). *What Are Accountability Measures?* Retrieved February 22, 2014, from http://www.jointcommission.org/about/JointCommissionFaqs.aspx?CategoryId=31#174.

Moen, R., and Norman, C. *Evolution of the PDCA Cycle.* Retrieved February 22, 2014, from http://pkpinc.com/files/NA01MoenNormanFullpaper.pdf.

Smith, Jim. (2009). Remembering Walter A. Shewhart's Contribution to the Quality World.

chapter 8

Adoption of Electronic Health Record Systems among U.S. Non-federal Acute Care Hospitals: 2008–2013. (May 2014). ONC Data Brief, No. 16. Retrieved from http://www.healthit.gov/sites/default/files/oncdatabrief16.pdf. The most recent adoption statistics are available at Health IT Dashboard. http://dashboard.healthit.gov.

HIMSS. *Early CHINS and HIE Organizations: Lessons for the Next Evolution.* http://www.himss.org/ResourceLibrary/GenResources.aspx?ItemNumber=22067.

HIMSS. (2013). *HIMSS Dictionary of Healthcare Information Technology Terms, Acronyms and Organizations,* 3rd ed. Chicago: Healthcare Information Management Systems Society.

Use and Characteristics of Electronic Health Record Systems among Office-Based Physician Practices: United States, 2001–2013. (January 2014). NCHS Data Brief, No. 143. Retrieved from http://www.cdc.gov/nchs/data/databriefs/db143.htm.

chapter 9

Centers for Disease Control and Prevention. (2003). *HIPAA Privacy Rule and Public Health.* Retrieved April 1, 2014, from http://www.cdc.gov/mmwr/preview/mmwrhtml/m2e411a1.htm.

Department of Health and Human Services. *Breach Notification Rule.* Retrieved April 4, 2014, from http://www.hhs.gov/ocr/privacy/hipaa/administrative/breachnotificationrule/index.html.

Health IT.gov. *Security Risk Assessment.* Retrieved April 5, 2014, from http://www.healthit.gov/providers-professionals/security-risk-assessment-tool.

HITECH Act Summary. (2013). *HIPAA Survival Guide.* Retrieved April 4, 2014, from http://www.hipaasurvivalguide.com/hitech-act-summary.php.

Office of Civil Rights. *Standards for Privacy of Individually Identifiable Health Information.* Retrieved March 31, 2014, from http://aspe.hhs.gov/admnsimp/final/pvcguide1.htm.

Ollove, Michael. (February 7, 2014). The Rise of Medical Identity Theft in Healthcare. *Kaiser Health News.* Retrieved July 13, 2014, from http://www.kaiserhealthnews.org/stories/2014/february/07/rise-of-indentity-theft.aspx.

chapter 10

Agency for Healthcare Research and Quality. (2013). *A Next Generation Personal Health Record System Enhances Preventive Care.* Retrieved April 29, 2014, from http://innovations.ahrq.gov/content.aspx?id=3769.

Carmen, K. L., et al. (2013). Patient and Family Engagement: A Framework for Understanding the Elements and Developing Interventions and Policies. *Journal of Health Affairs, 32*(2): 223–231.

Guillford, M., Naithani, S., and Morgan, M. (2006). What Is Continuity of Care? *Journal of Health Services Research Policy, 11*(4): 248–250.

Krist, A. H., et al. (2012). Interactive Preventive Health Record to Enhance Delivery of Recommended Care: A Randomized Trial. *Annals of Family Medicine, 10*(4): 312–319.

Shoop, Ron. (2013). *Modern Healthcare Management Insights. How Can I Increase Patient Portal Usage?* Retrieved May 2, 2014, from http://www.medicalwebexperts.com/blog/increase-patient-portal-usage/.

Wearable Tech Regulated as Medical Devices Can Revolutionize Healthcare. Retrieved August 7, 2014, from http://www.mddionline.com/article/wearable-tech-regulated-medical-devices-can-revolutionize-healthcare-6-18-2014.

chapter 11

American Health Information Management Association. (2014). *Appropriate Use of Copy and Paste Functionality in Electronic Health Records.* Retrieved July 12, 2014, from http://library.ahima.org/xpedio/groups/public/documents/ahima/bok1_050621.pdf.

Cook, Jane. (2012). HIM's Expanding Role in Clinical Data Analysis and Mapping. *Journal of AHIMA.* Retrieved July 12, 2014, from http://www.ahimajournal-digital.com/ahimajournal/201209?pg=57&search_term=health data analysis&doc_id=-1&search_term=health data analysis#pg57.

HIMSS. (2013). *Dictionary of Health Information Technology, Acronyms and Organizations, 3rd ed. Chicago: Healthcare Information Management Systems Society.* Chicago.

Jacob, Julie A. (2013). HIM's Evolving Workforce: Preparing for the Electronic Age's HIM Professional Shake-Up. *Journal of AHIMA, 84*(8): 18–22.

Logan, Debra. *What Is Information Governance? And Why Is It So Hard?* Gartner, Inc. Retrieved July 16, 2014, from http://blogs.gartner.com/debra_logan/2010/01/11/what-is-information-governance-and-why-is-it-so-hard/.

Reno, D., and Kersten, S. K. (2013). Getting Serious about Information Governance. *Journal of AHIMA, 84*(5): 48–49.

US Department of Labor. (2014). *Occupational Outlook Handbook: Medical Records and Health Information Technicians.* Retrieved May 18, 2014, from http://www.bls.gov/ooh/healthcare/medical-records-and-health-information-technicians.htm.

Front Matter

Beth Shanholtzer author photo: Aaron Riddle Wedding and Portrait Photography; Gary Ozanich author photo: Lifetouch Portrait Studios Inc./JCPenny Portraits.

Chapter 1

Figure 1.1: National Library of Medicine; Fig. 1.2: John Greim/Getty Images; Fig. 1.3: Archives of the American College of Surgeons, Chicago; Fig. 1.4: Library of Congress Prints and Photographs Division[LC-USZ62-123278]; Fig. 1.6: U.S. Department of Health and Human Services; Fig. 1.9: exdez/Vetta/Getty Images.

Chapter 2

Opener: ERproductions Ltd/Blend Images LLC; Fig. 2.1: Silverstock/Digital Vision/Getty Images; Fig. 2.2: Tripod/Digital Vision/Getty Images; Fig. 2.3, Fig. 2.4: Take One Digital Media/McGraw-Hill Education; Fig. 2.5: Massachusetts General Hospital, Archives and Special Collections.

Chapter 3

Opener: Cerner Corporation; Fig. 3.6: Fancy Photography/SuperStock; Fig. 3.8: Blend Images/Ariel Skelley/Vetta/Getty Images; Fig. 3.9: Hero Images/Fancy/Corbis.

Chapter 4

Opener: Chris Ryan/OJO Images/age fotostock; Fig. 4.3, Fig. 4.6: Cerner Corporation; Fig. 4.10: Copyright © 2014, Mayline; Fig. 4.11: Corbis/Superstock.

Chapter 5

Opener: Robert Shafer/Getty Images; Fig. 5.6: © The Joint Commission, 2014. Reprinted with permission.

Chapter 6

Opener: Blend Images/Ariel Skelley/Vetta/Getty Images; Fig. 6.1-Fig. 6.7: Cerner Corporation; Fig. 6.9: Sandra Mesrine/McGraw-Hill Education; Fig. 6.10 (clockwise from left): James Gathany/Public Health Image Library/CDC; Vstock LLC/Tetra Images/Getty Images; Heath Korvola/Digital Vision/Getty Images; McGraw-Hill Education; Judith Haeusler/Cultura/Getty Images.

Chapter 7

Opener: numbeos/E-plus/Getty Images; Fig. 7.1: U.S. Centers for Medicare & Medicaid Service; Fig. 7.2: © The Joint Commission, 2014. Reprinted with permission.; Fig. 7.3: Catherine Karnow/Historical/Corbis.

Chapter 8

Opener: Microzoa/Getty Images; Fig. 8.8: HealthIT Dashboard.

Chapter 9

Fig. 9.2, Fig. 9.5: Cerner Corporation.

Chapter 10

Opener: imec.be; Fig. 10.1: HealthVault; Fig. 10.2: Humetrix; Fig. 10.3: Hero/Corbis/Glow Images; Fig. 10.4: Ariel Skelley/Blend Images/Getty Images; Fig. 10.5: FABRIZIO BENSCH/Reuters/Corbis; Fig. 10.6: Gavin Roberts/Tap Magazine/Getty Images; Fig. 10.7: Preventice; Fig. 10.8: Dexcom; Fig. 10.11: PatientsLikeMe, Inc.

Chapter 11

Opener: Sam Edwards/Caia Image/Glow Images.